The Filth Disease

Rochester Studies in Medical History

Series Editor: Christopher Crenner
Robert Hudson and Ralph Major Professor and Chair
Department of History and Philosophy of Medicine
University of Kansas School of Medicine

Additional Titles of Interest

Sickness in the Workhouse:
Poor Law Medical Care in Provincial England, 1834–1914
Alistair Ritch

Of Life and Limb:
Surgical Repair of the Arteries in War and Peace, 1880–1960
Justin Barr

The Hidden Affliction:
Sexually Transmitted Infections and Infertility in History
Edited by Simon Szreter

China and the Globalization of Biomedicine
Edited by David Luesink, William H. Schneider, and Zhang Daqing

Explorations in Baltic Medical History, 1850–2015
Edited by Nils Hansson and Jonatan Wistrand

Health Education Films in the Twentieth Century
Edited by Christian Bonah, David Cantor, and Anja Laukötter

The History of the Brain and Mind Sciences:
Technique, Technology, Therapy
Edited by Stephen T. Casper and Delia Gavrus

A complete list of titles in the Rochester Studies in Medical History series
may be found on our website, www.urpress.com.

The Filth Disease

Typhoid Fever and the Practices of Epidemiology
in Victorian England

Jacob Steere-Williams

UNIVERSITY OF ROCHESTER PRESS

First published 2020
Reprinted in paperback 2024

University of Rochester Press
668 Mt. Hope Avenue, Rochester, NY 14620, USA
www.urpress.com
and Boydell & Brewer Limited
PO Box 9, Woodbridge, Suffolk IP12 3DF, UK
www.boydellandbrewer.com

ISBN-13: 978-1-64825-002-6 (hardcover)
ISBN-13: 978-1-64825-081-1 (paperback)
ISSN: 1526-2715; v. 49

Cataloging-in-publication data available from the Library of Congress

.

For my mentors, John Eyler and Peter Vinten-Johansen

Contents

Acknowledgments   ix

Introduction: Typhoid Cultures and Framing the Filth Disease   1

1   A Royal Thanksgiving: Disease and the Victorian Social Body   30

2   A Good Working Theory: Water and the Methods of Outbreak Investigation Before 1880   77

3   Nature's Not-So-Perfect Food: The Epidemiology of Milk-Borne Typhoid   128

4   Soils, Stools, and Saprophytes: Epidemiology in the Age of Bacteriology   172

5   Typhoid in the Tropics: Imperial Bodies, Warfare, and the Reframing of Typhoid as a Global Disease   224

Conclusion: The Afterlife of Victorian Typhoid   271

Bibliography   285

Index   317

Acknowledgments

I began thinking about nineteenth-century British epidemiology as an undergraduate student at Michigan State University. An eccentric Dane with a ponytail and a passion for history, Peter Vinten-Johansen, allowed me, a pesky undergrad, to enroll in a graduate-level seminar on the history of epidemiology. Peter was finishing a collaborative intellectual biography on John Snow entitled *Cholera, Chloroform, and the Science of Medicine,* and the group of us in the class spent the semester reading mid-nineteenth-century epidemiological reports on cholera, mostly by John Snow, William Farr, and William Budd, but the readings also included a host of other characters unknown to me at the time. Peter sparked a fire. He taught me that history was a lot like detective work and that ferreting out the traces of the past, crafting a narrative, and engaging with others' arguments are not just about pursuing history but are also at the heart of epidemiology. Peter helped me navigate my way to graduate school at the University of Minnesota, where I was fortunate to work with John Eyler and Susan Jones, who I hope will see their kind mentorship and sage advice imprinted everywhere in this book.

One key moment for this book came in 2012 when I was talking to Michael Worboys in a Manchester coffee shop. I remember explaining my idea to Mick about typhoid as a lens through which to view nineteenth-century British epidemiology. He took a long sip of coffee, paused for what seemed like an eternity, and half-jokingly asked me how I was going to manage looking through hundreds of long and tedious government reports. Thinking back now, what Mick was telling me is that this book would take longer to finish than I thought. And of course he was right. Mick, along with the late John Pickstone, supported this project from an early stage, and I'm eternally grateful.

More than anyone else, Anne Hardy has helped to shape and sharpen my thoughts and interest in the history of British epidemiology. As a doctoral student many years ago, I spent a year at what used to be the Centre for the History of Medicine at the Wellcome Institute in London. It was a year I cherish with fond memories, not the least of which was frequently sitting in Anne's office chatting about typhoid. It's not a given that senior academics take time to mentor junior scholars, and Anne always made time to help when I was stuck, to provide redirection or fresh sources, or just to encourage me to trod along and keep writing.

I've never actually met Bill Luckin, but we've corresponded via email for years. Bill has been central to the pages that follow. Generous with his feedback, clever with a turn of phrase, and encyclopedic when it comes to typhoid in nineteenth-century Britain, Bill's a terrific and big-hearted historian. Over the time it took to write this book, I've probably spoken to Chris Hamlin more than anyone else about the intricate debates over nineteenth-century disease etiology, water analysis, and our mutual long-gone friend, Charles Murchison. No one is more passionate or tenacious than Chris about these topics, and he pushed me to write a better book. Other allies that I needed along the way were Graham Mooney and Chris Otter. Both read portions of the manuscript, and Graham in particular helped me to think through the publishing process in clear and insightful ways over phone calls, emails, and beers. Every scholar needs these kinds of friends.

In the last year, when I was completing the manuscript and undergoing the review process, I became close friends with Jim Downs. Jim was also working on similar project, on epidemiological thought and practice in the eighteenth and early nineteenth centuries, particularly the impact of race, geography, and colonialism. We've had many long talks about our respective books, and Jim's friendship and mentoring always came when I needed it most. A host of other friends and colleagues read a portion of this book and provided meaningful suggestions and advice. In particular I'd like to thank Charles Rosenberg, Mike Sappol, Eli Anders, Chris Otter, Tim Carens, and Nathan Crowe.

I wouldn't have finished this book without the support of Nathan Crowe. We became close friends in graduate school at the University of Minnesota as confidants, office mates, beer brewers, soccer players, and wannabe bicycle-club members (it was a club of two). After grad school we were lucky enough to land jobs in the same area of the country, have kids around the same time, and be moving simultaneously along career and life paths. It isn't uncommon for Nate and I to speak daily. Nate has been there for me professionally and personally for well over a decade through the frustrations, roadblocks, breakthroughs, and joys. His encouragement has meant the world to me. Another close friend who deserves special praise is Stephen Casper, who I believe is my longest-running history of medicine colleague. I met Stephen at the Wellcome when I was an undergraduate, and he's a friend and mentor extraordinaire.

I have a great deal to be thankful for at the College of Charleston, and my current and former students top the list. I could not have written chapter one without the help of undergraduate students in History 299, my historical methods course. Having collected archival material from a recent trip to London, we spent a couple weeks of the semester sorting through William Gull's case notes and the bulky and revealing files of the 1872 Thanksgiving Reception Committee of the City of London. Hundreds of students have sat through, listened to, and commented on my framing of nineteenth-century epidemiology. I've been fortunate to work with and mentor some really outstanding history of medicine graduate students as well, including Hannah Conway, Kristin Brig, Bradford Pelletier, and Madeleine Ware. CofC has been a hospitable academic home, and plenty of friends and colleagues made it that way, including Max Kovalov, Bea Maldonado, Ryan Milner, David Parisi, Carl Wise, Jason Coy, Irina Gigova, Lisa Covert, Gibbs Knotts, Jordan Ragusa, Rich Bodek, Cara Delay, Adam Domby, Tim Coates, Bill Olejniczak, and Brian Bossack. Fellow Victorianist Tim Carens read the first chapter and provided incisive comments about Victorian popular culture. Phyllis Jestice deserves special praise: even while serving as department chair and working on her own research on medieval history, she takes the time to carefully read and comment on colleagues' work. She read the entire manuscript and helped immensely. I wrote much of this book while on sabbatical in 2019. Dean Godfrey Gibbison of the Graduate School was kind enough to provide a quiet office on the north campus of our university, away from the hustle of downtown Charleston. It was there that I holed up and finished the manuscript. Several university research grants also allowed me to travel to international archives.

Along the way so many folks have helped me think about typhoid and epidemiology in new and unexpected ways. I started going to the annual meetings of the American Association for the History of Medicine my first year of graduate school, and I haven't missed a meeting yet. It's my intellectual refuge of sorts, and the organization has provided a deeply important sense of community for me. I've presented, tested, and tweaked many of the ideas that made it into this book, and formal questions and informal conversations were fundamental to pushing me to think harder about my project. At the AAHM, and a host of other professional meetings, many folks in particular have provided guidance, including Warwick Anderson, Gerry Oppenheimer, Margaret Humphreys, Dale Smith, Leonard Wilson, Dorothy Porter, Judy Leavitt, Ian Burney, Roger Cooter, George Weisz, Steve Palmer, Simon Szreter, David Lilienfeld, Al Morabia, Jeremy Greene, Guenter Risse, Pratik Chakrabarti, David Barnes, John Harley Warner, Neil Pemberton, Richard Keller, Michael Brown, Laura Kelly, Abigail Woods, Agnes Arnold

Forster, Sam Alberti, Richard Barnett, Jennifer Gunn, Joris Vandendriessche, Andrew Ruis, Jackie Duffin, Janet Golden, David Edgerton, Vanessa Heggie, Mark Harrison, Ryan Johnson, Jamie Stark, Claire Jones, Michael Sappol, Eva Ehren, Bill Bynum, Richard Barnett, Stephanie Snow, Christoph Gradmann, Rob Kirk, Neil Pemberton, Matthew Newsom Kerr, Kevin Siena, Alex Chase-Levenson, Justin Barr, Erika Dyck, Peter Kernahan, Emily Webster, Justin Barr, Robin Scheffler, Andy Hogan, Deborah Doroshow, Todd Olszewski, Louise Penner, Tabitha Sparks, John Rankin, Ian Miller, Christos Lynteris, Lukas Englemann, Chris Willoughby, Rana Hogarth, and many others that I'm probably forgetting.

Archivists, librarians, and staff of numerous archives made this project possible, especially the Wellcome Library, the British Library, the National Archives, Kew, the Royal College of Physicians, the Royal College of Surgeons, and the London Metropolitan Archives. I'd like to give a particular shout out to the heroics of Ross MacFarlane at the Wellcome and Brandon Lewter at the College of Charleston interlibrary loan office.

I started talking to Ted Brown several years ago about this project when Ted was still the Studies in Medical History series editor with University of Rochester Press. As I got closer to completion, Chris Crenner succeeded Ted, and I've worked closely with Chris over the past year in bringing the manuscript to completion. Chris is a tremendously talented editor: patient, incisive, fair, and encouraging. Editorial director at URP, Sonia Kane, has been superb throughout the process as well, and I can't say enough about Chris, Sonia, and the incredible staff at URP. I'd also like to thank the two anonymous reviewers who provided invaluable feedback.

This book is about the everyday practices of epidemiology in Victorian Britain, but it's important for me to reflect and acknowledge the everyday practices of researching and writing the damned thing. Together my wife and I have a large extended family, and over the years it's been helpful to have family members ask about the project and prod me to continue. My father-in-law, Mike, a retired English teacher, read most of the manuscript, asking tough questions along the way and always reminding me to write more clearly. It's been my wife, Abby, and two children, Langston (five "and a half" he'll tell you) and Simon (two), who have helped me the most. I've tried over the years to be mindful of the ways that a project of this magnitude asks a lot of them. I went on numerous research trips, attended loads of conferences, and stayed up late writing more nights than I can remember. There was real and meaningful labor that supported this book by Abby, our family members, close friends, and even babysitters. It's important for me to acknowledge that labor. My family kept me going: Abby asked questions when I needed them and was relentless with her patience and her love. Langston has an odd curiosity about miasma theory, domestic plumbing, and all things poop related, so he was a natural collaborator and kept me laughing. Simon deserves some kind of medal for the chillist kid ever. Thanks, fam.

Lastly, I'd like to thank the publishers of the following articles for their permission to reproduce here revised portions of previously published material: "The Perfect Food and the Filth Disease: Milk-Borne Typhoid and Epidemiology Practice in Late Victorian Britain," *Journal of the History of Medicine and Allied Sciences* 65, no. 4 (October 2010), 514–45; "Performing State Medicine During its Frustrating Years: Epidemiology and Bacteriology at the Local Government Board, 1870–1900," *Social History of Medicine 28*, no. 1 (Spring 2015), 82–107; "Bloeming-Tyhpoidtein: Epidemic Jingoism and the Typhoid Corpse in South Africa," in *Post-Mortem Contagions: Infectious Corpses and Contested Burials*, edited by Christos Lynteris and Nicholas Evans. Medicine and Biomedical Science in Modern History Series (London: Palgrave, 2018).

Introduction

Typhoid Cultures and Framing the Filth Disease

"In the subject-matter of Preventive Medicine . . . Enteric Fever, with the diseases which are allied to it in mode of origin, must necessarily, I think, stand as first topic."[1] Thus began John Simon's most influential report as Victorian Britain's leading health authority. Titled *Filth-Diseases and Their Prevention*, named after the nineteenth century's most enigmatic infectious disease, typhoid fever, the report was first issued in 1874 as a supplement to Simon's annual report as medical officer of the local government board. *Filth Diseases* laid out a striking vision for British public health, whereby the incidence of typhoid stood as a litmus test for the health of a particular area. And a particular kind of epidemiology, outbreak investigation, was the central weapon in preventing the disease through local sanitary surveillance.[2] This book takes its title, *The Filth Disease*, from Simon's well-known report. Its subject is how overlapping and sometimes conflicting cultures of typhoid—popular, scientific, and political—dominated public health debates in Victorian Britain.

John Simon was the longest-serving chief medical officer in British history. He led centralized public health activities for twenty-one years, from 1855 to 1876, overseeing the health of the people of England and Wales and influencing a number of landmark health acts, including the Sanitary Act of 1866 and the Public Health Acts of 1872 and 1875. Together the acts compelled local authorities to provide municipal sanitation systems and to hire a medical officer of health (MOH). The acts also established a national sanitary surveillance system led by Simon and his team of inspectors at the Medical

---

1   Simon, *Filth-Diseases and Their Prevention*, 5.
2   Armstrong, "Medical Surveillance"; Armstrong, "The Rise of Surveillance Medicine."

Department.[3] A surgeon and pathologist by training, holding a long-term post at St. Thomas's Hospital, Simon broke into public health as the City of London's first MOH, a position he held from 1848 to 1855.[4] There he saw firsthand the grim realities of urban environmental degradation wrought by the Industrial Revolution. In his nearly decade-long trial by fire in the unprecedented role of the MOH, Simon called for wide-ranging reforms in water supply, sewerage, housing, cemeteries, and food adulteration, first publishing reports in the *Times,* and then in 1854 having them collated and sold separately as *Reports Relating to the Sanitary Condition of the City of London.*[5] In 1855 Simon accepted an offer from Benjamin Hall to lead the General Board of Health, replacing the outspoken and obstinate barrister Edwin Chadwick. The move shifted Simon's sanitary gaze from metropolitan London to the entire nation. Hiring a widely respected metropolitan surgeon and health officer ushered in a new era of public health in Britain, "a medical monopoly of state medicine," one scholar has recently noted.[6] The post was made permanent in 1858, when Simon and his small team of clerks and temporary inspectors were transferred to the Privy Council, where they were rebranded as the Medical Department and Simon the chief medical officer, and where they remained until further reorganization in 1871

---

3   As Christopher Hamlin has noted, while the acts of 1866 and 1875 provided legislation to compel local authorities to ensure sanitary services, "these were rarely applied." Hamlin, "Muddling in Bumbledom."

4   William Henry Duncan was the first appointed MOH in Liverpool. See Laxton, "Fighting for Public Health." The Metropolis Local Management Act of 1855 required all of London's vestries to appoint a MOH, the following year, 1856, all forty-eight metropolitan MOsH formed the Metropolitan Association of Medical Officers of Health. Simon was their first president. See letter May 6, 1856, Society of Medical Officers of Health, Wellcome Archives, London, SA/SMO/G2/1/1. The period from 1850 to 1870 was uneven in the establishment and activism of MOsH throughout Britain, as Anne Hardy has shown. See Hardy, "Public Health and the Expert." It was not until the Public Health Act of 1872 that MOsH were required throughout England and Wales, and even then many local MOsH bemoaned lack of adequate money or support. For a contemporary perspective see Davies, "The Trials and Difficulties of a Health Officer," and Dyke, "The Work of a Medical Officer of Health."

5   For context on the administrative and legal aspects of midcentury sanitary reform, see Hanley, *Healthy Boundaries.*

6   Goldman, *Science, Reform, and Politics in Victorian Britain,* 186.

transferred the department to the Local Government Board.[7] The Medical Department remained at the Local Government Board until 1919, when further reorganization created the Ministry of Health.

The newly established Medical Department had two central functions: to manage public vaccination throughout the roughly 3,500 vaccination districts in England and Wales and, when necessary, to conduct local investigations of epidemic disease.[8] It was a vague and mostly permissive mandate, combining the features of a standing administrative office with a royal commission, that central figure of Victorian governance.[9] Simon privately admitted that Parliament had little "definite notion of what I was to do," and this vagueness initially worked to his advantage.[10] Simon slowly increased the size and scope of the department, so much so that by the early 1870s there were ten permanent inspectors—mostly young aspiring doctors who had served as local medical officers of health (MOsH)—who were annually conducting fifty to eighty outbreak investigations.[11] In the two decades that he spent as chief medical officer, Simon developed an increasingly centralized vision of public health, whereby local authorities could be compelled to enact sanitary legislation: if not through parliamentary legislation then through surveillance, persuasion, and education.[12]

Simon defined state medicine as "the supposition that, in certain cases, the Body-Politic will concern itself with the health-interests of the people—will

---

7   This general process is covered in Porter, *Health, Civilization, and the State,* chapter 7.

8   John Simon, Confidential Report to Local Government Board President, November 30, 1867, National Archives, Kew, MH 113/2, 2. Alison Bashford has noted that "obsessed with dirt and cleanliness" as much as he was with "purity and pollution." Bashford, *Purity and Pollution,* xi. On nineteenth-century political debates over vaccination see Brunton, *The Politics of Vaccination.* For more on the even approach to compulsory vaccination see Williamson, *The Vaccination Controversy.*

9   Frankel, *States of Inquiry;* Prest, *Liberty and Locality.*

10 John Simon, Confidential Report to the President of the Local Government Board, November 30, 1867, National Archives, Kew, MH 113/2, 2.

11 Simon, "Statement Respecting the Inspectorial Staff of the Medical Department," n.d. National Archives, Kew, PC8/170. For more on the Medical Department staff see John Simon, draft of obituary of Robert Lowe. John Simon Papers, Royal College of Surgeons, England, 12.

12 For background on Victorian interventionist policies, see Baldwin, "The Victorian State"; Harling, "Powers of the Victorian State."

act, or command, or deliberate, or inquire, with a view to the cure or the prevention of disease."[13] Social policy, in other words, should be built on the technocratic knowledge of a "special class of experts" who would provide "a scientific basis for the progress of sanitary law and administration."[14] Simon Szreter has shown that such a statist, expert-driven ethos was at the center of the late Victorian public health movement, particularly at the General Registrar's Office (GRO), initiated during the tenure of its superintendent William Farr, one of Simon's close allies.[15] "Through its weekly and quarterly bulletins of comparative death-rates," Szreter argues, the GRO "fought a relentless campaign to heighten local awareness of preventable death."[16] Taken together, the Medical Department and the GRO were built upon the principle that "leading public and professional medical opinion" should direct social policy "through the didactic analysis of the nation's vital statistics."[17] But Simon's version of state medicine was distinct from that of Farr, and often scholars have conflated the kind of epidemiology that Farr and his successors practiced—the marshalling of statistics to make informed policy decisions and cajole local authorities—with the type practiced at the Medical Department, which featured field-based, experiment-driven epidemiological outbreak investigations.[18] Mortality and increasingly morbidity data gleaned from the GRO was critical to Simon's rhetorical and practical administrative strategy, and his, too, was a "major propaganda campaign" but only insofar as the demographic data provided a metropolitan starting

---

13 Simon, "Address Delivered at the Opening of the Section of Public Medicine," 287. The term "state medicine" emerged in the second half of the nineteenth century a galvanizing concept in medical and administrative circles. It owed its origin to Henry Rumsey, a physician from Cheltenham and vocal supporter of a centralized system of public health, from sanitation to housing, burials, and forensic medicine. Rumsey, *Essays on State Medicine*. See also MacLeod, "The Anatomy of State Medicine," 66–68.

14 Simon, "Address Delivered at the Opening of the Section of Public Medicine," 287.

15 Civil Registration of births, deaths, and marriages began in England and Wales in 1837. For historical context on Farr, see Eyler, *Victorian Social Medicine*.

16 Szreter, *Health and Wealth*, 242.

17 Szreter, *Fertility, Class and Gender in Britain*, 251.

18 The tradition of seeing Farr as emblematic of all Victorian epidemiology began with mid-twentieth- century epidemiologists writing the history of their discipline. See Greenwood, "President's Address: The General Register Office."

point to identify local districts where death rates surged or stagnated and where inspectors from London could be sent to investigate.[19]

In the second half of the century the Medical Department became the "nucleus of a genuine Public Health Department," even if its effect on local authorities was often limited to inspection and persuasion.[20] Simon created a unique and lasting culture at the department; it was the first governmental office to centralize the practice of epidemiological outbreak investigation in directing public health policy.[21] Interacting with local officials and residents, central inspectors almost daily played out what Patrick Joyce has called an "active public performance," displaying "objectivity and neutrality of . . . the new technoscientific state."[22] The four chief medical officers who followed Simon, Edward Cator Seaton (1876–79), George Buchanan (1880–92), Richard Thorne Thorne (1892–99), and William Henry Power (1900–1908), were all part of his team in the 1870s and roughly aligned with his vision of state medicine. The nationwide scope of disease surveillance Simon initiated lived well into the twentieth century; the idea is indeed a central part of today's modern public health systems.

Rethinking Simon's career at the Medical Department provides a launching point for this book. Scholars have had mixed views on Simon and the Medical Department's impact on British public health. Simon's first modern biographer, Royston Lambert, lauded Simon's achievements, placing him at the beginning of a long line of successors whose achievements led in time to the creation of the Ministry of Health, and situating Simon vis-à-vis a number of influential studies about the growth of nineteenth-century government associated with the work of Oliver MacDonagh.[23] Revisionist accounts have been more skeptical of Simon and the department's activities; Roy MacLeod has argued that while Simon's insistence on expertise marked an important stage in British public health, after his resignation in 1876 the department

19   Szreter, *Health and Wealth*, 244.

20   "The Scientific Aspects of Epidemics," *Sanitary Record* 2 (19 June 1875): 404.

21   Mervyn Susser has argued that Simon's greatest achievement was in directing a team of inspectors who pioneered the population survey approach, leaving "an indelible mark on the content of the modern discipline of an epidemiologically based public health." See Susser and Stein, *Eras in Epidemiology*, 106.

22   Joyce, *The Rule of Freedom*, 10.

23   Lambert, *Sir John Simon*. MacDonagh, "The Nineteenth Century Revolution in Government." The most recent reinterpretation of the MacDonagh thesis is a number of interesting articles in MacLeod, ed., *Government and Expertise*.

fell into decay, hampered by the bureaucratic weight of Gladstonian economic restriction. This period saw increased sanitary duties and tighter Treasury control over expenditure and salaries, which MacLeod characterizes as a "frustrating" one in the history of British public health.[24] The criticism was not lost on contemporaries. Ernest Hart, outspoken editor at the *British Medical Journal (BMJ)*, feared in 1878 that the Medical Department was "being strangled by red-tape and starved to death by the cold neglect of its unappreciative foster-parent [the Local Government Board]."[25] By numbers alone, in the years immediately after Simon's departure, the total number of outbreak investigations declined. And even Arthur Newsholme, chief medical officer from 1908 to 1919, was still frustrated by many of the administrative reasons that Simon had endured.[26] Even more critical of Simon is Christopher Hamlin, who goes so far as to say that much of Simon's work was "fruitless," and that the department's local investigations were "dubious" because "Simon's inspectors were in no position to compel local authorities to take remedial measures."[27] Instead, he and others have argued, local authorities in the provinces and municipalities, adopting a new "civic gospel" and considering the new professionalizing power of MOsH, ushered in major improvements in municipal sanitation that directly contributed to the decline of the major infectious diseases that plagued the Victorians.[28] Central bureaucrats like Simon, it seems, have been shelved as noisy figureheads who said a lot and did very little.

Such uneven interpretations tell us a good deal about the changing historiographical approaches scholars have used to understand Victorian public

---

24   MacLeod, "The Frustration of State Medicine." Lambert, *Sir John Simon*, chapter 23. Brand, "John Simon and the Local Government Board Bureaucrats."

25   Hart, "The Decadence of the Medical Department," 565.

26   On Simon's departure in 1876, see Brand, "John Simon and the Local Government Board Bureaucrats." On Newsholme, see Eyler, *Sir Arthur Newsholme and State Medicine*.

27   Hamlin, "John Simon," Oxford Dictionary of National Biography. Hamlin, "State Medicine in Great Britain," 148–50.

28   Hamlin, "Muddling in Bumbledom." Szreter, "The Importance of Social Intervention." It was a view generally adopted in Wohl, *Endangered Lives*. On the impact of local medical officers of health, see Watkins, "The English Revolution in Social Medicine." The conclusion that local over central interventions were most critical to the mortality decline continues to dominate the scholarly consensus by epidemiologists as well. See Vandersloot, et al., "Water and Filth."

health: a 1950s and 1960s political, administrative, and sometimes whig-gish set of histories of top public health leaders gave way to a critical revi-sionism in the 1980s and 1990s that stressed the work of local officials and questioned the very nature of public health as progressive improvement. Scholarship in both traditions has tended to see the Medical Department in isolation, focusing more on the internal politics of what the department was saying and virtually ignoring what they were actually doing.[29] Against this backdrop, *The Filth Disease* provides a new way to think about the Medical Department and its role in Victorian public health—not in isolation but rather as one important node in a network of public health practices.

Employing the concepts of practice, performance, and persuasion, and using a disease-centered approach, this book makes three claims. The first generation of professional epidemiologists, working at the Medical Department and as medical officers of health, I argue, placed typhoid at center stage and as a testing ground of state medicine. Victorian epidemi-ologists framed typhoid as the most pressing disease in order to persuade local officials to implement municipal sanitation and prevent the spread of disease. In the process, I demonstrate that in the second half of the nine-teenth century, epidemiologists forged a new kind of professional identity and gained a new kind of cultural authority. It was in this period, for exam-ple, that those practicing epidemiology—certainly not new to the Victorian era—began to call themselves epidemiologists and started to think in socio-logical, institutional, and even historical terms about their status as a dis-cipline.[30] Epidemiological research on typhoid at the Medical Department was central to that historical process, and inspectors were key members of groups such as the Epidemiological Society of London, the Medical Officers of Health Association, and the Social Science Association.[31] In the period when debates over disease causation, sanitary technology, and the provision of municipal sanitation were anything but unified, a particular kind of epi-demiology—outbreak investigation—was the chief science of state medicine. But despite the optimism of the Victorians that environmental problems

---

29 One exception has been the comparative analysis of Peter Baldwin, who argues that Simon was able to intervene at the local level while maintaining a politi-cal alliance to local self-government and the general politics of laissez-faire in Victorian Britain. See Baldwin, *Contagion and the State in Europe.*

30 Smart, "Introductory Address." For an early 1880s example see Buchanan, "Aids to Epidemiological Knowledge."

31 Goldman, *Science, Reform, and Politics in Victorian Britain,* chapter 6.

could solved through sound science and rational governance, this study lastly unravels the way that typhoid was protean throughout the second half of the nineteenth century. Typhoid was a tricky disease to diagnose, typhoid statistics were often untrustworthy, typhoid's etiology was hotly contested, and the disease even went by different names. In pushing for a model of preventive medicine with typhoid as a model disease, networks of British epidemiologists often came into intraprofessional conflict with a wide range of medical scientists—clinical physicians, pathologists, veterinarians, chemists, engineers, and bacteriologists—who in their own way used, understood, or ignored typhoid for very different scientific or political reasons. Broader cultural politics obfuscated any clear understanding and approach to the disease as well; even the British public feared typhoid in very different ways than the scientists who studied it.

A broader question at the heart of this book is why some problems of health and the environment are feared and framed as public health problems of immediate concern, while others are neglected, downplayed, or (as in the case of Victorian tuberculosis), romanticized by the public, policymakers, and the media.[32] Why was typhoid fever so important to Victorian Britons in the second half of the late nineteenth century? Why, for example, did the Medical Department, in the period from 1860 to 1900, investigate local outbreaks of typhoid more than any other infectious disease? Typhoid was not the only disease-related threat, nor was it even the leading national cause of death for England and Wales in the years between 1869 and 1900.[33] The disease was mostly on the decline in this period, rapidly in some areas like metropolitan London, while only stubbornly receding in others like the north of England.[34]

---

32 Tuberculosis, for example, annually killed more Britons than typhoid, yet the dominant cultural frame, as Carolyn Day as argued, was one of a "consumptive chic," a romanticizing of the disease. See Day, *Consumptive Chic.* Bashford has argued that the three most significant disease threats in Victorian popular culture were cholera, puerperal fever, and typhoid. Bashford, *Purity and Pollution,* 73.

33 Typhoid was only separately listed in the annual reports of the General Register's Office from 1869. For a general demographic analysis of mortality patterns in Victorian England, see Woods and Woodward, eds., *Urban Disease and Mortality in Nineteenth century England,* and Woods, *The Demography of Victorian England and Wales.*

34 Mercer, *Infections, Chronic Disease, and the Epidemiological Transition,* chapter 6.

A good starting point is Simon's 1874 report *Filth Diseases*, where, as we saw, he called typhoid both a "first topic" of public health and a "preventable" disease.[35] He also more poignantly called typhoid a litmus test of the "sanitary civilisation" of a local community.[36] Here the "why typhoid?" question comes into sharper focus, helping us to understand how the disease was recognized and rationalized, to borrow a phrase from Charles Rosenberg.[37] To reform-minded sanitary authorities like Simon, rates of typhoid could be used to see how well a local authority had taken up projects of sewerage and water supply and to look into the activities of a local MOH. "The prevalence of enteric fever in any district," Simon warned, "will prima facie impugn the sufficiency of the local administration."[38] Simon's style was deliberately wide ranging, literary, and moralistic, and he sought to connect Whitehall bureaucrats with members of the medical profession and the general public.[39] In some cases his rhetorical style was meant to deliberately shame what he saw as incompetent local authorities.[40] *Filth Diseases* was an exposé of the continuing problems of health administration in England and Wales; filth continued to plague urban city centers and rural environments, causing preventable sickness and death. Simon lamented that air, water, food, and soils were widely contaminated by fecal matter, and the cause was clear: improperly constructed middle- and upper-class house drains, faulty municipal sewerage systems, and the long-standing excremental soil pollution from rural cesspools and privies. Simon called the situation "an administrative scandal" and an "utter bestiality of neglect."[41] As Hamlin eloquently put it long ago, "It was not conditions that were at issue, but perceptions of them." The battle that Simon and contemporary public health reformers sought to

---

35 Szreter has argued that the GRO also rhetorically used the category of "preventable death" in calling for public health reform at the local level. See Szreter, *Health and Wealth*, 257.

36 Simon, *Filth-Diseases and Their Prevention*, 18.

37 Rosenberg, "Framing Disease: Illness, Society, and History."

38 Simon, *Filth-Diseases and Their Prevention*, 23.

39 For a contemporary study of how the politics of filth influenced ideas of public health in nineteenth-century France see Aisenberg, *Contagion*.

40 For a broader survey of the term filth in Victorian Britain, see Jackson, *Dirty Old London*.

41 Simon, *Filth-Diseases and Their Prevention*, 14, 17.

win in framing typhoid as a model disease "was over public sensibilities."[42] What was needed, he argued, was greater integration and oversight between central and local officials as well as health education for the general public.[43] In other words, the largely permissive Sanitary Act of 1866 and the Public Health Act of 1872 were failing. Simon had identified a wide range of environmental factors responsible for the spread of waterborne diseases. We can applaud his vision, even if it was not fully realized in the Victorian era.

Simon's 1874 *Filth-Diseases* was characteristic of the rhetorical style and political agenda adopted at the Medical Department. Annual reports were political weapons; each started with a broad-based review of the health of the nation, marshalling quantitative statistics and qualitative descriptions of key trends and highlights from local outbreaks.[44] The bulk of each report, however, was made up of the appendices, which contained handpicked epidemiological reports by the team's inspectorate. *Filth Diseases* quickly took on a life of its own. It was published as a separate pamphlet in Britain in 1875 and in America in 1876 under the title *Filth-Diseases and Their Prevention*.[45] Members of the State Board of Health of Massachusetts, led at the time by Henry Bowditch, for example, called it a "masterly essay . . . that could save hundreds of lives now annually doomed to destruction."[46] In other words, typhoid became a model cause of the public health movement in

---

42 Hamlin, *Public Health and Social Justice in the Age of Chadwick,* 11. Monica Garcia has recently shown that public health reformers in nineteenth-century Colombia also framed typhoid fever in a similar way. Garcia, "Typhoid Fever in Nineteenth-Century Colombia."

43 On the Victorian strain between local and central administrative politics, see Bellamy, *Administering Central-Local Relations.* On contemporary ideas of health education, see Buchanan, "Citizenship in Sanitary Work."

44 Simon stated three aims of the annual reports: to inform Parliament of the latest scientific research in order to improve sanitary law; to provide the public with knowledge about the spread of disease; and to keep local sanitary officials updated with the latest research on disease. See John Simon, *Confidential Report to the Local Government Board President,* November 30, 1867. National Archives, Kew, MH 113/2, 4. E.H. Greenhow's *Papers Relating to the Sanitary State of the People of England,* which Simon directed and for which he provided an introduction, set the stage for the type of nationwide epidemiological investigation that was to follow in the next several decades at the Medical Department.

45 Simon, *Filth-Diseases and Their Prevention,* 1875.

46 Simon, *Filth-Diseases and Their Prevention,* 1876.

late Victorian Britain because it fit the political agenda of reformers such as Simon, who believed that preventable deaths could be overcome through local municipal sanitation efforts, central surveillance, and epidemiological expertise.

But there were at least three other reasons that typhoid took center stage at this time, and not everyone—centrally, locally, or internationally—adopted Simon's vision for state medicine. Firstly, typhoid was a serious and persistent health threat in the second half of the nineteenth century. Annual sickness rates for England and Wales were 100,000 to 150,000, and deaths each year were sometimes as high as 20,000. In other words, we should take seriously the practical imperative to curb what was increasingly being understood as a preventable disease. But the demographic data alone do not sufficiently account for why typhoid fever dominated public health discourse in the second half of the nineteenth century. The second reason, as this book explains, is because of a national outcry against the disease among the British middle class, particularly after the 1861 death of Queen Victoria's husband, Prince Albert, from typhoid, and the severe attack of typhoid suffered by their son and heir to the throne, Prince Albert Edward, in 1871. Public discussions about health in the period from 1860 to 1880 were at a nationwide fever pitch. Popular fears of typhoid were further accelerated in this period by widely reported local epidemiological studies at the Medical Department that linked typhoid outbreaks to middle- and upper-class British homes that had adopted domestic sanitary technologies. Finally, typhoid was a model disease in late Victorian Britain for scientific reasons. Typhoid, a protean and hotly debated disease, was a research opportunity for a wide range of professionalizing fields, not only epidemiology (the focus of this book) but also clinical medicine, vital statistics, pathology, chemistry, veterinary medicine, and bacteriology.

In thinking through the complex and contingent ways that typhoid was a model disease for the late Victorian public health movement, this book further corroborates the view that the influx of insanitary environmental conditions—the sheer amount of filth—did not by itself constitute the central thrust of public health intervention.[47] Instead, in the case of typhoid fever, particular typhoid cultures influenced public health activities in this period as a result of state medicine's calculated political rhetoric, influenced

---

47 The so-called intolerability thesis is usually credited to Oliver MacDonagh; Christopher Hamlin critiqued it in *Public Health and Social Justice in the Age of Chadwick.*

to a great extent in Britain by Simon and followed by his close allies. They created a unique kind of culture that prioritized and defended a particular kind of epidemiology— outbreak investigation—to a broad spectrum of public and professional audiences. Public health in Victorian Britain, then, can usefully be conceived in terms of rhetoric and public persuasion if we examine the way that reformers pursued epidemiological analysis over other plausible modes of explanation.

Scholars have long been interested in how outbreaks of disease—their demographic impact and the cultural fear they produce—galvanize public health action. In examining Victorian Britain, historians have long adopted the view that epidemic cholera provided the central impetus for spurring public health reforms in municipal sanitation.[48] Examining late nineteenth-century sanitary reforms in four British towns, Hamlin has argued that "projects requiring years of sustained effort, such as waterworks or sewerage systems, are unlikely to have been responses to epidemics."[49] Hamlin's skepticism makes sense if we only focus on cholera, as the last major cholera epidemic in Britain occurred in 1866. Although during last three decades of the century health authorities would continue to fear another outbreak. Evaluating the impact of typhoid in this historical process is not only more complicated but also more fruitful. Typhoid was an endemic disease in the Victorian period, and although outbreaks seemed isolated, they were often explosive and almost always framed as the result of neglect. Some scholars have suggested that local epidemiological studies led by the Medical Department were not influential because the chief medical officer and his team of inspectors could not directly compel local authorities to act.[50] Judged only by results, in a kind of winner's history of public health, we might rightly be disappointed by the impact of local epidemiological investigations.

The Filth Disease provides insight into the more subtle (but often just as impactful) forms of persuasion available to John Simon and the inspectorate Medical Department in their quest to implement a system of disease surveillance. Often local epidemiological inquiry by Medical Department inspectors convinced local authorities to act; Simon's attempts at what he called

---

48 Winslow, *The Conquest of Epidemic Disease*; Brand, *Doctors and the State;* Rosenberg, *The Cholera Years;* Briggs, "Cholera and Society." Cholera in the nineteenth century has also been fruitfully used as an index of cultural ideologies. See Gilbert, *Cholera and Nation.*

49 Hamlin, "Muddling in Bumbledom," 59.

50 Hamlin, "State Medicine in Great Britain," 148–50.

"moral pressure" could be effective when combined with local outbreak investigation by a department inspector assisted by a local medical officer of health. But that was hardly the only pattern; at other times, local political or public works officials and tradesmen denied responsibility in a waterborne or milk-borne outbreak, or they ignored the advice of central inspectors.[51] This book shows that in giving weight to either the powerful voices of central public health leaders like Chadwick or Simon or the efforts of local officials, we have been asking unnecessarily narrow questions and missing the broader, more complicated networks between central and local health reform. Historians Bill Luckin and Anne Hardy, along with evolutionary biologist Paul Ewald, have conclusively shown that creation of a major sanitary infrastructure of clean water and effective sewerage systems, the safeguarding of adulterated food, and improved personal hygiene were central not only to the decline of typhoid fever by the early twentieth century but also to the overall improvement of the health of Britons.[52] The stakes are still high, in other words, when we assign causes to such a major demographic change in modern history.

"Everyday Epidemiology": Practice, Performance, Persuasion

A major theme of this book is how epidemiological knowledge was produced, defended, and debated in the Victorian period. In tracing outbreaks of typhoid to upper-class urban drains and water closets; to rural wells, rivers, and dairy farms; and to colonial bodies and environments, British epidemiologists confronted a number of critical contemporary debates about citizenship, governance, and public health that were at the heart of the admittedly uneven modernizing process of the Victorian period. This study provides a salutary reminder of the cultural milieu in which infectious diseases strike populations and how scientists study them.

Despite the long-standing scholarly interest in public health and the history of disease in Victorian Britain, there has not been much written about epidemiology, "The science," one Victorian contemporary explained, "which treats of the spread of disease."[53] In a 1993 historiographical essay, Gert

---

51 Lambert, *Sir John Simon*, 427.
52 Luckin, *Death and Survival in Urban Britain*, chapter 3. See also Hardy, *Epidemic Streets*, and Ewald, *Plague Time*.
53 Blaxall, "The Relations of Bacteriology to Epidemiology," 154.

Brieger remarked that "very little has been published about the development of epidemiology as a discipline."[54] Anne Hardy, the leading historian of British epidemiology, noted in her pathbreaking 2015 study, *Salmonella Infections*, that not much has changed: "The history of epidemiology remains largely unexplored, even by epidemiologists, still less by historians."[55] Historians and especially epidemiologists have tended to frame the history of epidemiology as statistical analysis springing from the work of William Farr at the GRO.[56] Epidemiologist Alfredo Morabia has gone some way in remedying the glaring omission by studying the practices and professionalization of late nineteenth- and early twentieth-century epidemiology, but Hardy still concludes that historians have "neglected" the subject.[57]

We know a good deal about so-called famous leaders in British public health, with biographies of Edwin Chadwick, John Snow, William Budd, and William Farr.[58] Scholars have acknowledged the origins of the Epidemiological Society of London in the early 1850s as a signpost in the history of the discipline, but much of the history of epidemiology remains wedded to what Hardy calls the "epidemiological mythology" of these classic figures and to a biographical and institutional set of histories.[59] Most scholars have suggested that British epidemiology "hibernated" in the second half of the nineteenth century, "overshadowed" by bacteriology until the early

---

54   Brieger, "The Historiography of Medicine," 33.

55   Hardy, *Salmonella Infections*, 9.

56   This is the classic view of epidemiologists, enshrined in textbooks like *Lilienfeld's Foundations of Epidemiology*. See also Lilienfeld, "Celebration: William Farr." P. Bingham, et al., "John Snow, William Farr and the 1849 Outbreak of Cholera," calls Farr "the dominant epidemiologist of the day."

57   Morabia, *Enigmas of Health and Disease*. See also Hardy, "Methods of Outbreak Investigation," 200.

58   Historical interest in Budd has probably been less than that of Chadwick, Farr, or Snow. E. W. Goodall in 1932 called Budd "a Forgotten Epidemiologist," and we still lack a critical scholarly biography of Budd's career. See Goodall, "William Budd: A Forgotten Epidemiologist."

59   Hardy, "Methods of Outbreak Investigation," 200; Finer, *The Life and Times of Sir Edwin Chadwick;* Hamlin, *Public Health and Social Justice in the Age of Chadwick;* Lambert, *Sir John Simon;* Vinten-Johansen, et al., *Cholera, Chloroform, and the Science of Medicine;* Dunnill, *William Budd: Bristol's Most Famous Physician.* The early history of the Epidemiological Society of London has been understudied. The original meeting books are located at the Royal Society of Medicine, London, Archvies, ESL/B/1 Meeting Minutes.

twentieth century, when biostatistics resuscitated and professionalized the practice.[60] Szreter, looking at the work of the GRO, has argued that "once the leading edge of aetiological debate had moved into the field of bacteriology" in the 1880s, "the techniques of medical epidemiology were temporarily eclipsed."[61] Perhaps that was true of the type of statistical work practiced at the GRO, but as I demonstrate in this book, bacteriology did little to eclipse or obscure the kind of epidemiological outbreak investigation practiced at the Medical Department and by local MOsH.

Apart from biographical accounts, scholars have tended to frame the history of epidemiology in terms of changing theories of disease causation, with impressive intellectual histories of disease concepts in the mid-nineteenth century by Margaret Pelling and in the late nineteenth century by Michael Worboys and K. Codell Carter.[62] Central to these recent debates is a scholarly assessment of the long-supposed pivotal role of the germ theory of disease in the late nineteenth century, a theory that would dominate ideas about infectious disease in the twentieth century. In this book I agree with a growing body of scholarship that views acceptance of the germ theory as less of a rupture in scientific discourse or public practice than has generally been assumed.[63] Linda Nash, for example, studying the daily practices of sanitary engineers and entomologists in the late nineteenth-century American West, shows how the germ theory "obscured as much as it revealed," and how a wide range of medical scientists remained wedded to environmental, antireductionist thinking about disease, medicine, and the body.[64] David Barnes puts this another way in his case study of sanitary ideas and practices in late nineteenth-century France: "The germ theory of disease changed everything and nothing at all."[65]

The Filth Disease argues that nineteenth-century epidemiology is best understood as a field science of outbreak investigation. In other words, in

---

60 Lilienfeld, "The Greening of Epidemiology," 526.

61 Szreter, *Health and Wealth*, 266.

62 Pelling, *Cholera, Fever, and English Medicine*; Worboys, *Spreading Germs*; Carter, *The Rise of Causal Concepts*. Worboys has recently called for more examination of the practices of public health. Worboys, "Practice and the Science of Medicine."

63 Worboys, "Was there a Bacteriological Revolution?" For a classic account of the bacteriological revolution see Porter, *The Greatest Benefit to Mankind*.

64 Nash, *Inescapable Ecologies*, 7.

65 Barnes, *The Great Stink of Paris*, 2.

order to understand epidemiology we need to think seriously about practice.[66] This framework builds on the work of Anne Hardy and William Coleman, who have shown that nineteenth-century epidemiology was primarily field based and observational and that epidemiologists only cautiously sought confirmation from the laboratory sciences of chemistry first and later bacteriology.[67] We often think of nineteenth-century epidemiology as population centered, only narrowing to a focus on individuals in the early twentieth century. But examining what I call "everyday epidemiology," referring to the routine practices of outbreak investigation at the Medical Department and by local MOsH, reveals that late Victorian epidemiologists also sought to understand the movement of individuals at a granular level through intricate case tracing. By the 1870s, for example, there was a consensus among the leaders in British epidemiology that solving the riddle of a local outbreak was dependent on discovering the index case. This book demonstrates that the hallmark of Victorian epidemiology was outbreak investigation: part an epidemiological way of knowing that characterized the public health movement of the second half of the nineteenth century and epitomized the way in which epidemiology began to professionalize in that period.[68]

By closely following the practices of epidemiology as a field science of outbreak investigation, this study reveals a wider range of epidemiological methods than scholars have typically discussed. Late Victorian epidemiologists used statistics, as we know, but they also relied on interviews, canvassing, case tracing, and experimentation. In order to persuade local, national, and professional audiences of their findings, epidemiologists also used various techniques of data visualization. We often think of spot maps, particularly John Snow's famous spot map of the outbreak of cholera in London, as the central visual tool used to explain the spread of epidemics.[69] Tom Koch has recently drawn attention to the rhetorical power of mapping disease more

66   There is a long-standing scholarly interest in practice as an analytical category stemming from the work of Pierre Bourdieu's *Outline of a Theory of Practice.* One recent example of thinking through practice in the history of medicine is Nolte, "Protestant Nursing Care."
67   I build on William Coleman's assertion that nineteenth-century epidemiology was field based, observational, and environmentalist. Coleman, *Yellow Fever in the North.* Downs's forthcoming *Empire's Laboratory* employs a similar framing to early nineteenth-century epidemiology.
68   Pickstone, *Ways of Knowing.*
69   Vinten-Johansen, et al., *Cholera, Chloroform, and the Science of Medicine.*

broadly in making the discreet reality of illness a public health event.[70] Spot maps were important tools in visualizing typhoid in the second half of the century, but we have tended to overemphasize their importance. They do not accurately represent the everyday practices of epidemiology. That is not to say that visual tools were inessential to knowledge production and its defense— and to maintaining and defending an epidemiological way of knowing.[71] Statistical charts were fundamental visual tools. The most important way of understanding typhoid and uncovering its epidemiology was through diagrams. This book contains numerous examples of such diagrams, which were used extensively to visualize the built and natural environment, such as the location of wells, water pipes, and drains in relation to houses and sick or dead individuals. In the everyday practices of epidemiology, diagrams were key visual aids in understanding how typhoid spread throughout the population. Sometimes these diagrams were granular and hyperlocalized, as in the examples detailed in chapters 2 and 3. By the end of the century, epidemiological maps sought to encompass larger geopolitical boundaries spatially; Frederick Barry and H. T. Bulstrode's typhoid maps, explored in chapter 4, are prominent examples.

The Victorian epidemiologists studied in this book used detailed case studies to disseminate their findings from local outbreak investigation. Taking their work as a methodological cue, *The Filth Disease* employs granular case studies. We often forget that nineteenth-century epidemiologists used narrative techniques: they told richly descriptive stories as part of the process of producing and defending epidemiological knowledge. This book privileges that story-making process, and many of the narratives of outbreak investigation in the pages that follow read like detective work.[72] There were hundreds of outbreak investigations of typhoid in the second half of the nineteenth century; the case studies drawn on here are admittedly not exhaustive but rather representative of the work of everyday epidemiology.

70 Koch, *Disease Maps.*

71 Pratik Chakrabarti has made a similar argument for studying cholera in British India, noting that "epidemiology provided cartographic visibility and statistical clarity to the disease [cholera], which was essential to the purposes of power and governmentality." Chakrabarti, *Bacteriology in British India*, 21.

72 "The Sherlockian Method in Epidemiology," *British Medical Journal* 228 (1936): 639.

As a way to capture the everyday practices of Victorian epidemiology, in this book I employ the term "epidemiological gaze."[73] The term borrows from Foucault's notion of biopower and recognizes the way in which epidemiologists worked within bureaucratic systems of governmental inspection that sought to regulate the broader cultural notions of middle-class respectability.[74] But like Tom Crook, whose recent *Governing Systems* has argued for a systems-based approach to understanding Victorian public health, epidemiological practice was often less about viewing the public as passive *objects* than as active *subjects* of public health reform.[75] This mirrors what Graham Mooney has recently said of the uneven implementation of disease notification strategies in the late Victorian period.[76] Mooney's notion of infectious disease surveillance is probably the most apt characterization of public health practices in this period.[77] The use of the epidemiological gaze extends the idea of surveillance and provides a useful term to define a specific approach to knowledge production. It also helps us to understand the complex ways in which epidemiologists defended their ideas to multiple audiences—members of the public, government officials, and other scientific practitioners—which was central to the professionalizing aims of epidemiologists in this period.

This book shows that the Medical Department was a key site of epidemiological practice and discipline formation in the second half of the nineteenth century. The inspectors at the department were the first full-time, state-sponsored epidemiologists whose sole duty was outbreak investigation. One contemporary in the *British Medical Journal* wrote that the inspectors served "a dangerous public duty" and "expose themselves, at every visit into an infected district, to the attacks of an unseen enemy, whom they track

---

73   Foucault, *The Birth of the Clinic.* I draw on Warwick Anderson's idea that tropical medicine saw the tropics and colonized peoples as research objects, and David Arnold's notion that a "traveling gaze" dominated British botanical attitudes toward understanding the early nineteenth-century Indian landscape. Anderson, "'Where Every Prospect Pleases and Only Man is Vile'"; Arnold, *The Tropics and the Traveling Gaze.*

74   Kerr's *Contagion, Isolation, and Biopower in Victorian London* presents the most recent and comprehensive example that incorporates Foucault's notion of biopower into nineteenth-century public health.

75   Crook, *Governing Systems,* 139.

76   Mooney, *Intrusive Interventions.*

77   Another good example of thinking about practice in this way is Stark, *The Making of Modern Anthrax.*

into his hiding-places, and seek to expel from his strongholds."[78] But the inspectors at the department did not exist in a vacuum, and this book uncovers how Medical Department inspectors were part of complex networks of epidemiological theory and practice across Britain and the British colonies in this period.[79] What is clear from this study, however, is that by the end of the century the epidemiology practiced in England was continuing a tradition largely established at the Medical Department.

By the end of the nineteenth century, the inspectors at the Medical Department had laid the groundwork for epidemiological study and had routinized its practice, which George Buchanan described as "the minute observations of particular outbreaks."[80] Shirley Murphy, in his inaugural address as president of the Epidemiological Society in in 1894, noted that the Medical Department's "investigations have provided definite object lessons for epidemiologists throughout the country. They have indicated the subject matter to which attention should be directed and the method of its investigation."[81] Edward Cox Seaton echoed Murphy and Buchanan, saying that the inspectors were a "rising school of epidemiologists" who provided "exact studies of outbreak of epidemics."[82] It was "epoch-making work," another contemporary noted, in "practical epidemiology."[83]

A Protean Disease

In framing typhoid fever as a model disease for preventive medicine and the science of epidemiology, British public health reformers had to contend with an elusive, protean disease. The history of typhoid has received relatively little scholarly attention compared to its Victorian counterparts: cholera,

---

78 The article was written after the death of Gwynne Harries. See "Killed in the Service of the State," *British Medical Journal* 672 (November 15, 1873): 578.

79 Secord, "Knowledge in Transit."

80 Buchanan, "On the Dry Earth System of Dealing with Excrement," 97.

81 Murphy, "On the Study of Epidemiology," 4. By the 1890s there were even standardized forms for outbreak investigation. See Medical Department Inspectorate form, titled "Costs of Inquiry," National Archives, Kew, MH113/34.

82 Seaton, "A Discussion on the Etiology and Epidemiology of Typhoid (Enteric) Fever," 169–75.

83 "Obituary of John Simon," *Transactions of the Epidemiological Society of London* 23 (1904): 257.

tuberculosis, and diphtheria. In Lloyd Stevenson's classic account, typhoid was an "exemplary disease" across debates in epidemiology, clinical medicine, and disease nosology.[84] Nigel Richardson's case study of the constrained local politics of public health reform in Uppingham provides a useful and interesting approach that situates typhoid at the center of contemporary political debate.[85] But few studies have unpacked all the ways that typhoid was a unique product of the Victorian period, produced by and mutually intelligible to historical actors of the nineteenth century.

Typhoid was ubiquitous, insidious, and omnipresent in the Victorian period, fulminating in explosive, localized outbreaks. Charles Murchison, England's renowned fever expert and longtime physician at the London Fever Hospital and St. Thomas's Hospital, crowned typhoid "the endemic fever of England."[86] In English upper-class homes the disease lurked in sewer gases, wafting from untapped drains and newly installed water closets. In English water pipes it bubbled away, waiting to strike its next victim from the next jolt of a pump handle or a glassful of refreshment. The disease found a nidus in England's most perfect food, milk: that ideal, rural, lacteal mainstay of the middle and upper classes. Typhoid prowled English soils, too, leaching into shoddy wells and inciting fecal-oral horror. And, of course, it was in English bodies, producing fevered sweats, delirium, and diarrhea. It debilitated young soldiers in the British colonies, and sometimes it even sat there silently and without symptom, called in the Victorian period "ambulatory typhoid," long before those historical icons of the disease, "Mr. N. the Milker" and "Typhoid Mary."[87] It all added up to a palpable public anxiety of the kind visualized on the cover of this book: a strikingly gothic representation of typhoid by Richard Tennant Cooper produced in 1912.

The name typhoid did not emerge until 1829, and the disease was long confounded with the broader group of early modern "fevers" and especially lumped together with typhus and often labeled "simple continued fever." In the Parisian dissection rooms of the Hotel Dieu in 1829, famed clinician and pathologist Pierre Louis provided a name: *Fièvre typhoïde*. The term was popularized in A. F. Chomel's *Clinical Lectures on Typhoid Fever* (1834) and by the 1840s was well known throughout western Europe and North America. From the 1830s there was a nosological maelstrom in naming the

---

84   Stevenson, "Exemplary Disease."

85   Richardson, *Typhoid in Uppingham*.

86   Murchison, *A Treatise on the Continued Fevers of Great Britain*, 412.

87   Leavitt, *Typhoid Mary*; Mortimer, "Mr. N. the Milker," 1354–56.

disease, a lack of agreement on its clinical symptoms in patients, and heated debates over its origin and spread. "Typhoid" was probably the worst name for the disease, a point lost on modern observers. It not only sounded like "typhus," but it literally meant "like typhus," a kind of nosological irony from which it was trying to escape. The English polymath physician Benjamin Ward Richardson, for example, lamented in the 1890s that calling the disease "typhoid" led to "the absurdest confusion, particularly by the ordinary people."[88] And so typhoid cynics came up with alternatives. To many English observers the term "typhoid" was too French.[89] Murchison favored his own term, "pythogenic fever," meaning "bred of filth," which was yoked to his name and popular in England until the late nineteenth century. But other monikers came and went in both the medical lexicon and scattered across the public sphere. Some, like Edwin Chadwick, interchangeably used epidemiologically specific terms such as "drain fever," "night-soil fever," and "cesspool fever." Across the British Empire, colonial doctors, often denying that the typhoid in Europe was the same disease seen in tropical environments, used a host of terms, from "colonial fever" to "typho-malarial fever."[90] A popular English attempt to escape the etiological uncertainty was the emergence of the name "enteric fever," which stripped away the marriage to typhus and focused exclusively on the intestinal lesions that seemed to distinguish the disease from other fevers. "Enteric fever" was the most popular English alternative to "typhoid" throughout the nineteenth century, but often the two were used interchangeably. The Royal College of Physicians in 1869, for example, updated their official disease classification scheme and listed the two as synonyms, designating "a continued fever, characterised by the presence of rose-coloured spots, chiefly on the abdomen, and a tendency to diarrhea, with specific lesion of the bowels."[91] But use of "enteric" waned in the early twentieth century, confusingly taking on a new meaning to describe the broader *Salmonella* family, of which typhoid was only one variety.

By the 1860s, when this book begins, there was at least agreement in Britain that typhoid was a specific disease, one striking between 100,000 and 150,000 individuals each year in England alone, according to the GRO.

88   Richardson, *Vita Medica*, 88.
89   Stevenson, "A Pox on the Ileum." For a general history of French pathological anatomy, see Maulitz *Morbid Appearances*.
90   Christison, "President's Address in the Public Health Department"; Smith, "The Rise and Fall of Typhomalarial Fever."
91   Royal College of Physicians, *The Nomenclature of Disease*, 5.

This was due to the confirmatory work of Alexander P. Stewart and William Jenner. The pathologists who correlated the outward symptoms of the disease with the internal lesions produced the first of many visualizations of typhoid, corporealizing and materializing the disease in hand-drawn illustrations of archetypical typhoid patients with ulcerated intestines.[92] Contemporary artistic representations of typhoid, like the vivid watercolor illustrations of Thomas Godart, librarian and artist at St. Bartholomew's Hospital (figures I.1 and I.2), came to represent the key features of the disease, especially when matched with clinical descriptions. T. J. MacLagan, a well-known Scottish physician practicing in London, described a prototypical typhoid patient in terms that might just as well have been a description of one of Godart's illustrations: "sunken and depressed" affect; "moist clammy skin"; "listless expressionless eye"; "sordes-coated teeth and lips"; "Dry brown tongue"; "the feeble flickering of the pulse"; the "low muttering delirium"; the "involuntary evacuations"; and the "rose-coloured spots."[93]

In order for epidemiological research to flourish on typhoid, the disease had to be made a stable target. The outward symptoms in patients were untrustworthy, mimicking other diseases in the early stages, or like the rose spots, known today to be bacterial emboli to the skin, only seen in about a third of all cases. It was only after 1870 that the GRO officially listed typhoid in its annual returns. But statistics tended to obscure rather than clarify the disease's cause and communication.[94] Outbreaks of typhoid were sudden and sporadic, leaving well-known London physician A. P. Stewart to declare in exasperation, "With regard to the producing cause of typhoid fever, all is vague and uncertain."[95] Typhoid's randomness led many physicians to argue that the disease originated spontaneously out of fermenting excremental filth: that gratuitously descriptive yet moralizing environmental accumulation of dirt and disgust that Simon was fighting against in his

---

92   For context on the history of pathological illustration, see two new works: Meli, *Visualizing Disease,* chapter six; Wils, et al., *Beyond Borders.* On Godart see "Obituary for Thomas Godart," *British Medical Journal* 1413 (28 January 1888): 220.

93   MacLagan, *Fever,* 80–81.

94   For an excellent study of statistics in early nineteenth-century Paris, see La Berge, "Medical Statistics at the Paris School."

95   Stewart, "Some Considerations," 295.

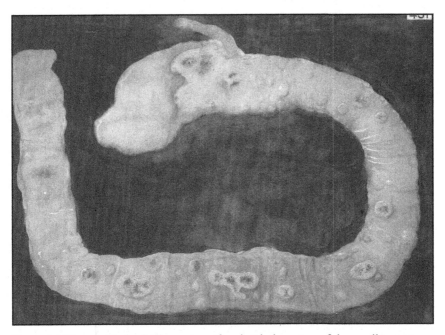

Figure I.1 Thomas Godart's illustration of typhoid ulceration of the small intestine, in an early stage of the disease. St. Bartholomew's Hospital Archives and Museum. Image courtesy of the Wellcome Library, London. Creative Commons Attribution license CC BY 4.0.

1874 report.[96] Though contemporaries spoke of filth diseases in a generalized sense, typhoid was most commonly heralded as the prototypical filth disease. Charles Cameron, leading Irish public health authority, exemplified contemporary opinion in 1868: "Filth is a prolific source of almost all kinds of diseases, and is the chief carrier of contagia. No town, no house, no man, can remain unclean, and be healthy."[97] Framing typhoid as a general filth disease continued until the late nineteenth century, particularly among rural medical officers of health and medical practitioners, who held eclectic views on the spread of typhoid.

Charles Murchison was the most vocal advocate for the spontaneous origin of typhoid in Victorian England. His 1862 *Treatise on the Continued Fevers*

96 For a broader conceptualization of filth and modernity, see Cohen and Johnson, eds., *Filth*.
97 Cameron, *Lectures on the Preservation of Health*, 159.

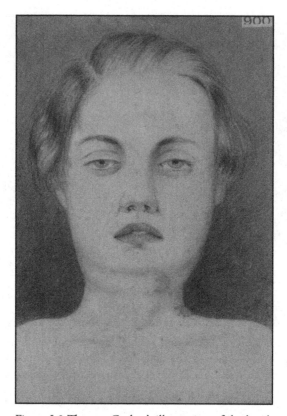

Figure I.2 Thomas Godart's illustration of the head and neck of a patient suffering from typhoid fever. St. Bartholomew's Hospital Archives and Museum. Image courtesy of the Wellcome Library, London. Creative Commons Attribution license CC BY 4.0.

of Great Britain, updated in 1873, was based on both an unprecedented statistical study of cases at the London Fever Hospital and Murchison's military service with the East India Company.[98] He argued that typhoid was spread via a poison carried in excreta that spontaneously ferments in the environment—sometimes in the soil but especially in drains. Murchison's

---

98   There is a great deal of literature on nineteenth-century fever hospitals, particularly their role in sanitary reform in London. See Pickstone, "Dearth, Dirt and Fever Epidemics"; Bynum, "Hospital, Disease and Community"; Kerr, *Contagion, Isolation, and Biopolitics.*

model dovetailed with William Farr's influential zymotic theory, which held that specific poisons, originating from decomposing and fermenting animal or vegetable products, were the chief cause of infectious disease.[99] The key to Murchison's typhoid theory was its eclectic flexibility in explaining the widespread existence of the disease and its contingent acknowledgment of spontaneous generation. It is no surprise that successive discoveries of the etiology of the disease—its spread through water and food and its bacterial existence—could be easily adapted to fit Murchison's theory.

A critical alternative to Murchison's theory of typhoid came from William Budd, although Continental observers often mistakenly associated both Murchison and Budd with an "English school" or approach.[100] A Bristolian physician who in the late 1820s studied the pathology of typhoid in Paris under Broussais, Budd turned to outbreak investigation and comparative analogy to explain typhoid's spread in the population.[101] The bulk of Budd's epidemiological work on typhoid in Devonshire was conducted in the 1850s and 1860s, collated into one typhoid tome, *Typhoid Fever: Its Nature, Mode of Spreading, and Prevention and* published in 1873 three months before Murchison released his expanded second edition. Typhoid was a specific, self-propagating, communicable disease, Budd argued, spread only via the fresh fecal discharges of typhoid patients, which mixed with air and water. There was no fermentation process needed, and Budd was decidedly against the theory of spontaneous generation.

Although both Murchison and Budd were widely influential in British medical practice and preventive medicine circles, Budd's model for the spread of typhoid came to dominate the type of epidemiological outbreak investigation that emerged at the Medical Department in the 1870s. Budd's ideas were instrumental in focusing epidemiologists on the minute details of the spread of typhoid, particularly the search for an index case. Using a well-known Victorian-era phrase that echoed in the pages of books and articles on typhoid, Budd stated that the drain was a continuation of the intestine. It was a powerful metaphor, allowing one to visualize how typhoid linked the body with the body politic.[102]

---

99   Eyler, *Victorian Social Medicine,* chapter 5.
100 De Pietra Santa, "An Address on Typhoid Fever in Paris," 947.
101 Pelling, *Cholera, Fever, and English Medicine.*
102 Porter, *Bodies Politic.* See also Sigsworth and Worboys, "The Public's View of Public Health."

Organization of the Book

Each chapter of *The Filth Disease* is organized around an epidemiological medium at the center of Victorian practices on typhoid. The book follows a roughly chronological unfolding of knowledge of the spread of the disease via air (chapter 1), water (chapter 2), milk (chapter 3), soil (chapter 4), and bodies (chapter 5). The book begins with a powerful example of how typhoid was yoked to middle-class anxieties about citizenship and respectability. Hospital clinicians like Murchison had argued that the disease had a proclivity not for the urban poor but for the middle and upper classes. From the 1860s the epidemiological gaze of the Medical Department had narrowed to the spread of the disease among the well-to-do, who breathed in the disease via dangerous sewer gases that wafted from newly installed drains and water closets. Outbreak investigation was beginning to reveal some uncomfortable truths, in other words, about the supposedly progressive and class-designating domestic sanitary technologies of water closets and drained homes. The fear of sewer gases intensified after 1871, most famously when Queen Victoria's son and heir, Prince Albert Edward, nearly died from typhoid. This episode forms the basis for chapter 1. During the prince's attack and later recovery (marked by a National Thanksgiving Day service in London), typhoid was in the spotlight, imprinting on the Victorian social body the realization that typhoid was endemic among both rich and poor.[103] In the words of Alfred Haviland, delivering a lecture on typhoid in 1872 at St. Thomas's Hospital, the disease became "a national disgrace," which he argued "ought not to rest until we reduce it to one simply local or personal; its existence will then become punishable."[104]

The decade that followed the prince's attack was the most prolific period in English epidemiology, no doubt spurred by the cultural moment of the filth disease being pervasive in public debate. From 1870 to 1880, before the discovery of *B. typhosus*, "a science of epidemiology" had emerged, discovering "new truths" about the food- and waterborne nature of the disease.[105] Chapters 2 and 3 cover this critical period in the history of disease and the development of epidemiological practice by focusing on water- and milk-borne typhoid, respectively. By 1880, studies of waterborne typhoid

---

103 This builds on a bulk of scholarship on identity and nationalism. See Anderson, *Imagined Communities*; Hobsbawm, "Language, Culture, and National Identity."

104 Haviland, "The Geographical Distribution," 148.

105 MacNalty, *The History of State Medicine in England*, 34–35.

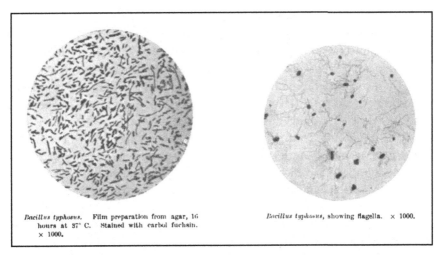

Figure I.3 Microphotographs of B.typhosus from George Newman, Bacteriology and Public Health (Philadelphia: Blakiston's Son & Co., 1904), 302. Orphan work in public domain.

demonstrated two uncomfortable truths: that typhoid was pervasive in rural areas as a result of the contamination of local wells, and it struck in urban and suburban locations due to faulty municipal sanitation projects. The epidemiological investigation of milk-borne typhoid did even more to cement the filth disease into popular anxieties, showing that the health of the urban middle classes—the principal drinkers of cow's milk—very much depended on complicated food pathways and the sanitary habits of rural farmers. Chapters 2 and 3 provide new ways of understanding the broader process of the development of epidemiological methods and the growth of public health infrastructure in the Victorian period, particularly the way that central inspectors at the Medical Department unevenly interacted with local officials.

Chapter 4 turns to the epidemiological study of typhoid after the discovery of *B. typhosus* (figure I.3). Initially, bacteriology did little to influence outbreak investigation, which relied on what was by the 1880s an established tradition and set of practices of epidemiological outbreak investigation. This chapter confirms what a number of scholars have recently said about the impact of the bacteriological revolution.[106] But in the 1890s, building on

106 Wall, *Bacteria in Britain;* Hardy, "Methods of Outbreak Investigation"; Worboys, "Was There a Bacteriological Revolution"; Engelmann, et al., *Plague and the City.*

epidemiological knowledge that typhoid could exist outside of the body in the soil, bacteriologists at the Medical Department, especially Edward Klein, began to contribute in important ways to a nascent ecological understanding of the disease, seeing typhoid across geopolitical and environmental boundaries. By the end of the century there was a model for a combined approach to outbreak investigation that involved the laboratory and the field, one that was later taken up in studies of food poisoning.

As the nineteenth century came to a close there was unbridled optimism in the fight against the filth disease. In 1886 George Buchanan crowed that epidemiology had been successful in connecting typhoid with the excremental pollution of food and water and "has been an important factor in the sanitary improvements made during the last 20 years, which have resulted in the extinction of fully one-third of the mortality from that disease in the whole of England and Wales."[107] By 1900 the incidence of the disease had been even further reduced, concentrated in the north of England and localized to sporadic outbreaks. The death rate in England and Wales had fallen from 21.8 per 1,000 per year in 1868 to 18.1 in 1,000 1888, and 14.8 in 1908.

But before the end of the Victorian era typhoid once again took center stage in popular discourse, this time during the South African War (1899–1901) in the single biggest outbreak of the disease. Chapter 5 explores the palpable anxieties that once again rose to the surface, extending the filth disease from an English problem to one of the British Empire. Epidemiological studies of typhoid in South Africa brought to the fore a trenchant debate among colonial medical practitioners about the existence of typhoid in the tropics, particularly in British India and Africa. While two products of the laboratory—the Widal Test and Almroth Wright's antityphoid vaccine—promised an end to "tropical typhoid," neither they nor epidemiological practices in the military effectively curbed typhoid abroad. By 1900, however, there was at least agreement that typhoid was a global disease spread via food and water, a point long made by English epidemiologists. Pratik Chakrabarti has recently argued that bacteriology "ushered internationalism in colonial medicine," and chapter 5 shows that epidemiology was also central to that globalizing process.[108]

As the Victorian era ended, epidemiological approaches to typhoid still dominated public health interventions across the nation and throughout the

---

107 George Buchanan, "Memorandum as to the Duties of the Board's Medical Department," 1886, National Archives, Kew, MH 78/1.

108 Chakrabarti, *Bacteriology in British India*, 16.

British Empire as a whole. To contemporaries the success was obvious.[109] J. Lane Notter, for example, in 1898 claimed that "epidemiology offers even to the non-professional man many features, not only of interest but also of study . . . to master the rules of life which will allow us to guide and govern an empire on which the sun never sets."[110] Notter's was a powerful trumpeting for the kind of everyday epidemiology that was domesticated into popular culture and public health in the twentieth century. Despite the disastrous incidence of the disease during the South African War, typhoid had declined in England from 1870 to 1900, even if, as Bill Luckin has shown, the last precipitous decline of the disease only truly began in the first decade of the twentieth century.[111] The first two decades of the twentieth century saw bacteriological approaches begin to influence the study of typhoid alongside outbreak investigation, not only with the discovery of the healthy carrier state but also in refining the diagnostic test for the disease and Wright's vaccine.

In the years after 1900, the typhoid of the Victorians disappeared. Or, rather, it became fragmented and disjointed by laboratory science into the broader *Salmonella* group.[112] Today we know typhoid to be the most virulent of 2,600 known serotypes, continuing to strike about twenty million people each year, killing about two hundred thousand individuals annually, predominantly in the Global South. Evolutionary biologists tell us that the disease has long been affecting human populations.

This book recovers the history of the disease during the Victorian era.[113] The Victorian approach to typhoid had a lasting impact on British public health, both on the central ideas that came to dominate the provision of municipal sanitation as well as on the broader concept of disease surveillance. Just as important were the complex ways that epidemiological research on typhoid in the second half of the nineteenth century helped to refine and standardize the methods of outbreak investigation that became central to twentieth-century epidemiology, a topic to which we will return in the conclusion.

---

109 George Buchanan, "Memorandum as to the Duties of the Board's Medical Department as at Present Constituted," 1886, National Archives, Kew, MH 78/1.

110 Notter, "International Sanitary Conferences of the Victorian Era."

111 Luckin, *Death and Survival in Urban Britain*, chapter 3.

112 Hardy, *Salmonella Infections*, 6.

113 Rosenberg, "Disease in History: Frames and Framers."

Chapter One

A Royal Thanksgiving

Disease and the Victorian Social Body

On a bright and sunny February day in 1872, Britons and foreigners alike, rich and poor, packed the troop-lined London streets. Buckingham Palace to St. Paul's Cathedral was awash with people jostling to catch a glimpse of a carriage whose occupants included Queen Victoria and her son, the thirty-year-old heir to the throne, Prince Albert Edward (later Edward VII). The occasion was one of the most grandiose public spectacles of the nineteenth century, providing a model for Queen Victoria's 1887 Golden and 1897 Diamond Jubilees. But whereas the latter two events marked continued rule and expanding empire, the 1872 outpouring of British nationalism was a celebration of restored health. It was a victory, popular rhetoric pronounced, against one of the Victorian period's most feared infectious diseases. Queen Victoria had declared the date, February 27, as a National Thanksgiving— to celebrate the recovery of her son after his prolonged bout with typhoid fever. The event was, the *Illustrated London News* remarked, "an occasion for the grandest outburst of unanimous popular emotion witnessed here since the age of the Tudors."[1] The Thanksgiving was an extravagant celebration. It was a promise of the future of the monarchy, no doubt, but also spoke to the health of a nation. The public spectacle, in other words, was not only a physical and spatial coming together but also a sentimental cultural gathering. At no other point in nineteenth-century British history had a disease, "a

---

1   "The Thanksgiving Day," *Illustrated London News*, March 2, 1872, 206. But the Thanksgiving also fit within the context of contemporary aristocratic funerals. See Jalland, "Victorian Death and Its Decline," 244; Sinnema, "Anxiously Managing Mourning."

most insidious, treacherous, and threatening disorder," left such an indelible mark on British national identity.[2]

The 1872 Thanksgiving provides a vivid lens through which to view the broader contemporary discourse on typhoid fever. Such a focus affords a unique opportunity to investigate the history of infectious disease, one that illuminates the connections between the personal, clinical, and cultural realms of sickness. The first half of the chapter focuses on the prince's sickness, his recovery, and the February Thanksgiving. The events are a powerful example of how a private sickbed became popularized and commodified by a new English middle-class culture. The public nature of the sickness, furthermore, wrought object lessons for how the nation should grieve but also how it should celebrate recovery from disease. It also threw into question the relative merits of private physic versus public prayer. More important was the way in which the royal sickness ignited epidemiological debates over the spread of typhoid, particularly by sewer gases, explored in the second half of the chapter.

An ever-expanding press elevated the popular discourse on typhoid well outside of the immediate realm where the disease was principally discussed: in medical societies, journals, lecture courses, and within the confines of institutions such as fever hospitals. The royal sickness came at a time of intense debate in the medical community over the etiology of the disease, as discussed in the introduction. Although most practitioners routinely distinguished between typhoid and typhus, the GRO, for example, only officially distinguished the two diseases in 1869. But that did not end the bevy of etiological questions surrounding the origin of the disease and how it spread, queries that dominated British public health in the last three decades of the nineteenth century and provided a model for understanding the new science of germs.

The aftermath of the Royal Thanksgiving brought to light a series of entrenched and sometimes esoteric debates about whether typhoid was spread via sewer gases or infected water, whether it was directly or indirectly contagious, and whether the disease arose spontaneously, *de novo*, or only from a previous, ancestral case of the disease. The public nature of the prince's sickness and the events surrounding the 1872 Thanksgiving, both

---

2   "The Illness of H.R.H. The Prince of Wales," *British Medical Journal* 572 (December 16, 1871): 699. The 1872 Thanksgiving was a key moment in what Mary Poovey called "the consolidation of a national identity" in Victorian Britain. See Poovey, *Making a Social Body*, 55.

extensively reported in the press, combined with a series of debates on the transmission of typhoid fever to create a fever pitch in late Victorian Britain. This furor set the stage for the epidemiological research discussed in the chapters that follow. Typhoid was elevated to the most important infectious disease from the early 1870s, taking the inglorious title from epidemic cholera, which last struck English shores in 1866. The last three decades of the nineteenth century and the first decade of the twentieth—due to the virulent incidence of the disease during the South African War—was the most visible period for typhoid fever in British history. The royal typhoid attack became deeply imprinted in British cultural memory.[3] And although it had been endemic before, after 1872 a wider range of large-scale metropolitan and small-scale rural outbreaks of typhoid garnered national, governmental, and medical attention. The majority of these outbreaks were investigated by local medical officers of health and inspectors at the Medical Department. As William Stewart, honorary surgeon to the Beckett Hospital in Barnsley, put it in 1877, typhoid was universally prevalent "in town and country, in the houses of the rich and the hovels of the poor."[4] Chapters 2 and 3, respectively, offer ample demonstrations of this flurry of epidemiological activity. What drove what we might call this golden age of field-based epidemiological inquiry was physicians' deep-seated thirst for intimate knowledge about the disease and how it behaved in the community. But it was also a public impetus, a cultural moment that arrived after the decoupling of typhoid from typhus, not to mention the spectacle of the next king of England falling prey to the filth disease.

We should be cautious in overstating the importance of a singular historical event. But what we can say is that in the years after 1871, typhoid gained a greater degree of public visibility as a result of the royal sickness. It also produced a palpable fear in the hearts and minds of Britons—if the future king could succumb, so could middle- and upper-class Britons. Samuel Sneade Brown, a former colonial administrator and Bristol resident, for example, noted in 1861 that the prince's father, Albert, "perished in the prime of life [from typhoid] like a common Terling peasant," and this kind of public sentiment was recharged in 1871.[5] But the prince, after all, had recovered, and within his convalescence—encoded in the 1872 Thanksgiving—was a national hope that typhoid could be overcome by the nation too.

---

3   Carpenter, *Health, Medicine, and Society,* 10–11.

4   Stewart, "A New Theory of the Origin of Typhoid Fever," 289.

5   Brown, *A Lay Lecture on Sanitary Matters,* 35.

Clinical Encounters at the Royal Sickbed

Prince Albert Edward, the future king of England, labored under the feverish spell of the food- and waterborne bacterial infection in the late months of 1871 and into early 1872. During much of this time, he was subject to fits of delirium and delusion. He had a raging fever, headaches, dyspnea, and leg pain. What was intended to be a private sickbed, his Jacobean, red-brick country estate, Sandringham House, proved to be anything but isolated. His symptoms were, according to contemporary medical authorities, "characteristic of a rather severe attack of typhoid fever."[6] The Norfolk mansion had been purchased in 1861, somewhat ironically, the same year Albert Edward's father, Prince Albert, had died of the same disease. The similar attacks on father and son—ten years apart nearly to the day—made the events all the more gripping for the British public but especially for the royal family. In her diary entry for November 29, 1871, for instance, Queen Victoria described walking into the dimly lit sickroom only to hear a painful, audible wheeze. She saw her son "lying rather flat on his back, breathing very rapidly and loudly."[7] "It reminded me so vividly and sadly," she lamented "of my dearest Albert's illness!"[8] After Albert's death in 1861 Victoria began an almost decade-long period of private mourning, stricken with chronic grief.[9] Here she was again faced with the deadly filth disease.

Two well-known elite London physicians, William Withey Gull (1816–90) and William Jenner (1815–98), treated the sick prince. Jenner had been one of Victoria's court physicians from 1861 when he was called from private practice to the Royal Household by Dr. James Clark, physician-in-ordinary, to assist in the prince consort's losing battle with typhoid. By 1871 Jenner had himself risen to the rank of physician-in-ordinary, the highest for a court physician. Perhaps Jenner thought Gull could do better with the son than he had a decade earlier with the father. Gull and Jenner's professional lives intersected throughout their careers. The two were born a year apart, obtained medical degrees from the University of London, and held longtime appointments as royal physicians. Jenner's early fame in distinguishing typhoid from

6   "The Prince of Wales," *Lancet* 101 (December 2, 1871): 790.
7   Buckle, *The Letters of Queen Victoria,* 171.
8   Ibid.
9   Homans, in *Royal Representations* argues that Victoria's decade of mourning and private detachment from formal political life helped to encourage the growing middle class and an expanding electorate.

typhus and relapsing fever in the mid-1840s made for a quick rise on the London medical scene. But their paths continued to intersect. The very meeting where Jenner read his famous paper on the subject to the Royal Medical and Chirurgical Society (RMCS) in December 1849, for example, Gull was inducted to the organization. They each later served as presidents of both the RMCS and the Pathological Society and were two of the earliest members of the Epidemiological Society of London.

Gull did the lion's share of clinical treatment and case management for the prince in 1871. He came from a middling background and rose to medical fame—amassing what was by Victorian doctoring standards a small fortune. Born at Colchester, Gull lost his father, a barge owner, when he was ten years old. He studied medicine first at Guy's Hospital, then obtained a medical degree from the University of London in 1846, where he studied under pioneer epidemiological thinker Benjamin Guy Babington.[10] Gull practiced at Guy's for decades, first serving as a pupil of the London clinician Thomas Addison. In 1854, during the same cholera outbreak in London that John Snow traced to an infected water supply, Gull was part of the Cholera Committee of the Royal College of Physicians. By 1871 he had stepped down at Guy's as a consulting physician to focus on a lucrative private practice. It was during this time that he increasingly took on professional leadership roles in the metropolitan medical elite, for example, as president of the Clinical Society of London. For his service to the royal family, Gull was given a series of honors. He received a baronetcy in 1872 and was appointed physician extraordinary. In 1880 he became physician-in-ordinary to Queen Victoria. Although already well known in London medical circles as a result of his treatment of the Prince of Wales, Gull thereafter became an iconic public figure and one of London's leading physicians. One biographer noted that Gull's treatment of the prince was "the principal event" of his life.[11] So apt was this characterization that the satirical magazine *Punch*, for instance, parodied Gull in their "Fancy Portraits" caricatures in 1882 (figure 1.1). The

10   Babington, presumably, introduced Gull to the society, and in the 1850s Gull sat on the society's council. See Archives of the Epidemiological Society of London, Royal Society of Medicine, Archives, ESL/B/1 Meeting Minutes. The first biographical sketch of Gull, which includes many of his published writings, was begun by close friend and contemporary, Oxford physician Henry Acland. Acland never finished the task, however, and it was left to his son, Theodore Dyke Acland, who coincidentally married Gull's daughter, Caroline. See Acland, ed., *A Collection of the Published Writings of William Withey Gull.*

11   Wilks and Bettany, *A Biographical History of Guy's Hospital,* 264.

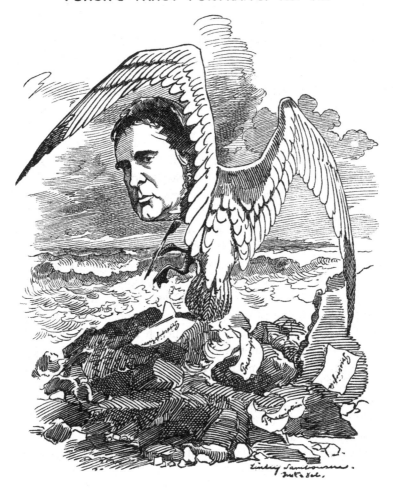

SIR WILLIAM WITHEY GULL, Bart., M.D., D.C.L., F.R.S.

THE CLEVER BIRD WHO ADDED A PRINCE OF WALES'S FEATHER TO HIS PLUMAGE.

Figure 1.1 "Sir William Withey Gull, Bart., M.D., D.C.L., F.R.S. The clever bird who added a Prince of Wales's feather to his plumage," from Punch 1882. Copyright permission by Topham Partners LLP.

illustration, by prominent *Punch* draughtsmen Edward Linley Sambourne, featured Gull's head attached to a seagull's body, with the line, "the clever bird who added a Prince of Wales's feather to his plumage."[12] Gull's public career was thus yoked to his care of the prince. Gull was close with many members of England's medical aristocracy, and as Harry Marks has noted, he was part of a small group of elite doctors—including George Humphrey, Henry Acland, Samuel Wilks, and James Paget—who were passionate about the role of pathological anatomy in clinical medicine but interested in studying disease through a broader lens: what became known in the 1880s as the "collective investigation" of disease.[13]

While not a prolific medical writer—his best-known research outside of an interest in typhoid was on the etiology of anorexia nervosa and on hormones—Gull was active in clinical practice. His attention to detail and painstaking care for patients are characteristics that reappear in each of his contemporary biographical accounts.[14] "Never forget," he was fond of telling his students, in an aphorism illustrative of his vision of generalized patient care, "that it is not a pneumonia, but a pneumonic man who is your patient. Not a typhoid fever, but a typhoid man."[15] Giving the annual oration at the Hunterian Society in February 1861, Gull proclaimed that "we may indeed say that a man has a fever, but in reality he is the fever."[16] Gull noted in an address before the British Medical Association in 1868, for example, that "the clinical physician knows that the phenomena of disease are not explained by the knowledge of healthy textures, nor by the action of healthy organs," but instead by a general investigation of the body.[17] He combined, as Christopher Lawrence has argued, "a physiology peculiarly English in its relations with the natural theological tradition," and was embedded in what George Weisz has called the "gentlemanly" culture of elite London hospital physicians, who, as Weisz notes, "prided themselves on clinical skill and 'gentlemanly' personal and cultural attributes rather than on the methodical,

---

12 "Sir William Withey Gull," *Punch* 82 (February 25, 1882): 94.

13 Marks, "Until the Sun of Science." The term "collective investigation of disease" meant a collaborative study of the origin and spread of disease combined with intimate knowledge of family history. Gull, "An Address on the Collective Investigation of Disease."

14 For more on Gull's research on anorexia, see Brumberg, *Fasting Girls.*

15 Acland, *A Collection,* xxiii.

16 Acland, *A Collection,* 30.

17 Acland, *A Collection,* 37.

empirical research that promoted specialization elsewhere."[18] He was, in the terms that Stephen Casper and Rick Welsh have recently articulated, a "generalist."[19]

Gull's penchant for personalized patient care and the primacy of interpersonal skills was fully apparent in his careful treatment of the prince. *The Times*, for example, lionized Gull, noting that he "combined energy that never tired, watchfulness that never flagged; nursing so tender, ministry so minute, that in his functions he seemed to combine the duties of physician, dresser, dispenser, valet, nurse."[20] Like his views on politics, Gull's position on therapeutics was conservative, and he followed what historians have referred to as "therapeutic skepticism."[21] Gull's obituarist noted, for example, that "he was never tired of exposing the absurdity of much of the traditional polypharmacy" and preferred to let disease, particularly fever, run its course without much pharmacological intervention.[22] His treatment of the prince followed these therapeutic beliefs of supportive care. He rarely deviated, for example, from hourly combinations of chicken broth, milk and seltzer, arrowroot, beef tea, port wine, sherry, and brandy. Only occasionally did he turn to laudanum-laced starch enemas, popular at the time for treating typhoid and other bowel complaints, and camphorated tinctures of opium, an antidiarrheal that Charles Murchison, lecturing at St. Thomas's Hospital, noted was of "great use."[23] Gull's therapeutic approach might have earned scorn from the likes of Murchison, who quipped in his authoritative *A Treatise on the Continued Fevers of Great Britain* that "the tendency of modern practice in England . . . is not to starve fevers, but to overfeed them."[24] To Gull's mind, simple restorative therapy had saved the prince's life and

---

18   Weisz, *Divide and Conquer,* 27. Lawrence, "Incommunicable Knowledge."

19   Casper and Welsh, "British Romantic Generalism." Gull's contemporary biographer went as far as to note that Gull was "one of the foremost men of mark of his time . . . due to his extensive and thorough acquaintance of every subject in medicine." Wilks and Bettany, *A Biographical History of Guy's Hospital,* 266.

20   Acland, *A Collection,* xviii.

21   Warner, *The Therapeutic Perspective.*

22   "Obituary for William Withey Gull," *Guy's Hospital Reports* 47, no. 3 (1890): xxxiii.

23   T. D. Acland, Lecture Notes of Charles Murchison at St. Thomas's Hospital, 1877, Wellcome Library, GB 120, MSS 3652.

24   Murchison, *A Treatise on the Continued Fevers of Great Britain* (London, 1884), 289.

held a critical lesson for the British public. After the prince's recovery, Gull remarked: "One thing I am thankful Jenner and I have together succeeded in doing," is that "we have disabused the public of the belief that doctoring consists in drenching them with nauseous drugs."[25]

And although Gull did the lion's share of the future king of England's treatment in late 1871, Jenner was rarely far from the case. This is hardly surprising considering that he was both a royal physician, and, alongside Murchison, considered one of the key fever experts in Britain. Renowned for his investigation two decades earlier into over a thousand cases of febrile disease at the London Fever Hospital, Jenner was not the first but was certainly the most prominent physician in Britain to distinguish typhoid from typhus and relapsing fever. Jenner's confirmation of the separate identities of typhoid and typhus not only served as a springboard for his illustrious career, but it was also a finding deeply entrenched in the history of epidemiology. Jenner's sometime correspondent, John Netten Radcliffe, one of the outspoken leaders of British epidemiology, went before the Epidemiological Society of London, for example, on November 11, 1875, and gave a speech entitled "The Progress of Epidemiology in England." There Radcliffe called Jenner's unraveling of fever "the true starting point of all epidemiological knowledge."[26] Like Gull, Jenner was deeply tied to the establishment of clinical medicine and held a position in the highest ranks of professional society. As Sir James Barr celebrated in his *Treatment of Typhoid Fever (1892)*, Jenner was "the Sydenham of our day."[27] Like Gull, Jenner adopted a therapeutic skepticism, particularly in cases of typhoid fever. "I have never known a case of typhoid fever cut short by any remedial agent—that is cured," he noted in *the Lancet*.[28] His early research on typhoid, no doubt, combined with his treatment of the prince, made him an often celebrated figure in the formation of British epidemiology. Like Gull, although he practiced very little of what was emerging as epidemiological inquiry, he was one of its champions, even serving as the president of the Epidemiological Society of London.

The case of the prince's sickness was full of drama and intrigue. Gull's detailed case notes reveal the intimate side of doctoring in nineteenth-century England. While certainly not representative (in terms of class, race, or

---

25 Acland, *A Collection*, xxv.

26 "The Epidemiological Society," *Medical Times and Gazette* 2 (November 20, 1875): 580.

27 Barr, *The Treatment of Typhoid Fever*, 32.

28 Jenner, "An Address on the Treatment of Typhoid Fever," 715.

gender) of everyday doctoring of the masses, the case is testament to what John Harley Warner has called "workaday activity at the bedside" of the aristocracy. Gull's extensive clinical case notes and correspondence offer a unique window into the emotional experience of both doctor and patient.[29] We should reflect here on the emotional effects of such clinical encounters between the medical community and the public, particularly the emotional ordeals of doctors treating typhoid and the patients suffering from it, as these encounters are often omitted from the historical record. Mediated through Gull, we see glimpses of the prince as a typhoid patient in case notes. Gull's notes offer an example for the flourishing field of the history of emotions currently being explored by historians of medicine such as Michael Brown, who has shown new fruitful lines of historical inquiry studying the emotional landscape of nineteenth-century surgery.[30]

At a time before clinical case notes were standardized, Gull's notes were a mixed bag of illness narrative, personal reflection, hand sketches—attempts to visualize the disease through clinical observation—and ardent though unsuccessful attempts at objectifying, measuring, quantifying, and standardizing the patient record. Gull's case notes are an interesting blend of emotionally driven narratives of doctor-patient interaction from the early to mid-nineteenth century, to what Warner argues became "the *formal* transformation of the patient record." Joel Howell has shown that by the early twentieth century this transformation was defined by regimentation, visualization, standardization, and shortening of the patient record to a blank form.[31] Gull's clinical hybridity in prioritizing the prince's language, feelings, and emotions was tempered by the potential unreliability of these clinical semiotics, necessitating in his mind an incorporation of technologies of quantitative measurement and visualization.

The private notes reveal in detailed and unedited fashion each prescription Gull gave to the prince, time-stamped updates on the prince's condition, and personal reflections on the patient's progress. They move us beyond the afterthought descriptions printed in contemporary medical journals, and beyond what Gull and others said about treating typhoid patients, to his actual "clinical creativity," which Warner calls the "least explored use of

---

29   Warner, "The Uses of Patient Records," 101.

30   Brown, "Surgery, Identity and Embodied Emotion"; Boddice, *The History of Emotions.*

31   Warner, "The Uses of Patient Records," 109; Howell, *Technology in the Hospital.*

patient records."[32] Gull's notes, furthermore, demonstrate the delicacy of communicating to family members, colleagues, and the public about the reality and prognosis of typhoid in this period; he frequently wrote to Queen Victoria throughout the prince's sickness, typically providing brief, measured updates on the prince's condition. Gull's private diary was more candid in offering admissions, whereas his letters to family members and daily bulletins meant for public consumption revealed much less of the reality of what was occurring at Sandringham. Gull also wrote to Jenner and other physicians, using language and tone not found in his personal case notes, an interesting example of intraprofessional culture among elite English physicians. The case notes, in other words, form one example of the layered intricacies of Victorian medical culture.

The prince first showed signs of typhoid fever on November 13, 1871, and was taken to Sandringham House on November 14, initially under the care of Dr. John Lowe, the resident Sandringham physician who occasionally assisted Gull throughout the prince's illness.[33] It was popularly believed that the prince contracted typhoid via inhaling dangerous sewer gases at Londesborough Lodge, Scarborough, where he went to join one of his frequent hunting parties, from October 30 to November 4. The suspicion thrown on Scarborough was intense enough to warrant a special commission set up by the leading English medical journal, *the Lancet*, which conducted a full epidemiological inquiry, explored below. The sewer gas suspicion raised both popular alarm and public anxiety but also brought into the popular consciousness debates over the etiology of typhoid fever.

Gull's case notes are filled with hourly jottings of his treatment of the prince as well as detailed qualitative and quantitative observations of the prince's condition. "The anxiety of the House-hold, high and low, is intense . . . those in the inner royal circle 'feel very anxious,'" the duke of Cambridge noted in his diary for November 23.[34] There was good reason to be anxious. In addition to noting the languor, chills, delirium, wheezing, sputum, vomiting, diarrhea, and headaches, Gull made careful note of what the prince looked like, how he felt, and what he said. What was more, Gull thrice daily

---

32 Warner, "The Uses of Patient Records," 109.

33 Gull was first contacted about the case on November 15. See Letter to Gull, November 15, 1871, Wellcome Archives, MS5873 F/2.

34 Diary of the Duke of Cambridge, November 23, 1871. See Edgar Sheppard, ed., *George Duke of Cambridge*, 302.

recorded the prince's pulse, temperature, respiration, and the actions of his bowels.

Gull visualized the prince's illness in a series of hand sketches. Two are particularly revealing. Figure 1.2, for example, is Gull's rather unique version of a late Victorian fever chart. The u-shaped chart showed the chronology of the prince's fever, bounded on the top side of the curve with the day of the month (from the onset of typhoid on November 13, 1871) and the bottom side with the day of the fever. Along the simple curve—meant to track change over time and any deviations—Gull recorded temperature, pulse, and respiration rates, as well as the prince's qualitative symptoms (the period of delirium, for example, from November 24 to 27, or the appearance of the rose spots on November 22).[35] The addition of qualities to the fever chart represent what Bill and Helen Bynum have called "a throwback to an older qualitative tradition felt by the hand," demonstrating the intimate side of doctoring before the standardization of clinical practice in the twentieth century.[36] Figure 1.3 illustrates how Gull combined central quantitative measurements of the prince's illness (pulse, temperature, breathing) into one visual aesthetic that mirrors a standard Victorian fever chart. Similar to the clinical creativity featured in figure 1.2, in figure 1.3 Gull jotted down important clinical features—such as the appearance of the rose spots—as well as the dual chronological metrics of day of the month and day of the fever.

Gull's was a pathophysiological approach. With the use of the clinical thermometer to quantify the prince's sickness, coupled with his hand-drawn fever charts, he was attempting to visualize typhoid as a way to make it easier to understand in living people. For at least two decades, typhoid was most readily recognized only from the postmortem pathological analysis of the Peyer's patches on the victim's small intestine. Thankfully for the queen— and for Gull's subsequent career—the prince's cadaver was not available to Gull in late 1871, so he instead turned to detailed case tracing, observation, and new technologies of measurement, such as the clinical thermometer. The latter was slowly introduced into practice in Europe after Carl Wunderlich's well-known 1868 treatise, *On the Temperature in Disease*, and in Britain after Leeds physician Clifford Allbutt designed an easy-to-use (and shorter) six-inch thermometer.

---

35   The standard contemporary medical opinion was that typhoid had an incubation period of twelve to fourteen days. See Charles Murchison, *A Treatise*, 435.

36   Bynum and Bynum, "Object Lessons," 359.

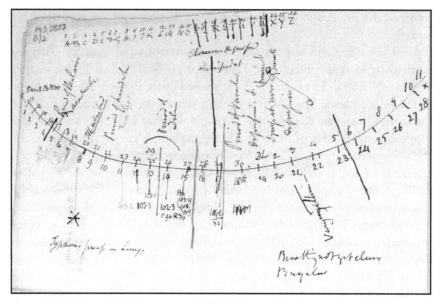

Figure 1.2 William Gull, fever chart, n.d. Wellcome Archives. MS 5873/B/2. Wellcome Library, London. Creative Commons Attribution license CC BY 4.0.

Christopher Hamlin has recently argued that the "dictatorial thermometer" of the late nineteenth century signified a shift in the understanding and treatment of fever. He suggests that the thermometer moved the clinical encounter away from both the patient's lived experience of fever and the narrative, emotional understanding of sickness, to a "militantly physiological view of disease."[37] Gull's clinical case notes do not fully substantiate this view but instead reveal that he was in the liminal zone of this transition. He was eager to incorporate new diagnostic tools but not at the expense of what he—particularly from his perch as a conservative, urban-elite practitioner—understood to be the sound clinical practices of close bedside observation of the patient's feelings and the qualities of his symptoms and outputs of breath, phlegm, urine, and feces. Yet for all of his penchant for generalism and genteelism, Gull was adept at incorporating new clinical technologies that were increasingly considered to embody a new "science" of medicine,

37   Hamlin, *More Than Hot*, 11.

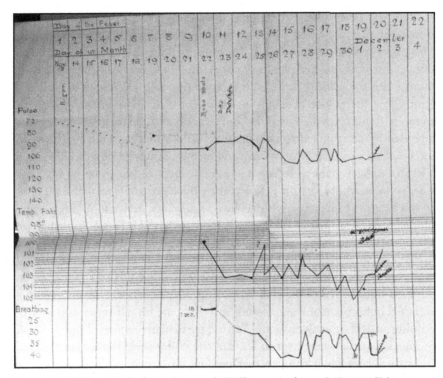

Figure 1.3 William Gull, fever chart, n.d. Wellcome Archives. MS 5873/B/2.
Wellcome Library, London. Creative Commons Attribution license CC BY 4.0.

in spite of the fact, as historians agree, that English physicians were slow to embrace experimental science.[38]

The last month of the prince's case was turbulent. Throughout late November his fever hovered around 103 degrees Fahrenheit. He was getting worse, and many close to the royal family, including his physicians, believed he would perish. In his private notes Gull used the word, "anxious," but writing on December 2 to his son, Willie, who was studying at Eton, he was optimistic that "our good Prince is soon I hope to be better and when he is I shall come home."[39] But his optimism was tested the following week.

---

38   Lawrence cites Samuel Wilks, one of Gull's closest allies, as noting that the clinical thermometer came into use at Guy's Hospital only in 1870. Lawrence, "Incommunicable Knowledge," 515.

39   William Gull to Willie Gull, December 2, 1871, Wellcome Library, MS5873/I/4.

So, too, was Bertie's wife, Alexandra. In early December the princess was so distraught that she asked the local Sandringham reverend vicar, Mr. Luke Onslow, to prepare for a funeral. The prince's fever had spiked to over 103 degrees for days, so her plea was not without medical evidence. Nearly a month into the prince's battle with typhoid fever, on December 8, Gull and Jenner saw the prince through an imminent crisis. The prince was at his worst, with his fever measured by Gull at noon and 2 p.m. at 105.4 degrees, attended by coughing fits, hallucinations, and vomiting. Gull had tried to intervene all morning with brandy and arrowroot but to no avail.[40] Queen Victoria was telegraphed to come at once from Windsor to be by her son's side, perhaps for the last time. When the prince dozed off around 2:00 p.m. at the height of his battle with typhoid, Gull and Jenner took a few spare moments to clear their heads and take in some fresh air in the Sandringham garden before Victoria's scheduled arrival at 4:00 p.m. "Well if he lives till 4," Jenner lamented, "I shall be satisfied." Not satisfied and ever the clinical optimist, Gull replied: "That will not satisfy me."[41] Gull's was, however, an outward optimism that needed rehearsing. December 10, for instance, he sketched in his notebook a makeshift seal that bore his self-prescribed motto, echoing an 1854 *Punch* cartoon: "You are particularly requested not to speak to the man at the wheel . . . fear is a bad councillor [*sic*]."[42]

The prince made it through that perilous December night, lightened by Gull's hourly prescriptions of brandy, but his slightly improved condition did not last long. By December 11 he had a second episodic fit, and again Gull messaged Queen Victoria to come at once, as, Victoria noted in her diary, "at any moment dear Bertie might go off," from "threatening paroxysms."[43] Gull sent updates to Victoria three times a day, but even that was not enough to keep the queen's mind at ease; she lamented to Gull in a telegraph at 9:00 p.m. on December 22, 1871, that she wished Gull would send one more message that night, as "it is so long to wait till tomorrow morning."[44]

---

40   William Gull case notes, Wellcome Library, MS5873/B/5.

41   William Gull, untitled draft, April 29, 1889, Wellcome Library, MS 5873 J/3.

42   William Gull notebook, December 10, 1871, Wellcome Library, MS 5873/b/23.

43   William Gull casebook, December 10, 187, Wellcome Library, MS5873/B/23. See also Buckle, *The Letters of Queen Victoria*, vol. 5, 176.

44   Telegraph from Queen Victoria to William Gull, December 22, 1871, Wellcome Library, MS 5873/E/3.

By mid-December the prince's condition seemed to keep him away from death's doorstep, but he was only slowly on the mend. Whereas his telegraphs to Queen Victoria often abruptly noted "Prince still sleeping," Gull's private diary was more explicit. On December 16, for example, when the press was reporting a splendid recovery, Gull reflected that the prince "mistakes his identity; thinks someone else is coughing." Gull's entry for December 22 noted that the prince's "mind wandering, confused this morning . . . thinks himself in an American Hotel . . . he cannot realize that the pain in his leg is his."[45] "At times," Gull expressed in a phrase common to his case notes, "I am anxious," allowing for a rare glimpse into the emotions of Victorian doctors.[46] But by December 18 Gull confidently wrote from Sandringham to his colleague and friend Dr. W. N. Thursfield, medical officer of health for Shropshire, that "my anxious duties here are coming to an end so that now for the first time I am looking forward to return to my routine duties."[47] At Christmas, Gull stayed at the bedside of his royal patron, writing to his son, Willie, on Christmas Eve, expressing his sorrow that he could not be with his family but optimistic that "England will have a happier Christmas tomorrow as the Prince is better."[48]

The first few days of January saw the prince still having feverish spells, leaving Queen Victoria to ask in exasperation, "What can be the cause of the return of fever in the afternoon and evening?"[49] By January 8, Gull's last full day of treating the prince at Sandringham, the queen was "truly rejoiced at good accounts but terribly afraid of imprudence," as the prince had not walked, read, or dressed himself in nearly two months.[50] And though Gull left Sandringham to return to the rigors of London life, he received multiple

---

45 William Gull diary, December 16, 1871, Wellcome Library, MS5873/B/36. See also William Gull diary, December 22, 1871, Wellcome Library, MS5873/B/46.

46 William Gull diary, December 16, 1871, Wellcome Library, MS5873/B/36.

47 William Gull to W. N. Thursfield, December 18, 1871, Wellcome Library, MS8375/6.

48 William Gull to Willie Gull, December 24, 1871, Wellcome Library, MS5873/I/5.

49 Queen Victoria to William Gull, January 5, 1872, Wellcome Library, MS 5873/E/8.

50 Queen Victoria to William Gull, January 5, 1872, Wellcome Library, MS 5873/E/12.

updates on the prince's condition.[51] Queen Victoria, writing to Gull from Osborne on February 12, 1872, lamented, "I think he shows how *ill* he has been."[52] Gull checked in on the prince several times at Osborne, and as the preparations began for the February Thanksgiving Day, the queen remained worried that the prince might not be up for the celebration. She turned to Gull for advice. Writing on February 3, 1872, she said, "If every one [*sic*] here and the Govt quite of our opinion about the going to St. P. hope you will put that straight. It has worried me a good deal."[53] Victoria continued to worry about the prince attending the event, begging Gull and Sir James Paget to visit the prince again on February 24 at Osborne to ensure that he was rested and recovered enough for the Thanksgiving events.

The near two-month clinical encounter between Gull and the prince at Sandringham offers a few suggestions. First, Gull's normative preaching in printed works and lectures about therapeutic conservativism played out in private practice, where he mostly fed the prince a supportive diet. Secondly, analysis of the case demonstrates that elite practitioners such as Gull were often Janus faced in the late nineteenth century in examining and caring for their patients' emotions (and reflecting on their own) and in mediating that narrative encounter with new technologies of measurement and visibility, such as the fever chart. A third and final suggestion from the prince's illness speaks to the clinical nature of suffering and caring for typhoid fever in the Victorian era. Too often both our historical accounts as well as contemporary epidemiological studies, such as the ones found in the chapters that follow, are devoid of the clinical encounter. This is because Victorian epidemiology by and large was only conducted once an epidemic had already occurred, when patients were either dead, recovered, or convalescing. The prince's case, then, is a reminder of the emotional toll the disease took on both doctors and patients, as well as on their family members. But in some cases, such as the one explored here, the private sickbed had an even greater impact on a nation.

---

51   Princess Alexandra to William Gull, January 24, 1872, Wellcome Library, MS5873/G/7/1–2.

52   Queen Victoria to William Gull, January 5, 1872, Wellcome Library, MS 5873/E/29/1; emphasis in the original.

53   Queen Victoria to William Gull, January 5, 1872, Wellcome Library, MS 5873/E/24.

Contesting the Royal Sickbed in the Victorian Press

More than a private space of monarchical and elite medical worry, the future king of England's sickbed was a public spectacle, an "all absorbing topic of thought and conversation."[54] In an age when the press and the printed word would become the medium of the public sphere, and when new forms of capitalism manifested an intensely commodified culture, news of the prince's illness spread not only throughout Britain and its imperial networks but also throughout the world. "Never before that we can remember," noted an editorial in the *Lancet,* "has the bearing of all classes exhibited the strength of that common band of sorrowful sympathy which we are all bound together as a nation."[55] Gull's thrice daily updates were telegraphed to London, where they were printed, sent to local police stations, and then posted by newsboys at key sites in London, such as Mansion House and Marlborough House. The *Echo* and the *Globe*, in London, went as far as issuing morning, midday, and evening updates with news of the prince, a topic, as one journalist noted, that "now engages all pens, tongues, and hearts."[56] Gull's bulletins, not surprisingly, bore only a slim resemblance to his intricate bedside case notes. For example, his bulletin of Thursday, December 7, read:

> 9 a.m.—His Royal Highness the Prince of Wales has passed a quiet night. The decline of the symptoms continues regularly. 5 p.m. His Royal Highness has passed a quiet day; there is no material change in the symptoms.

That is not to say, however, that Gull deliberately deceived the public in his bulletins. On Friday December 8, the day Gull described as an "imminent crisis," his bulletin was more explicit and took a graver tone, giving concern to the entire nation:

> Friday, 8 a.m.—His Royal Highness has passed a very unquiet night. There is a considerable increase in the febrile symptoms. 1 p.m. The Prince of Wales has slept at intervals during the morning, but there is no abatement of the graver symptoms. 5.30 p.m. His Royal Highness continues in a precarious state. The exacerbation of the symptoms which began late last evening has been attended by a great prostration of the strength. 9.30 p.m. The Prince has slept, but still

---

54 "The Prince of Wales," *Illustrated London News*, December 16, 1871, 567.

55 "The Progress of H.R.H. The Prince of Wales," *Lancet* 101 (December 16, 1871): 857.

56 "Editorial," *Illustrated London News*, December 16, 1871, 570.

continues in a prostrate condition. Night, 1 a.m. His Royal Highness continues in the same condition as at 9.30 p.m.

Notice that Gull's public bulletin lacks the kind of intimate details he privately pored over in the prince's case, notably the emotional state of the prince and the measurable qualities of the case—the prince's temperature, pulse, and respiration. The contemporary medical community praised Gull's bulletins. *The Lancet,* for instance, applauded the bulletins for not "entering into unnecessary details, or endeavouring to veil the facts by the use of technicalities."[57] The *British Medical Journal* also stated that "by avoiding unnecessary details," Gull's bulletins "have afforded almost as accurate a clinical record as if the thermometric figures and the bedside observations had been published."[58] The populist *Times,* meanwhile, was more critical, noting to its readership that Gull's bulletins were "guarded" and that when Gull wrote that "the fever is strong and the nights are unquiet," what he really meant was that "there is more or less of delirium, and that the affection is acute."[59]

So engrossing was news of the prince's condition that only the fervor for news during the Crimean War and the Indian Mutiny matched it. "It was as though the door of the sick-room had been left ajar," the *Illustrated London News* noted, "and the entire population of the kingdom had been assembled in the ante-room to catch, in breathless anxiety, the smallest intimation of the alterations of that mortal contest which was going on within . . . it will doubtless take its place in history as an event unprecedented."[60] The press coverage, in other words, turned a private sickbed into a public event, commodified and ingested by the English public. And this commodification was not just in metropolitan London but throughout Britain, the Empire, and Continental Europe. *La France* noted that "political life is suspended in England. One sole anxiety absorbs all minds—the health of the Prince of Wales."[61] Throughout Britain events were cancelled, such as the Education Conference of the Nonconformists in Manchester and a meeting of Roman

---

57   "The Prince of Wales," *Lancet* 98 (December 9, 1871): 824.
58   "The Illness of H.R.H. The Prince of Wales," *British Medical Journal* 571 (December 9, 1871): 671.
59   "Court Circular," *Times,* November 19, 1871, 7.
60   "The Convalescence of the Prince of Wales," *Illustrated London News,* January 20, 1872, 54.
61   Ryle, *What Good Will It Do?,* 38.

Catholics in Dublin. The coverage of the sickness accomplished two ends: to make the disease more visible in the public sphere than ever before and to enshrine the work of the prince's physicians, principally Gull. The *Illustrated London News,* for example, in its December 23, 1871 edition, featured a full page with images of Jenner, Gull, and Lowe. The article included biographical details of each doctor but centered on Gull, using an excerpt from the *Times* that extolled his "watchfulness that never flagged—nursing so tender, ministry so minute."[62] The hyperbolic rhetoric of the mainstream press coverage of the prince's recovery and his doctors stressed that Britons were coming together as one nation to join a common cause.

But the rhetoric of the nation grieving as one at the royal sickbed—praying for the prince, the royal family, and for the future of the monarchy—irked some members of the English medical community. The *Medical Times, British Medical Journal,* and the *Lancet* all closely followed the prince's sickness and reported on the case, poring over the clinical details. But as the prince began to convalesce in late December, and although the *Illustrated News* had prominently featured Gull, Jenner, and Lowe, the *Lancet*

> wondered whether the public ever for a moment considered the position and responsibilities of his medical advisers. The care of life is at all times an anxious thing, but the charge of such a life, exhausted by a month of typhoid, and jeopardised by paroxysms of dyspnea, with a whole nation looking on, and a whole profession critcising and constructing bulletins, means a strain of all the powers of body and mind which cannot be realized fully by many, even of professional men.[63]

This kind of professional grandstanding for cultural authority was seen in a number of *Lancet* articles that covered the prince's sickness. "For once medicine was in the ascendant. It was a State institution . . . neither men nor women would read anything but the bulletins of the doctors at Sandringham," a December 30 editorial proudly announced.[64] The public nature of the sickness brought to the fore unanswered questions about how the nation should grieve and to whom sympathies were due. The medical community's clamor was partly a response to what many doctors saw as a

---

62   "The Prince of Wales' Physicians," *Illustrated London News,* December 16, 1871, 597.

63   "The Prince's Physicians," *Lancet* 101 (December 23, 1871): 893.

64   "The Annus Medicus," *Lancet* 101 (December 30, 1871): 925.

neglectful coverage of the diligent work of the royal physicians. It was also a product of a short-lived but intense debate on the value of prayer for the sick.

On December 9, the day of the imminent crisis, William Gladstone wrote to the archbishop of Canterbury, Archibald Campbell Tait, asking for some kind of clerical intervention. That day Tait prepared an address, a special prayer that was printed and circulated to every church in England and Wales and immediately that night to the London churches. As the prince's condition slowly improved, many in England believed that steadfast and earnest prayer had saved the prince's life. By Sunday, December 17, for example, Archbishop Tait—who was also one of Gull's patients—rejoiced in his diary that "the Prince has wonderfully rallied in answer to the prayers of the whole country."[65] To many church officials there was a lesson in the prince's recovery: that more focused prayer was needed going forward. As the archdeacon of Buckingham implored, "Loyal subjects and faithful Christians, be encouraged by these things to more diligent and fervent in prayer."[66] Again in mid-January, the Privy Council ordered that a prayer of thanksgiving be offered in the churches of England and Wales, foreshadowing the public events of the February Thanksgiving Day, which culminated in a service at St. Paul's Cathedral, where Archbishop Tait was called on once again to give the sermon. And while no doubt local clergy were acknowledging the prince's condition in their weekly November and December sermons, the *Illustrated London News* allowed readers across the nation to peer into the local church service in Sandringham, which Princess Alexandra attended on Sunday, December 10, at the height of the prince's sickness. "The intense anxiety" of the nation, the article began, resembles a "family affliction" to the people of Sandringham.[67] Speaking two weeks later, when the prince seemed close to death, the archdeacon of Buckingham, as reported in the high Tory Sunday magazine *John Bull*, closed his sermon by saying that "for the moment men talked of nothing else. Business was arrested. Political and religious differences were laid aside; and this great nation, as one man, was prostrate in prayer."[68] Queen Victoria even addressed the nation as the prince was convalescing, in a letter widely published in the press: "We have just passed through

65   Davidson and Benham, eds., *Life of Archibald Campbell Tait*, 106.

66   "The Prince of Wales," *John Bull*, December 30, 1871, 908.

67   "Illness of the Prince of Wales," *Illustrated London News*, December 16, 1871, 597.

68   "The Prince of Wales," *John Bull*, December 30, 1871, 908.

a period of anxiety," she began, using that word so common to the events surrounding her son's sickness. "The expression of emotion during the illness of the Prince of Wales," she continued, "the earnest prayers during the crisis of the fever, and the universal joy and thanksgiving for his recovery, mark the earnestness of the British character."[69] Here the queen was performing the kind of bourgeois morality—showing that the royal family was susceptible to death and grieving just like common Britons—that made the last decades of her reign popular. Just as Britons saw typhoid "as a personal affliction to the nation," so, too, they had collectively grieved.[70] Although the overwhelming focus on prayer and religious intervention had vexed some English doctors, this spiritual angle also created a stir in the scientific community.

The "prayer-gauge debate," as it was colloquially known, began shortly after and as a result of the prince's recovery and public Thanksgiving. Numerous high-ranking church officials, such as Archbishop Tait, openly and publicly argued that it was the power of collective prayer that had saved the prince. Following the February 27 Thanksgiving, in early March the *Guardian* published a lengthy editorial, praising the "brotherhood among men" and the "universal participation" that led to such steadfast prayer that aided in the prince's recovery. The editorial proclaimed that it was

a distinct National Proclamation of Fate in the reality of special and personal Providence. The thousands whose eyes involuntarily turned to the face of the Prince—worn, but refined, by illness-as the special Thanksgiving was offered, really felt that he had been brought back to them from the very threshold of death, not by some abstract 'Law of Health,' not merely by human skill and tenderness, but by the mercy of the God who hears and answers prayer.[71]

It was both a bold assertion for the power of prayer, and another call to British nationalism, as the article ended: "It ought to be our exhortation to a greater and truer unity of class with class, and of man with man . . . we may at least desire and hope that the united Thanksgiving to the Father of all may do something to influence that tone, and rekindle a desire which will not fail to find its means of accomplishment."[72] *The Guardian* article was a not-

---

69   "The Prince of Wales," *John Bull*, December 30, 1871, 908.

70   "The Annus Medicus," *Lancet* 101 (December 30, 1871): 925.

71   "The Religious Press on the Thanksgiving at St. Paul's," *Public Opinion* 21 (March 2, 1872): 262.

72   Ibid.

so-subtle knock on the royal physicians' care of the prince. Historian Frank Turner has gone as far as to call the affront "still another blow to the ambitions" of English physicians.[73] Recall, for example, that a December *Times* article had praised Gull's "tenderness" in treating the prince. But to famed Victorian scientist and Royal Institute professor John Tyndall, the national focus on prayer in healing the prince was an attack on natural law and scientific materialism. In July 1872 Tyndall sent an anonymous letter, later attributed to surgeon Henry Thompson, to *the Contemporary Review*. Titled "The Prayer for the Sick: Hints towards a Serious Attempt to Estimate Its Value," the letter included an introduction by Tyndall.[74] In the piece Tyndall and Thompson—vocal skeptics of the power of prayer to intervene in the material world—proposed a way to settle, scientifically, whether prayer influenced the course of disease in an individual. The idea was in vogue with the kind of experimental science of which Tyndall was a leading advocate: a hypothetical clinical case study in which patients could be found in a single ward of a hospital, suffering from the same disease under similar conditions. Over a longitudinal study of at least three to five years, they suggested, the sick should receive special prayers. The patients' care, they urged, should be under leading physicians and surgeons, and after enough experimental time has passed it would be "exhaustive and complete" to compare death rates against historical data as well as rates at contemporary institutions. Although it is clear that Tyndall and Thompson were not serious in proposing such an experiment, the article created a stir, with mentions in newspapers and magazines across Britain. It was, as one correspondent noted, "the sensation of the season."[75] Historian Robert Bruce Mullin has argued not only that Tyndall faced public backlash against his plan to test the efficacy of prayer but also that the prayer-gauge debate was "perhaps the high-water mark of Victorian scientific naturalism," sparking debate about the bounds between divine intervention and scientific materialism and opening the door for more rigorous debate about the scientific method and psychical research.[76] For my purposes, the prayer-gauge debate is another telling example of the kind of public discourse created by the prince's sickness with typhoid fever.

---

73   Turner, *Contesting Cultural Authority*, 167.

74   Tyndall, *The Prayer-Gauge Debate*.

75   Tyndall, *The Prayer-Gauge Debate*, 3.

76   Mullin, "Science, Miracles, and the Prayer-Gauge Debate," 223.

The story of the prince's bout with typhoid, and the intense public debate that ensued, sheds light on the politics of grieving in the Victorian period.[77] Pat Jalland has suggested that the Victorian culture of death was much more complex than exercising funeral rites. Instead, Jalland has shown, religion-inspired practices of grief played a central role from when a family member was ill to funerary practices and later memorialization.[78] Recently, scholars have shown how such grieving practices played out even in working-class families, but we know much less about collective acts of popular grieving in the Victorian period.[79] The case of the prince's sickness presents an opportunity to investigate such practices of collective grief. While the Victorian press created a discourse in which the prince's sickbed could be commodified, the Thanksgiving Day on February 27, 1872, further materialized that cultural process, ensuring that celebrating recovery from disease was also central to Victorian practices of death.

The Public Spectacle of Celebration

Queen Victoria officially announced plans for the Royal Thanksgiving in a speech at the opening of Parliament on February 6, 1872, although she had already in late January ordered William Lawley, of the Corporation of London, to convene and head a Royal Reception Committee (RCC) to plan the event.[80] The committee numbered nine aldermen and thirty-one members of the House of Commons. Thankful for "the deliverance of my dear son the Prince of Wales from the most imminent danger . . . during the period of anxiety and trial," the queen, speaking before the House of Lords and shifting her rhetoric away from the subject of her son's recovery, added that the Thanksgiving was to celebrate the good fortune of the entire nation.[81]

---

77 Strange, *Death, Grief and Poverty in Britain.*
78 Jalland, *Death in the Victorian Family.*
79 Strange, *Death, Grief and Poverty in Britain.*
80 Notice of Motion by William Lawley, January 26, 1872, LMA MISC MSS 328/1. See also Royal Reception Committee, *Report to the Court of Common Council on the Thanksgiving for the Recovery of his Royal Highness the Prince of Wales*, February 27, 1873, 5, LMA, MISC MSS 328/3.
81 Queen Victoria's speech, *Hansards,* February 6, 1872, vol. 209, cc2–6.

There was a frantic energy to the RCC's planning, which officially began on February 1, 1872.[82] Given that they had less than a month to plan the entire Thanksgiving, "the arrangements were carried out under extreme pressure," Lawley noted in a private memo.[83] Lawley's committee turned to historical precedent and to English tradition, modeling the prince's public service on a General Thanksgiving on April 23, 1789, to celebrate the "happy recovery" of King George III, which also culminated at St. Paul's Cathedral.[84]

The Corporation of London erected special seats for the ceremony—at the expense of over £3,000—at St. Dunstan's Church, lining Fleet Street, on vacant ground in the Old Bailey, in the yard at the Sessions House, and on both sides of the Holborn Viaduct, adjoining the church of St. Sepulchre.[85] These were used for distinguished guests, set aside among the three thousand tickets issued by the RCC.[86] The Metropolitan Board of Works erected a special covered seating pavilion in Hyde Park near Marble Arch for the use of the Corporation of London, various vestries, and members of district boards for the return trip.[87] At St. Dunstan's and St. Sepulchre, special seats were allotted for charity children of each parish.[88] Well-known architect Horace

---

82   See the RCC's official notebook, LMA MISC MSS 328/2.

83   Royal Reception Committee, *Report to the Court of Common Council on the Thanksgiving for the Recovery of his Royal Highness the Prince of Wales*, presented February 27, 1873, 15, LMA, MISC MSS 328/3.

84   *General Thanksgiving, 1789.* London Metropolitan Archives, MISC MSS 328/3. The RCC of 1872 expressly stated that they were "guided much" by the 1789 Thanksgiving. See Royal Reception Committee, *Report to the Court of Common Council on the Thanksgiving*, 6. LMA, MISC MSS 328/3.

85   For a list of expenses on seating, see Royal Reception Committee, *Report to the Court of Common Council on the Thanksgiving*, 19, LMA, MISC MSS 328/3.

86   Admittance ticket for Thanksgiving Day, LMA, MISC MSS 328/3. Those with tickets for the special seats were not admitted after 10:00 a.m., and carriages were not allowed to pass after 8:00 a.m. Each group of seats was arranged in blocks, similar to what was done at the opening of Blackfriars Bridge and the Holborn Valley Viaduct. Seating was so important to the event that the RCC appointed a special Seats Committee, with William Lawley as the subcommittee's chairman.

87   Royal Reception Committee, *Report to the Court of Common Council on the Thanksgiving*, 13, LMA, MISC MSS 328/3.

88   Thomas Hodges, St. Dunstan's churchwarden, to RCC, February 12, 1872, LMA MISC MSS 328/1.

Jones designed special hoardings on the bridge over Farringdon Street, meant to protect the voluminous crowds.

The RCC's planned procession was a seven-mile journey in all, from Buckingham Palace through Stable-Yard Gate and then via Pall-Mall, Charing Cross, the Strand, Fleet Street, and Ludgate Hill to the west entrance to St. Paul's Cathedral. The entire route was decorated "to make the Ceremonial as imposing as possible"; lampposts were repainted and decorated along the route, and the RCC spent £500 constructing lamps and over £50 in flags to mark the way.[89] According to the *Illustrated London News*, the route was teeming with people: "The streets along the whole route were lined with a dense throng of people . . . every shop, every window, upper and lower, every doorstep, portico, and balcony, and the roofs of many houses were occupied by eager spectators . . . Banners, streamers, and strings of flowers stretched across from house to house.[90] The royal entourage—which included the royal family, the lord chancellor, the Speaker of the Commons, the great officers of the Royal Household, and the Household in Waiting—assembled at Buckingham Palace, arranged in precise carriage order. There were nine carriages in all; Queen Victoria occupied the ninth and final carriage, drawn by six horses, flanked by the equerry in waiting and field officer escort. The first eight were occupied by elite nobles, such as the Duke of Cambridge and Silver Stick in Waiting, Colonel Duncan J. Baillie. The procession followed a direct route to the cathedral, with military regiments lining the streets and parks along the route; a battalion of four hundred petty officers and seamen of the Royal Navy guarded Waterloo Place alone.

---

89 Royal Reception Committee, *Report to the Court of Common Council on the Thanksgiving* 14, LMA, MISC MSS 328/3. The residents of Ludgate Hill were especially keen to assist in the preparations, due in part to what they called the "unsatisfactory way in which Ludgate Hill was decorated on the occasion of the Entry of the Princess of Wales." See *Memorial of the Inhabitants of Ludgate Hill*, February 6, 1872, LMA MISC MSS 328/1. Only days before the Thanksgiving, a committee of Ludgate Hill residents bemoaned the RCC's decorating of lamps, which they claimed destroyed "the harmony of our decoration." Residents asked the RCC for permission to decorate without the assistance of the RCC, although with financial assistance. See Ludgate Hill Committee to RCC, February 20, 1872, LMA MISC MSS 328/1. The RCC agreed and moved the lamp decorations to the Holborn Viaduct. See RCC memo, Decoration of Lamp Posts, February 21, 1872, LMA MISC MSS 328/1.

90 "The Thanksgiving Day," *Illustrated London News*, March 2, 1872, 206.

As the procession neared Temple Bar, Sir Christopher Wren's imposing gateway to the City of London, Mayor of London Sills John Gibbons, the sheriffs of London and Middlesex, and a deputation of aldermen from the City of London, preceded by four trumpeters, approached the queen's carriage. The gate was flanked by twenty-two horses of the Royal Artillery, ornamented with scarlet saddle cloth bordered with gold, each with a trooper attendant directed by the Duke of Cambridge.[91] Consistent with what was called the Temple Bar Ceremony, the mayor presented to the queen—and then received back—the City Sword of State, a custom to designate when a sovereign enters the City of London. As the procession entered the City of London, it next met an architectural wonder designed for the occasion by Horace Jones and constructed by the building firm of Trollope and Sons. It was a massive triumphal arch (figure 1.4), which stood at the junction of Fleet Street and Ludgate Hill and had cost the City of London £4,000.

The workmen—gasfitters, carpenters, and decorators—were at work putting finishing touches on the arch until the very last moment.[92] The inscription on the Gothic-style arch—86 feet wide and 70 feet high—was "God Bless the Prince of Wales." To further memorialize the occasion, the RCC commissioned commemorative medals, from the design of J. S. and A. B. Wyon, chief engravers of Her Majesty's seals.[93] The medals (figure 1.5) were sent to members of the court and various public libraries, available in gold at the cost of £25 each.

Proceeding past the arch, east through the lavishly decorated Ludgate Hill, the group landed at the steps of the grand west entrance of St. Paul's, where the bishop of London and the dean of the cathedral met the queen's carriage. Entering St. Paul's, George Cooper, the organist of Chapel Royal, St. James's, played until the queen, the prince, and the princess of Wales were seated in the royal pew in the center of the cathedral (figure 1.6).

The cathedral—refitted for the occasion to hold over thirteen thousand people, teemed with foreign and domestic dignitaries from both Europe and the

---

91 Royal Reception Committee, *Report to the Court of Common Council on the Thanksgiving*, 7, 12. LMA, MISC MSS 328/3.

92 Horace Jones to RCC, March 11, 1872, LMA MISC MSS 328/1.

93 J. S. and A. B. Wyon to Willam Lawley, January 31, 1872, LMA MISC MSS/328/1. See also J. S. and A. B. Wyon to Royal Reception Committee, September 10, 1872, LMA MISC MSS/328/1. See also London Common Council Order for Medal, June 27, 1872, LMA MISC MSS/328/1. The medals were not completed until late December 1873.

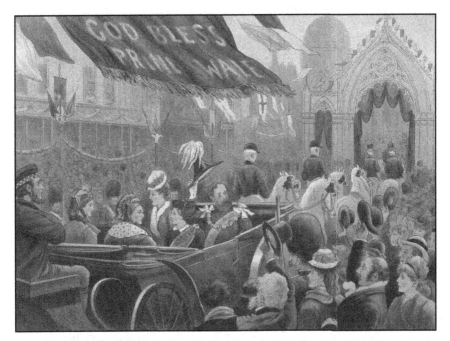

Figure 1.4 Thanksgiving Day, 1872. Alfred Johnson in "The Silver Wedding." Copyright permission by Mary Evans Picture Library LTD.

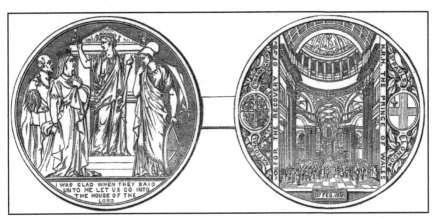

Figure 1.5 City medal for the Royal Thanksgiving in St. Paul's. Image courtesy of the Wellcome Library, London. Creative Commons Attribution license CC BY 4.0.

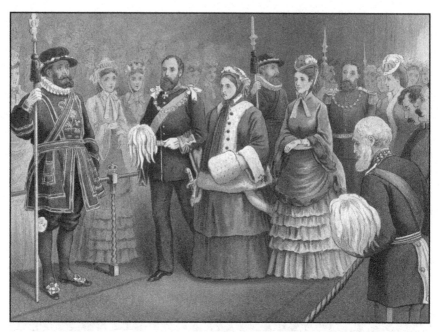

Figure 1.6 Thanksgiving Day, February 27, 1872: The procession in St. Paul's Cathedral. Alfred Johnson in "The Silver Wedding." Copyright permission by Mary Evans Picture Library LTD.

far reaches of the British Empire. In attendance near the queen were international representatives, the Maharajah Duleep Singh, Prince Higashi-Fushimi-No-Miya of Japan, Prince Hassan of Egypt, the Nawab Nazim of Bengal, and Prince Soliman-Kudr-Vahid-Ali-Bahadoor.[94] Lord lieutenants, high sheriffs, university professors, physicians, and mayors from across Great Britain filled the seats. There were 324 seats alone allotted for officers of the Court of Common Council.[95] Middle- and working-class Britons were there too. An express goal of the RCC, stated as early as their report of February 8, 1872,

94   Lord Chamberlain, *Ceremonial, Thanksgiving at St. Paul's Cathedral*, LMA, MISC MSS 328/3, 11.

95   Royal Reception Committee, *Report to the Court of Common Council on the Thanksgiving*, 6, LMA, MISC MSS 328/3.

was to admit "the largest number of persons possible into the Cathedral, and the claims of the Citizens for a fair share of those admissions."[96]

Archbishop Tait's sermon echoed the nationalist rhetoric that dominated the discourse of the prince's sickness and recovery. He implored that "all the people of this United Kingdom—the whole British race everywhere, all of every blood who own allegiance to our Queen—joined in prayer as one family, a family wide as the world, yet moved by one impulse, watching over one sick bed, yearning with one heart for one precious life." [97] While the word "typhoid" was never used at the Thanksgiving service at St. Paul's, J. H. Coward, warden of the College of Minor Canons, was relieved that God had "heard the prayers of this nation in the day of our trial . . . for that thou hast raised thy Servant *Albert Edward* Prince of Wales from the bed of sickness."[98] The choir at St. Paul's numbered two hundred voices and included singers from Westminster, Windsor, Canterbury, Warwick, and Eton. At the conclusion of the service, guns were fired at the Tower of London and in St. James's Park.

After the service, those in the procession returned to their carriages and headed back to the palace via Ludgate Hill, north past Old Bailey, and west near the Holborn Viaduct, which held three hundred children from the Foundling Hospital in specially constructed seats.[99] They continued west along Holborn and Oxford Street, reaching Marble Arch, where they headed south along the east side of Hyde Park and then returned to Buckingham Palace via Constitutional Hill just before 4 p.m. The return route, longer than the initial journey, had been "graciously consented to" by the queen "in order to meet the loyal wishes of Her Subjects."[100] Two days after the Thanksgiving, William Gladstone, then first lord of the Treasury and leader

---

96 Royal Reception Committee, *Report to the Court of Common Council on the Thanksgiving*, 5, LMA, MISC MSS 328/3.

97 "The Thanksgiving Day," *Illustrated London News*, March 2, 1872, 206.

98 Thanksgiving Service Form, in Royal Reception Committee, *Report to the Court of Common Council on the Thanksgiving*, 27, LMA, MISC MSS 328/3.

99 Only days before the Thanksgiving, on Monday, February 19, 1872, the City Lands Committee warned that the proposed route would have to pass Newgate Prison and would thus be unsuitable. See H. Heath, Chairman of City Lands Committee to RRC, February 19, 1872, LMA MISC MSS 328/1

100 Lord Chamberlain, *Ceremonial, Thanksgiving at St. Paul's Cathedral*, LMA, MISC MSS 328/3, 9.

of the House of Commons, was confident that "the City of London has perhaps never witnessed one [a ceremony] more solemn or more satisfactory."[101]

The 1872 National Thanksgiving brought the monarchy into popular view in a way that had not been seen in a decade. The event also quieted a republican critique spearheaded by Charles Dilke's popular public lectures against the monarchy.[102] "It made us feel," *John Bull* reported, "that Royal persons are of the same flesh and blood, one with us; and it also made us feel, what is yet more important, that we are of the same flesh and blood with them."[103] This was, no doubt, a jingoist display of national pride, ceremony, and tradition. But it was also a way to connect British imperial spaces. The day was reserved as a national holiday in Calcutta, with Thanksgiving services being held in churches and chapels throughout India. In Bombay over one hundred thousand Indians gathered to rejoice in the recovery of the Prince of Wales. As one correspondent wrote, "In the broad circuit of the British Empire many joined in our prayers who scarcely knew the God to whom we prayed."[104]

Historians have successfully used the concept of jingoism—aggressive nationalism—to categorize late British imperialism, especially during the South African War, to contextualize monarchal rituals such as Queen Victoria's jubilees in 1887 and 1897, and her own funeral in 1901. Beneath the surface of aggressive displays of nationalism were deep-seated anxieties and insecurities about the imperial mission. But the events of 1872 were not just about monarchy and nation. Rather, they brought typhoid fever to the fore of English consciousness, sparking a debate about how the disease was spread and how to prevent it. This set the stage for the landmark Public Health Acts of 1872 and 1875, which not only made medical officers of health compulsory throughout Britain but also established a routine vaccination policy and increased funding for municipal sanitation projects.

101 W. E. Gladstone to Lord Mayor of London, February 29, 1872. Royal Reception Committee, *Report to the Court of Common Council on the Thanksgiving*, 15, LMA, MISC MSS 328/3.

102 Dilke, *On the Cost of the Crown*; Morris, "The Illustrated Press."

103 "The Prince of Wales," *John Bull*, December 23, 1871, 881.

104 "The Thanksgiving Day," *Illustrated London News*, March 2, 1872, 206.

Suspecting Sewer Gas and the Ascendance of Typhoid Fever

The popularization of the prince's sickness, as we have already seen, sparked several public debates, including the relative merits of prayer versus physic, and the nature of private versus public grieving. The events of late 1871 and early 1872 also intensified an important sanitary debate over the etiological role of sewer gas in spreading typhoid fever, which centered on three pressing and largely unanswered questions in late Victorian public health. The first was the class-based question of why there were so many middle-and-upper-class Britons succumbing to typhoid fever in spite of making seemingly effective and progressive strides in sanitary engineering, particularly providing houses with water closets and connecting drains to sewerage works. The second was a professional squabble over who best could detect and eliminate sewer gases from English homes—engineers, plumbers, or epidemiologists. The third was an epidemiological query—one of methodology—about how investigations of sewer gas–borne typhoid should be conducted.

Sewer gas fears undercut a series of class-based, morality-fueled debates over typhoid fever. From the early nineteenth century, typhoid was typically understood to be a disease of the poor, the metropolitan "great unwashed masses" huddling in fever dens. Kevin Siena has recently used the term "the moral biology of the British poor," to describe late eighteenth- and early nineteenth-century discourse that linked urban poverty, filth, disease, and morality.[105] Matthew Newsom Kerr, likewise, has shown that the early nineteenth-century origins of the London Fever Hospital had inherited the tradition of moralizing about urban disease and poverty. The beginning of the hospital, he shows, was an attempt to remove the putrid bodies of the urban poor out of their contaminated environment into a space for recuperation. The discourse of the fever den, a dangerous center of contagion in urban areas, maintained a stronghold in popular discourse throughout the Victorian period.[106] And while this sentiment was often normative and rhetorical—typhoid had been seen in rich and poor alike since its disentangling from typhus—the large-scale sanitary changes in Britain from the 1850s, ushered in and spearheaded by Chadwickian sanitarians, meant that the middle and upper classes had to contend with new disease threats. Typhoid was chief among them, to the extent that the *Times,* reflecting on the prince's illness on December 12, 1871, called the occurrence of typhoid among the

---

105 Siena, *Rotten Bodies,* chapter 1.
106 Kerr, *Contagion, Isolation, and Biopolitics,* 39.

middle and upper classes "among the recognised necessities of advanced civilization." What they had in common were habitations and institutions—villa residences, college buildings, new sewerage schemes "designed and constructed as if for the express purpose of cultivating typhoid fever."[107]

Sewer gas was in some ways was a product of the increasing reality of a Chadwickian pipe-bound city from the late 1850s, as Christopher Hamlin has shown. By the 1870s, London alone had over seven hundred thousand water closets, overwhelmingly in middle- and upper-class homes, and the same pattern could be found throughout Britain.[108] Modern domestic plumbing arrangements created what Tom Crook calls a "technological irony," whereby "the domestic water-closet doubled as a technology of privacy and detachment *and* as a technology of connection and publicity."[109] Moreover, the sewer gas controversy, combined with the high-profile nature of the prince's bout with typhoid in 1871, pointed to the reality that the middle and upper classes might be just as susceptible—maybe even more susceptible—to typhoid than the working classes. This had already been shown through epidemiological reports by the inspectorate of the Medical Department, explored below, but the public nature of the prince's sickness brought the matter to a full-blown crisis. "There can be no such thing as safety in modern houses," retired army surgeon Charles Mayo lamented, "until the unclean and dangerous fashion of laying on sewer-gas by means of pipes up to our very bedroom doors is abandoned."[110] As we will see in chapter 3, the threat of milk-borne typhoid, which also gained public attention in 1871, further intensified the class-based discourse on the disease.

Crook has argued that sewer gas generated a substantial amount of fear because it attacked the seemingly safe confines of domestic spaces and also because, while public health officials agreed that sewer gases were dangerous to health, there was little agreement as to the specific ways that sewer gas spread disease.[111] "It was a danger that was defined," Crook suggests, "as much by fear and dispute as expert 'rationality' and technical know-how."[112]

---

107 "Villa Residences and Typhoid Fever," *Times*, December 12, 1871, 12.

108 Crook, "Danger in the Drains,"110.

109 Crook, "Danger in the Drains," 117. Michelle Allen has likewise shown how the new sewerage systems were often understood as harbingers of the disorder of urban environments. See Allen, *Cleansing the City*.

110 Mayo, "Typhoid Fever," 3.

111 Crook, "Danger in the Drains."

112 Crook, "Danger in the Drains." 107.

Barbara Penner has extended this discussion to show how fears over sewer gas were particularly important for the aspirations of sanitary engineers and building professionals, who used new visual tools such as sanitary sections to augment their claims of expertise.[113]

Sewer gas was not a new preoccupation to either public health officials or sanitary engineers in 1871; it fit within long-standing fears of dangerous miasmas. But the prince's illness raised the profile of dangerous drain emanations, particularly through a public debate that played out in the pages of the *Lancet* and the *Times*, both of which extensively covered the prince's condition. Throughout late 1871 and into 1872 the *Lancet* used the prince's bout with typhoid to decry the high incidence of such a preventable disease, the general sanitary state of Britain, and the lack of legal oversight of sanitary matters. "As a nation we do nothing," the *Lancet* bemoaned, "and the result is that, on average, we have about *one hundred and twenty thousand cases of typhoid fever every year, from fifteen to twenty thousand deaths*, a terrible percentage.... It is, as we have said, a national scourge ... it is also a national disgrace."[114] Parliamentary reform was needed, particularly laws to prevent sewage from contaminating water and provision for the compulsory disinfection of excreta. A second editorial in the *Lancet* on December 9, 1871, further stated that the "etiology of typhoid fever" is of "an overwhelming ... national importance," as rich and poor alike were succumbing to the disease.[115] But the *Lancet's* grumbling was not just armchair sanitary grandstanding. The central issue at stake, in some ways, was how the prince contracted typhoid in the first place. The question had already risen to public interest when Lord Londesborough wrote to the *Times* on November 30, boldly stating that the suspicion that the prince had contracted typhoid at Scarborough was "entirely unfounded" and that he would initiate an investigation to clear the matter.[116] The *Lancet* responded by initiating a Lancet Sanitary Commission (LSC), led by J. H. Stallard, to investigate

---

113 Barbara Penner has argued that in the last two decades of the nineteenth century the "fight against sewer gas was feminised," citing a number of influential sanitary tracts, such as Harriette Plunkett's 1885 *Women, Plumbers, and Doctors*, about domestic hygiene geared toward women. See Penner, "The Prince's Water Closet," 253.

114 "Typhoid Fever," *Lancet* 101 (December 2, 1871): 788.

115 "Scarborough & Sandringham," *Lancet* 101 (December 9, 1871): 821.

116 "Editorial" *Times*, November 30, 1871, 9.

Londesborough Lodge, Sandringham House, and the general sanitary conditions of Scarborough and the Sandringham area.

The LSC's approach in investigating Londesborough Lodge was three-fold: first they examined the house's sanitary arrangements; second, they interviewed the people who were at the lodge during the royal visit, including questions about any sicknesses they had contracted; third, they surveyed the health and sanitary conditions of Scarborough, particularly the cases of typhoid that had occurred that fall, using mortality and morbidity records from the Scarborough Dispensary. It was already well known in the press that George Philip Stanhope, Earl of Chesterfield—who died of typhoid on December 1—had most likely contracted the disease while at Londesborough Lodge, but the LSC uncovered that several others present either came down with diarrhea, such as Lord Londesborough himself, or were afflicted with typhoid, such as the prince and Chesterfield. The latter included one of Londesborough's grooms, Blegg, who also died of the disease in early December. A critical fact of the case, according to the LSC, was that the prince's bedroom door opened onto an unventilated water closet, which connected to an old cesspool. As the tide rose, they surmised, unmitigated sewer gases were pushed into the prince's bedchamber. In the first of a series of leading articles on December 9, the LSC concluded that the bedroom was thus "placed upon the summit of a closed sewer, with nothing but a few inches of water to protect the sleepers from the probable source of their disease."[117]

A series of responses came in the *Times* on December 11, one by engineer George P. Dale, and another cosigned by a Scarborough group that included Dale, physician John William Taylor, architects Stewart and Bury, contractor William Peacock, clerk J. H. Carroll, and plumber Septimus Bland, all of whom had worked on and later investigated the sanitary system at Londesborough Lodge.[118] The LSC's report, they argued, was unfounded and inaccurate. An LSC rejoinder came in the *Lancet* on December 16, reexamining Londesborough Lodge with two new pieces of information: that a butler was suffering from typhoid during the prince's visit, undisclosed during the initial investigation, and that the certificate of Londesborough's architect and contractor, published in the *Times*, was misleading about the nature of the drainpipes, which were only trapped with syphon valves—to

---

117 "Report of the Lancet Sanitary Commission," *Lancet* 101 (December 9, 1871), 830.

118 Taylor Dale, et al., "Londesborough Lodge," *Times*, December 11, 1871, 5.

prevent backflow of sewer gases—after the prince's visit. "Painful as it must be to Lord Londesborough's feelings," the LSC concluded, "the evidence is irresistible."[119] The LSC's argument was a professional jab at the local sanitary engineers, who, they argued, were trying to cover up the sanitary conditions of Londesborough to protect the health-resort status of Scarborough. Physicians, the LSC insisted, "can alone appreciate the danger of sewer emanations, and estimate at their proper value the safeguards employed."[120]

And while the populist *Times* published the accounts of the local Scarborough sanitary engineers, it also joined with the *Lancet* in vilifying Scarborough's water supply and Londesborough Lodge's sanitary arrangements: "Londesborough Lodge . . . is nothing more or less than a vessel inverted over the mouth of a pipe, through which rises continually, sometimes with violence, a deadly vapour . . . the effluvia of Avernus, which the poet says killed the very birds that tried to fly over it, could not be more deadly than those which must be almost always rising up the funnel terminating in Londesborough Lodge."[121] Sewer gas fearmongering in the *Times* did not stop there. An article on December 12 made use of the fervent national spirit the royal sickness had created, arguing that typhoid killed twenty thousand people per year, which was "entirely preventable and unnecessary," echoing the stance John Simon was making at the Medical Department. From 1861 to 1871, the *Times* argued, two hundred thousand had died and millions had been made sick from the disease, costing Britain nearly £35 million in the last decade: "We have commemorated the blameless life of the father by statues and gilding; may it yet be given us to commemorate the recovery of the son by waging a successful war against the pest by which both have been stricken down!"[122]

The sewer-gas controversy intensified when William Henry Corfield, professor of hygiene and public health at University College London, published in the *Times* his own epidemiological investigation of Londesborough Lodge. Corfield was emerging as one of the leaders of English public health. Trained at Oxford in mathematics and natural science, he was a part-time

119 "The Cause of the Illness of H.R.H. The Prince of Wales," *Lancet* 101 (December 16, 1871): 857.
120 "The Cause of the Illness of H.R.H. The Prince of Wales," *Lancet* 101 (December 16, 1871): 857.
121 "The Report of the Lancet Sanitary Commission," *Times*, December 9, 1871, 9.
122 "Villa Residences and Typhoid Fever," *Times*, December 12, 1871, 12.

inspector at the Medical Department, a pupil of William Jenner, and an ally of William Budd in believing typhoid to be a specific disease spread via the fecal-oral route. Corfield had recently been elected medical officer of health for Islington upon Edward Ballard's move to the Medical Department and in 1870 had published an influential treatise, *The Treatment and Utilisation of Sewage*. He held a series of high-level posts in public health, including president of the Epidemiological Society, before his death in 1903. Corfield traveled to Londesborough from London, and, like Stallard with the LSC, examined the location and state of the drains in and around the lodge. But unlike the LSC, Corfield found very little amiss: no cesspool under the lodge or unventilated soil pipes. He also used an anemometer to conduct several plumbing experiments and found no currents of escaping gas from the pipes. He sent soil samples to his UCL colleague and chemist Alexander Williamson, who found no sewage leakage. Corfield concluded that the LSC's findings were "incorrect and exaggerated."[123] "It was not a case in which the disease was conveyed by sewer air," he said before the Royal Medical Chirurgical Society.[124] Thirty years later, in 1902, delivering the Milroy lecture before the Royal College of Physicians, Corfield sketched an entire history of research on typhoid fever, noting that the prince, Lord Chesterfield, and the others who came down with typhoid and diarrhea, had probably done so as a result of some infected food or drink—oysters or salad.[125] While the *Lancet* might have been the foremost professional medical authority in the 1870s, Corfield's was a powerful voice in the field, particularly among the burgeoning group of younger British epidemiologists. By the 1880s and 1890s he had carved out a special niche as the leading expert on house sanitation, catering to the sanitary reconfiguration of hundreds of country houses and writing several books on the subject.[126] No doubt his own career, like Gull's, had been marked by the royal sickness.

---

123 Corfield, "Londesborough Lodge," 4.
124 "Obituary for William Henry Corfield," *Lancet* 162 (September 12, 1903): 778.
125 Corfield, *Typhoid Fever and Its Prevention*, 109.
126 Corfield, *Foul Air in Houses;* Corfield *Dwelling Houses and their Sanitary Construction;* Corfield; *The Laws of Health;* Corfield, *Disease and Defective House Sanitation.*

Searching for Sewer Gas

The search for sewer gases as the culprit in spreading typhoid fever steadily increased in the 1870s, with most medical thinkers arguing, as George Buchanan and John Netten Radcliffe did in 1869, that typhoid was "the result of excremental pollution of air and water," which they maintained was "one of the best established facts of sanitary medicine."[127] This was anything but an antiquated view of miasma theory but rather looked to the first generation of epidemiologists investigating local outbreaks of typhoid fever. The sewer gas controversy opened up new questions not just about etiological theorizing but also about practical methodology.

There had been several local studies that linked typhoid to sewer gas prior to 1871. In 1852, for example, Croydon was an early center of public health tensions over sewer gas. In the summer of 1852 Croydon officials constructed a new sanitary works system of drainage, water supply, and sewage. The new stoneware pipes burst, however, and sewage drained into the surrounding soils. According to the investigation by General Board of Health inspectors Neil Arnott and Thomas Page, who were working under Edwin Chadwick, the sanitary mishap was the direct cause of a fulminating, or sudden outbreak of fever; in a town whose population was about 16,000 people, 1,800 were struck with fever, and 60 died.[128] Subsequent works tying sewer gas to the generalized notion of fever continued in the 1850s, and leading works such as *Sewage and Sewer Gases, and on the Ventilation of Sewers, written by* chemist and MOH for the City of London Henry Letheby in 1858, provided systematic coverage of the topic.[129] But it was concern for royalty— not unlike the later case in 1871—that piqued epidemiological interest in sewer gas. In the fall of 1858 Windsor was the site of an intense outbreak of typhoid; during the last months of the year over four hundred individuals were attacked and thirty-nine died. With cases on the rise, "exciting much alarm," physician to Queen Victoria, Dr. James Clark, asked that the newly established Medical Department of the Privy Council investigate.[130]

John Simon investigated the case himself, assisted by Henry Austin, a holdover expert on sewers from Chadwick's administration. Simon's first

---

127 Buchanan and Radcliffe, "On the Construction and Use of Midden Closets," 111.

128 Hamlin, *Public Health and Social Justice,* 322–27.

129 Letheby, *Report to the Honorable Commissioners of Sewers of the City of London.*

130 Simon, "Windsor," 17.

impression upon investigating the outbreak was that typhoid had largely struck middle- and upper-class residents.[131] In a shoe- leather style of house-to-house inspection that became the hallmark of outbreak investigation at the Medical Department, Simon walked around the town, finding the usual sanitary mishaps of mid-Victorian Britain, "extreme slovenliness," unregulated slaughterhouses, filthy pigsties, dung heaps, standing sewage, and offensive smells. These general observations of filth alone might presage an outbreak of typhoid, especially following Murchison's pythogenic theory, but Simon narrowed the investigation to a specific flaw of Windsor's public sewers: that they were unventilated and must have emitted gases into the houses connected to the works. Upon closer inspection of houses in Windsor, Simon found that many water closets were improperly trapped, which led, he argued, to a "habitual escape of sewer-atmosphere into houses."[132] But it was not all houses. Instead, there were geographic groupings where the disease arose and where specific sanitary defects could be found. The area around the sewage outfall, for example, was filled with modern middle-class homes, but with an east wind, he argued, sewer gases backed up from the main and into houses' water closets and sinks. In a low-lying area of Windsor, where houses were connected to the public works, water closets were mostly dried up, due to a long drought that fall that lowered the level of the Thames. Upon further investigation Simon found that Windsor's poorer neighborhoods were generally spared from the outbreak, a finding that ran against contemporary logic. Where the environmental accumulations of filth were perhaps worst, houses lacked indoor water, sewer drainage, and water closets. The sanitary arrangements and incidence at Windsor Castle threw even greater light on the investigation. The main part of the castle was drained separately from the town on its own system, and Simon found proper ventilation and drainage; the closets of the castle were flushed every morning with a special water supply. But two parts of the castle, the resident cloisters of St. George's Chapel and the mews, were connected to the town sewers. Typhoid struck no one in the castle, but several cases appeared among residents of the chapel and mews. To Simon, the facts of the investigation added up to a series of powerful conclusions: the local board of health, on the premise of improving the sanitary arrangements, were "breathing whiffs or streams of excremental effluvium into the houses which it pretends to make wholesome."[133] But there were

---

131 Simon, "Windsor," 17.
132 Simon, "Windsor," 19.
133 Simon, "Windsor," 21.

outspoken detractors. Charles Murchison, most prominently, reporting to the Epidemiological Society of London, argued that the Windsor outbreak was proof of his increasingly popular pythogenic theory, which held that typhoid was not contagious and that sewer air in particular was of imminent concern.

Together, the epidemiological investigations at Croydon and Windsor pointed, however indiscriminately, to sewer gas as the cause of the typhoid outbreaks. In the early 1860s the pattern continued at the Medical Department, largely spurred by Simon's new insistence on showing the sanitary defects of arrangements made after the Public Health Act of 1858. What had happened at Croydon and Windsor, Simon maintained to his inspectorate, might be more widespread than previously thought. Sometimes sewer gas was an easy scapegoat for a local outbreak when a more direct waterborne route could not be blamed. J. S. Bristowe, for example, investigating an outbreak of typhoid at Grantham in 1864, could not find fault with the local water supply and instead blamed sewer gases: "Known well as we do that typhoid fever has been shown over and over again to arise from the effluvia of accumulated human excrement and that throughout the whole town of Grantham such effluvia have prevailed there remains, I think, scarcely a doubt that the disease must be attributed to this cause."[134] But in the last few years of the 1860s, inspectors at the department increasingly focused on showing the precise ways that sewer gas could transmit typhoid. In the process, they began to consolidate a particular kind of epidemiological practice: an emerging epidemiological gaze.

George Buchanan, MOH for London's St. Giles from 1856, was an occasional inspector for Simon at the Medical Department until he was hired permanently in 1869. From 1865 to 1866 Simon commissioned Buchanan to undertake an extensive study of twenty-five towns in England that had undertaken substantial sanitary works to improve public health. Buchanan started by studying the mortality data from the GRO—"a method," he lamented, "in which there are certain confessed weaknesses"—before sanitary works of the Public Health Act of 1858 began, while they were being executed, and after their completion.[135] In numerous towns Buchanan found a marked decrease in mortality rates for typhoid fever. Salisbury's annual mortality rate, for example, had decreased from 7.5 per 10,000 to 1 per 10,000, while Stratford's had decreased from 12.5 per 10,000 to 4 per 10,000. This

---

134 Quoted in Corfield, *The Etiology of Typhoid Fever*, 36.
135 Buchanan, "Report on the Results," 40.

decrease in mortality can be linked to the drying of sewage-laced soil via cesspools, and a reduction in overcrowded houses, an ample supply of clean water. But above all, it was "the purification of atmosphere from decomposing organic matters that has been most uniformly followed by a fall in the prevalence of typhoid."[136] Yet in other towns such as Chelmsford, Penzance, and Worthing, typhoid deaths had actually increased. Worthing, where there was a 23 percent increase in mortality after the installation of sewage works, was the most striking example.[137] Moving beyond the analysis of mortality data from the GRO, Buchanan turned to outbreak investigation to unravel the cause of the increase in typhoid. Worthing, with a population of around six thousand, had undertaken sewerage, water supply, and paving projects between 1853 and 1856; four- or six-inch house drainpipes connected to six- to eight-inch street sewer pipes, which collected surface water and continued on to egg-shaped, brick-lined sewers that in turn led to a pumping works at the north end of the town. At the works, sewage entered a subterranean tank, where it was pumped by steam engine either to the sea or away from the town. Buchanan found that no ventilation system had been constructed for the sewers, which he argued was the chief cause of the mischief. With heavy rainfall, like what occurred during a virulent outbreak of typhoid in Worthing in the fall of 1865, the amount of sewage was greater than the engine could pump, creating a massive backup of sewage into houses: "Foul gases . . . had no means of escape but by bubbling up through the traps of sinks and waterclosets."[138] Moreover, the 1865 typhoid epidemic struck only the wealthier houses, which had water closets connected to the sewer system, not poor houses with cesspools and unconnected outdoor privies. Buchanan's survey was later called a "remarkable report" by Corfield and illustrates Simon's earlier vision for an epidemiological gaze that started in London, originated from examining GRO statistics, but relied on on-the-ground fieldwork that stretched geopolitical boundaries over the entirety of England and Wales.[139] Simon used local reports in Buchanan's to influence the Sanitary Act of 1866.

Local outbreak investigations in this period often inverted the traditional, class-based logic that typhoid was a disease of general environmental filth, localized to the poor. Often, as we saw above, wealthy inhabitants of an area

---

136 Buchanan, "Report on the Results," 44.

137 Ibid.

138 Buchanan, "Report on the Results," 195.

139 Corfield, *The Etiology of Typhoid Fever*, 36.

were struck with typhoid as a result of newly installed public sanitary systems. But that was not always the problem, and the inspectorate's investigations demonstrated that a variety of sanitary shortcomings could spread the disease. One key example was a sudden typhoid outbreak that occurred in 1870 outside of London, which was limited to the fast-growing suburban area of Forest Hill. Simon sent John Netten Radcliffe to investigate, and he found a similar, class-related relationship between domestic sanitary arrangement and the incidence of typhoid. Houses in Forest Hill that had connected to the public sewers with recently constructed drainage, Radcliffe observed, had minimum rates of typhoid; those connected to the estate sewers that linked with public sewers were often inferior in construction, and typhoid was common. But the worst incidences of typhoid, Radcliffe uncovered, were in houses where water closets were connected directly to cesspools. What was revealing for Radcliffe, what *the Times* called "shocking," was the way in which his Forest Hill study mapped disease onto class. *The Times* noted that "there is good reason for the belief that the well-to-do or wealthy population in the suburban districts which occupies villa residences unconnected with the public sewers, suffers, not uncommonly, to a much larger extent . . . from enteric fever, than the labouring population living in cottages similarly circumstanced."[140] Before the prince's attack, then, which raised popular alarm as to the dangers of new middle- and upper-class homes, epidemiologists had already started to prime the pump of popular fears of sewer gases and to vocalize the uncomfortable idea that typhoid was a disease that struck rich and poor alike.

After the prince's attack in 1871 and the controversy that played out in the *Times* and the *Lancet*, sewer gas received even closer scrutiny as a medium of typhoid fever. As Michael Worboys has argued, the late 1860s and early 1870s saw the most heated debates over germs.[141] Louis Pasteur's work on fermentation, Joseph Lister's ideas of antiseptic surgery, and John Tyndall's experiments on living organic matter floating in the air all contributed to a fervor in the medical community about the cause and communication of disease. John Burdon Sanderson, whose research was being funded by the Medical Department, was deeply engaged in this fray, and his research on germs provided an insider voice to epidemiological investigations.

---

140 Quoted in "Villa Residences and Typhoid Fever," The Times 27244 (12 December 1871), 12.

141 Worboys, *Spreading Germs*, chapter 4.

In epidemiological circles these were also the years when the methods for conducting outbreak investigation were becoming standardized. As the study of typhoid continued into the 1870s, sewer gas could fit into an emerging vision of professional epidemiological practice but only in a narrowly confined way as a specific medium of the disease. While Murchison's pythogenic theory of typhoid still held that the disease could arise *de novo* from accumulations of filth, Budd's more specific, fecal-oral theory provided a practice-based basis for outbreak investigation at the Medical Department. But there were still plenty of anomalies, and among general practitioners, MOsH, and especially hospital physicians, Murchison's theory that typhoid was essentially noncontagious still held enormous sway. As William Strange, physician to the Worcester Infirmary, noted in 1881, "Enteric fever has long been the battlefield for opposite parties to tilt at each other."[142] Examining the relationship between sewer air and typhoid on behalf of the Metropolitan Board of Works, for example, Joseph Bazalgette found that men and boys employed to flush and cleanse sewers were rarely attacked by typhoid.[143] Hospital physicians such as Strange also often remarked that nurses and doctors were rarely struck with typhoid. Such evidence was easily adapted to suit Murchison's theories. In the 1860s most epidemiologists at the Medical Department were undecided and hedged etiological bets with a kind of eclectic or contingent-contagionist view, although some, like Corfield and Radcliffe had aligned with Budd's theory that typhoid was a waterborne, fecal-oral disease.[144]

Budd's 1873 magnum opus, *Typhoid Fever*, marked a turning point in the epidemiological approach to studying typhoid, particularly as it related to how epidemiologists approached sewer gas in practice. Budd lamented both the scientific and community's obsession with sewer gas, which had "come to be looked upon as the actual and primary source of the disease," instead of the intestinal discharges of typhoid patients, which Budd insisted were chiefly to blame. The "great truth," Budd argued, was that "the sewer only owes its fatal influence to its connection with man . . . and only acts in the work of dissemination by opening a wider sphere to the contagious principle."[145] There it was, a theory of sewer gas consistent with the burgeon-

---

142   Strange, "Notes on the Origin and Diffusion," 507.

143   Metropolitan Board of Works, *Return Showing the Number of Persons*, 1–16.

144   Thorne, for example, said in the *British Medical Journal* in 1870 that typhoid "may occasionally have a spontaneous origin." Thorne, "The Propagation of Enteric Fever," 426.

145   Budd, *Typhoid Fever*, 162.

ing notions of epidemiological practice. Sewer gas might be important but only because it could be a medium in the spread of typhoid. Sewer gas itself was not the issue: it only became problematic when charged with the excreta of typhoid patients. Budd's work marked a steady move away in English epidemiological circles from Murchison's idea that typhoid could be produced spontaneously. While Murchison's name remained closely tied to typhoid, Budd's theories dominated public health practice in the last two decades of the nineteenth century.[146] A year after Budd's treatise was published, in 1874, before the Epidemiological Society of London, for example, Corfield was in the spotlight advocating for Budd's approach. He also implored epidemiologists to abandon the idea that even rural and seemingly isolated outbreaks of typhoid were produced spontaneously. Instead, Corfield explained, it was necessary to follow the people (those sick, and particularly visitors to an infected area, and index cases) and disease mediums: infected air, water, and milk.[147] Corfield here was following Radcliffe's advice, given at his 1868 address at the Epidemiological Society. From the mid-1870s this methodological turn was put into practice at the Medical Department, no doubt led by Radcliffe and orchestrated by Simon. Even as sewer gas remained in the spotlight, it became linked to finding the specific ways that typhoid-charged sewer air could either be breathed in, or, as became more likely, interacted with a fecally contaminated water supply and was then imbibed.

One important investigation of sewer gas by the Medical Department in this period was at Cambridge University. In early 1874 Simon sent George Buchanan to investigate a sudden increase in typhoid among students in Caius College. Buchanan found that the disease had struck fifteen students, twelve of whom were residents of one section of the college, Tree Court. Buchanan interviewed the sick residents as to the timing and duration of their attacks. He also hinted at the inductive process of his methodology: "It has been necessary to hold all the foregoing facts in view, and to choose among various hypotheses of causation, that which best explains all the occurrences," whereby typhoid-charged "excremental matter . . . have been presented to the lungs and stomachs of the persons attacked."[148] To Buchanan, following Corfield and Radcliffe, the three hypotheses were the media of air, water, or milk. Inductive in his approach, he ruled out milk as the vehicle

146 Wilson, *A Handbook of Hygiene and Sanitary Science*, 74–75.
147 Corfield, "On the Alleged Spontaneous Production," 493–502.
148 Buchanan, "Report to the Local Government Board on an Outbreak of Enteric Fever in Caius College, Cambridge," 65.

for the outbreak, although local physicians had suggested to him that milk might have been the cause. There had been cases of typhoid among other customers of the dairy that supplied Caius College, but the same milk was used throughout the entire college, Buchanan found, and only residents of Tree Court were attacked with typhoid.

To assist the investigation Buchanan used an 1873 ground plan of the college to map the location of water, sewerage pipes, and water closets. The visualization of the sanitary scheme of the college, included in his final report, was useful in tracing the localization of the outbreak to Tree Court. The college received its water supply in six different places; only one five-inch supply line, which ran under the Gate of Humility, was used for Tree Court. In his official report Buchanan noted that this was "a repetition, at least in essentials" of Blaxall's investigation of Sherborne.[149] Earlier that same year, Buchanan's colleague at the department, Frank H. Blaxall, had been sent to the Dorsetshire town of Sherborne, where between December 1872 and May 1873 nearly 250 cases of typhoid had exploded among the population of six thousand. The outbreak was localized to those who received public water supply, and Blaxall found that an intermittent supply, coupled with faulty traps, led to the intrusion of typhoid-laced sewer gas into the water supply. Buchanan's conclusions were much in line. He found that not only did the water closets of Tree Court receive water directly from the main supply—as opposed to the normal setup at the college with an individual cistern—but that several water closets in Tree Court had faulty traps. He traced the outbreak to drinking water that had intermixed with sewer air. Critical to both Buchanan and Blaxall's methodology was to figure out how the sewer air had been charged with typhoid. The problem was not just that it was sewer air but air charged with pathogenic typhoid, as Budd had explained in his 1873 treatise. Such was typical of investigations that involved sewer gas at the Medical Department in the mid-1870s and into the 1880s; Blaxall again pointed to such a route in an investigation of typhoid at Melton Mowbray and Selborne, and so, too, did Buchanan at Croydon, and Hurbert Airy at York.

While fears over sewer gas lingered, the last two decades of the nineteenth century saw fewer epidemiological investigations at the Medical Department tracing outbreaks of typhoid fever to sewer gas. As we will see in chapter 4, after the discovery of the typhoid bacillus, sewer gas fears shifted in the 1880s

---

149 Buchanan, "Report to the Local Government Board on an Outbreak of Enteric Fever in Caius College, Cambridge," 70.

and 1890s to an interest in the life of the bacterium outside the body, particularly in soil. In epidemiological investigations at the Medical Department, when it was in the spotlight, sewer gas became a kind of scapegoat: a "must-have-been" mode of communication if water or milk was ruled out. C. O. Stallybrass, in his 1931 *Principles of Epidemiology*, still lamented, for example, that "unconsciously" the sewer gas theory was still influential.[150] The idea of sewer gas was convenient because it could fit into a variety of etiological theories of typhoid and because it explained localized cases that could not be explained by infected food or water. What epidemiological studies had accomplished was to reframe sewer gas and its dangers and to point to the faults of domestic sanitation in the spread of typhoid.[151] This started with the impetus in the 1870s to show the specific ways that sewer gas, only when it was impregnated with the poison of typhoid, could spread the disease. That narrowing led to such breakthroughs as Buchanan and Blaxall's typhoid investigations, which argued that sewer gas was really only important when it was mixed with water. By the 1890s it was becoming clear that sewer gas was only symptomatic of faulty plumbing; it was not, as Budd had lamented in 1873, "the actual and primary source of the disease."[152] In practical outbreak investigation sewer gas was the canary in the coal mine, but late nineteenth-century bacteriologists had difficulty in definitively agreeing that it could transmit typhoid.[153] Yet, for all the uncertainty surrounding sewer air, as the century came to a close even Chief Medical Officer Richard Thorne Thorne, in a cholera memorandum, still hedged practical bets, warning the public of "the danger of breathing air which is foul with effluvia" from the specific discharges of the sick.[154]

The heating up of sewer gas debates resonated in new ways after the prince's typhoid attack in 1871 was traced to faulty plumbing at Londesborough Lodge. And while epidemiological research into sewer gas was the least successful method of inquiry in establishing strong causal claims—compared to research on water, milk, and soils—in determining the etiology of the disease, sewer gas research at the Medical Department accomplished two

---

150 Stallybrass, *The Principles of Epidemiology*, 8.

151 Davey, "The Prevention of Enteric Fever," 509.

152 Sanitary engineer H. Alfred Roechling had even designed a smoke test for sewer gas in the 1890s. See Roechling, *Sewer Gas*.

153 Parkes, "Reviews of Books," 143–52.

154 Richard Thorne Thorne, "Precautions Against the Infectious Cholera," August 26, 1892, National Archives, Kew. MH 113/29.

things. First, the transition from sewer gas as *prima facie* cause of the disease in the 1860s to a potential symptom of defective plumbing in the 1890s directed more detailed epidemiological research into the waterborne nature of typhoid. This topic is explored in chapter 2. Second, research into sewer gas often meant intruding into domestic spaces—like Londesborough Lodge, Windsor Castle, or Caius College, Cambridge—and into the homes of middle- and upper-class Britons.[155] The product was a new kind of epidemiological intrusion, which included digging up drainpipes under houses, taking apart water closets, and peering into the intimate details of the wealthier classes. The results were sometimes unflattering. As William Jenner once quipped, "The palaces of the rich were often found . . . to be as insanitary as the hovels of the poor."[156] Sewer gas fears thus ignited a new kind of class-based understanding of the disease, one that Alfred Haviland, MOH for Northamptonshire, cleverly defined in a new kind of class-based, epidemiologically specific way, whereby "the poor suffer from *drinking* the poison—the rich from *inhaling* it."[157] But just as the nation had come together to celebrate the recovery of a future king, they had to collectively suffer the filth disease and face the epidemiological gaze. Typhoid had become, as Haviland pronounced in 1873, a "national disgrace," a rhetorical admission that stemmed from the growing body of epidemiological research, as well as the cultural moment that raised the disease's profile after the royal attack.

---

155 Nancy Tomes has found a similar pattern in America. See Tomes "The Private Side of Public Health." And there was a longer, class-based history of understanding cholera. See Kudlick, *Cholera in Post-Revolutionary Paris.*

156 "Obituary for William Henry Corfield," *Transactions of the Epidemiological Society of London* 22 (1903): 162.

157 Haviland, "The Geographical Distribution," 232.

Chapter Two

A Good Working Theory

Water and the Methods of Outbreak

Investigation Before 1880

Months after seeing the Prince of Wales through the most sensationalized case of typhoid fever in British history, William Gull delivered a prophetic lecture on the disease at Guy's Hospital in June of 1872.[1] Calling typhoid by its colloquial name, the "filth fever," Gull foresaw that in 250 years typhoid would be "uncommon" and "comparatively rare."[2] Coming off of his successful treatment of the prince, Gull, aged fifty-seven, had an optimistic view that typhoid could be conquered. But the defeat of typhoid, according to Gull, was going to take more than the cautious clinical case management he showed at Sandringham. He went so far as to say that there was "no use tinkering with the disease if one does not try to prevent it, and it no doubt may be prevented." Prevention, Gull argued, was predicated upon knowledge of the etiology of typhoid. "The theory," he went on, "is that it is connected with germs which get into the blood; we know nothing about these germs— the air is full of them. There is an idea that they are imbibed by drinking water, and that they increase and multiply within the body." "Although this has not been demonstrated," Gull explained, "it is a good working theory."[3] By the early 1870s it was well accepted that typhoid was waterborne, even if, as Gull noted, the theory still needed further evidentiary proof. Sewer gases, as explored in chapter 1, had gained unprecedented attention as a medium

---

1   Gull, "A Lecture on Typhoid Fever," 896.
2   Gull, "On Typhoid Fever," 17.
3   Ibid.

of the disease after the sickness of the Prince of Wales. And as we will see in chapter 3, cow's milk exploded onto the scene as a conveyor of typhoid in 1871, expanding the epidemiological picture of the disease. But there were plenty of unanswered questions: about the nature of the "poison," or "germ"; about the alleged spontaneous origin of the disease; and about the uneven distribution of typhoid geographically and demographically. These queries would largely be settled in the last three decades of the nineteenth century through a combination of laboratory study, statistical analysis, and local outbreak investigation, which was spearheaded at the Medical Department.

This chapter explores the development of what Gull called "a good working theory." To the vanguard of British epidemiologists, Gull's working theory was at the center of a practical methodology of outbreak investigation. First established by studying cholera in the 1850s, the waterborne theory gained significant traction in the 1860s and 1870s through epidemiological fieldwork on typhoid conducted in both urban and rural areas by inspectors at the Medical Department and by MosH. The chapter begins with two remarkable epidemiological studies of cholera by John Netten Radcliffe during the last visitation of epidemic cholera in London in 1865 and 1866. Radcliffe's cholera studies marked a turning point in the validation of the waterborne hypothesis, and he was a key actor in shifting the epidemiological gaze at the Medical Department from cholera to typhoid. By the late 1860s Radcliffe had become a spokesperson for defining British epidemiology and a leading advocate for Budd's theory of the specific, fecal-oral spread of typhoid. The turn in outbreak investigation toward typhoid came partly out of practical necessity; typhoid outbreaks were on the rise by the 1870s and occurring throughout Britain, keeping Radcliffe and his colleagues busy all year round.

The period from 1865 to 1880, the subject of part two of the chapter, saw a flurry of epidemiological activity that linked typhoid to fecally contaminated water. This period is significant in the history of British epidemiology for two reasons. First, studies of waterborne typhoid expanded etiological knowledge of the disease at a time "when eminent men differ much in their opinion regarding the etiology of typhoid fever."[4] Outbreak investigations, particularly at the Medical Department, demonstrated how typhoid spread differently in urban and rural areas and how the contamination of deep versus shallow wells influenced the distribution of the disease. Department investigations revealed the inefficacy of numerous methods of excrement removal,

4   McNeill, "A Contribution to the Etiology of Typhoid Fever," 739.

sewerage, and waterworks construction. This suggested that remedial action was necessary, even if local officials did not always comply. Second, outbreak investigations of waterborne typhoid provided a testing ground for a number of qualitative and quantitative epidemiological methods, such as experimentation, case tracing, interviewing, statistical analysis, and visual strategies such as making diagrams and maps. From the 1870s, in other words, an expanding epidemiological toolkit was beginning to coalesce into a routine method for outbreak investigation at the Medical Department. It was during this period, for example, that an important rhetorical shift occurred: those practicing epidemiology first started to call themselves "epidemiologists" and to lay out, as Radcliffe, Corfield, and Budd did, the precise ways to go about outbreak investigation. The stylistic change was critical, particularly because the views and practices among MOsH in this period were still eclectic. The Medical Department–sponsored study of waterborne typhoid from the late 1860s to the early 1880s—two decades before the discovery of the typhoid bacillus—formed one of the most important periods in the history of British epidemiology.

Epidemiological Methods during "The Final Catastrophe": Part One—Rural Essex

In the summer of 1865 foreign reports flooded British newspapers that cholera was epidemic in Egypt. Fearful of the "scourge of the East," many Britons prepared, as a writer in *the Era* noted, for "at any moment [cholera might] extend its boundaries and spread, like wildfire, in any direction the winds or fortuitous circumstances may carry it."[5] With cholera approaching, John Simon, chief medical officer of the Medical Department of the Privy Council, hired John Netten Radcliffe to conduct a special investigation into the diffusion of cholera in the Mediterranean. Receiving pressure from Parliament, it was a chance for Simon to show the international breadth of the department and to respond to an impending crisis.[6]

---

5   "The Progress of Cholera in Egypt," *Era*, July 23, 1865, 9.

6   By 1865 Radcliffe had risen within the Epidemiological Society to be its secretary. For his final report, see Radcliffe, "Report on the Sources and Development of the Present Diffusion of Cholera in Europe." Radcliffe continued his study into the 1870s. See John Netten Radcliffe, "Recent Diffusion of Cholera in Europe," National Archives, Kew. MH/25/23.

Radcliffe was one of the Medical Department's experts on waterborne disease and foreign epidemics. He was, as Bill Luckin notes, an *"elite* within an *elite*," convinced of Snow and Budd's waterborne theory from the early 1850s. It was at that time, as an aspiring surgeon in Leeds, that Radcliffe was elected to the newly formed Epidemiological Society of London (ESL). A Yorkshireman, Radcliffe was educated at the Leeds School of Medicine. He qualified as a member of the Royal College of Surgeons in 1853 and served as a surgeon in the Crimean War. From there Radcliffe moved to London and was appointed medical superintendent of the Hospital for the Paralyzed and Epileptic in Queen Square, a position he obtained with help from his older brother, Charles Bland Radcliffe, a prominent London neurologist. But it was in epidemiology, not neurology, that Radcliffe found his passion. He quickly made a name for himself at the ESL, delivering early papers on "The Hygiene of the Turkish Army" and "Fever on Board the Turkish Line of Battleship Tesherfieh." It was at the ESL that Radcliffe met the most important professional contact of his life: John Simon.

Just as many had feared, in September cholera struck British shores, first in the port town of Southampton. The earliest recorded case was on September 17, and the first death occurred on September 24. Simon turned to Edmund Alexander Parkes, professor of military hygiene at the Army Medical Hospital, to investigate. Parkes found sixty cases of cholera and thirty-five deaths at Southampton.[7] Within a week, with Parkes still on assignment, Simon received word from Radcliffe, who was carefully following statistical reports from the GRO that a seemingly isolated outbreak had occurred in a small farming community in Essex, in the Epping Union parish of Theydon Bois. With rumors swirling about the spread of cholera, he sent Radcliffe to investigate. Such an assignment pattern, where statistics from the GRO indicated a spike in deaths (and later sicknesses), and then an inspector was sent to investigate the particular locality, became a staple of British epidemiology in the last three decades of the century.

Radcliffe's report, "On the Outbreak of Cholera at Theydon Bois, Essex, in 1865, With Special Reference to the Propagation of Cholera by Water as a Medium," was a masterful epidemiological study, indicative of the emerging practice of outbreak investigation in the 1860s. The isolated nature of the outbreak afforded Radcliffe a unique opportunity to discover the index case and carefully trace the outbreak back to Southampton and its importation

---

7   Parkes, "Report on the Outbreak of Cholera."

from Alexandria, Egypt. Already in the mid-1860s, Radcliffe was thinking globally about the spread of disease.

At Theydon Bois, twelve people were struck with cholera and nine died. It was precisely because of the virulent and localized nature of the outbreak that Radcliffe was able to isolate "the special localizing causes." Theydon Bois was a rural parish with a population of just over six hundred inhabitants. Like many parts of Britain in the Victorian period, Theydon Bois was, according to Radcliffe, in a dire sanitary state. His study began with the people attacked. Who were they? What age were they? Had they recently travelled? How did they interact with one another, and what were the dates that they first fell sick or died? Radcliffe visualized this data in a chart (figure 2.1), which was central in the statistical and spatial understanding of the outbreak. He narrowed the outbreak to a cluster of cases at Little Gregory's Farm. There he studied the sanitary condition of the farm and the personal habits of those affected.[8]

Radcliffe found the water supply, from a well, to be "very turbid and abominably fetid . . . it was clear that the water was laden with decomposing organic matter."[9] As was common at the Medical Department, Radcliffe sent a sealed sample of the farm's water to his London colleague William Allen Miller, professor of chemistry at King's College. In the period from 1860 to 1880 John Simon and his successors relied on a variety of chemists and early bacteriologists to conduct such work, including John Burdon Sanderson, August Dupre, J. L. W. Thudichum, and Edward Klein. Miller found traces of sulphuretted hydrogen and a large quantity of ammonia, remarking that there was definitely "some leakage from the cesspool into the well."[10] Christopher Hamlin has shown that even among analytical chemists like Miller there was little agreement over what constituted "pure" water until the very end of the nineteenth century.[11] This was not a point lost on epidemiologists of the 1860s and 1870s; as we will see later in this chapter, some members of the Medical Department, like Richard Thorne Thorne, often refused to send suspected water for analysis while on outbreak

---

8   Simon included shorter extract of the Theydon Bois report alongside his longer European cholera study. See, Simon, *Eighth Report of the Medical Officer,* 438–40.

9   Radcliffe, "On the Outbreak of Cholera at Theydon Bois Essex," 92.

10   Radcliffe, "On the Outbreak of Cholera at Theydon Bois Essex, 93. On Miller, see "Obituary for William Miller," *Lancet* 2 (October 8, 1870): 523.

11   Hamlin, *A Science of Impurity,* introduction.

Residence.	Name.	Age.	Date of attack.		Death.		Recovery.	
			Diarrhœa.	Cholera.	During collapse.	During consecutive fever.	From collapse.	From consecutive fever.
I. Little Gregory's Farm	Mrs. Groombridge	50 years	Sept. 26	Sept. 28	...	Oct. 11	...	...
„	Miss Emily Groombridge . .	8 years		Sept. 30	Sept. 30	...	...	...
„	James Bass	17 years	Sept. 30	Oct. 1	...	...	...	Oct. 14
„	Miss Kate Groombridge . . .	16 years	Oct. 2	Oct. 3	...	...	...	Oct. 17
„	Maid-servant	18 years	Oct. 5	Oct. 6 Relapse, Oct. 6	...	Oct. 19	...	...
„	Mr. Groombridge	49 years	Sept. 23	Oct. 6	Oct. 7	...	...	...
„	Mr. Charles Groombridge . .	20 years	Oct. 6	Oct. 7	...	...	Oct. 11	...
„	Mrs. Parcell	87 years	Oct. 6	Oct. 7	Oct. 14 Exhaustion	...	...	...
II. The Place, Epping .	Mr. McNab	74 years	Oct. 2	Oct. 2	Oct. 2	...	...	...
III. Bell Common	John Riley	34 years	Oct. 5	Oct. 7	Oct. 7	...	...	...
IV. Cottage near the toll-bar	Susan Saville	46 years	...	Oct. 10	Oct. 11 Syncope?	...	...	...
V. Cottage near the Bell public-house, and a little to the east of the toll-bar . . .	Henry Hagger	3 years	...	Oct. 31	Nov. 1	...	...	...

CHOLERA AT THEYDON BOIS.

Figure 2.1 Statistical chart of the distribution of cholera cases. From John Netten Radcliffe, "On the Outbreak of Cholera at Theydon Bois Essex in 1865, with Special Reference to the Propagation of Cholera by Water as a Medium," Transactions of the Epidemiological Society of London, 91. Orphan work in public domain.

investigation because of inconclusive and untrustworthy evidence from the laboratory. But Radcliffe in 1865 found value in Miller's tests; his field-based methods had suggested a connection between sewage and water. Miller's test had simply confirmed it.

Even with Miller's endorsement, Radcliffe was set on providing more proof for his hypothesis that the disease was carried by water. He turned to a simple experiment. Radcliffe had found two leaks at the farmhouse, one in the sink drain and one in the soil pipe. By pouring water into a drain in the house and examining the two leaks, he found that "the escaped matters penetrated downwards along the outer wall of the house, passed beneath the foundation, saturated the earth in the angle between the pump and the well, and so reached the latter. Water having been poured down the water-closet, in ten minutes a portion had passed along this tract and was dripping into the well."[12] Simple experimentation of this sort became a hallmark of epidemiological investigations at the Medical Department.[13] Through case trac-

---

12   Radcliffe, "On the Outbreak of Cholera at Theydon Bois Essex," 93.

13   In another early example of experimentation, Edward Cox Seaton, investigating an outbreak of typhoid at Page Green, Tottenham, in 1866, poured carbolic acid down a sewer drain he suspected was in contact with a shallow well.

ing, chemical analysis, and experimentation, Radcliffe was now satisfied that most cholera cases in Theydon Bois were caused by the drinking of water charged with the discharges of the index case. Yet Radcliffe still had not answered the question of how cholera had made its way to Theydon Bois in the first place. That he never turned to Murchison's pythogenic theory, which held that cholera could arise spontaneously at Little Gregory's Farm, is telling of Radcliffe's etiological views. He was determined to find the index case, which he traced to the owners of the farm, Mr. and Mrs. Groombridge. The couple, Radcliffe found, had recently traveled to Weymouth, briefly stopping at Southampton, the seat of the outbreak in England. They had come into contact with the disease there, perhaps at the train station, he surmised, and brought it back to Essex.

His final report went to the desk of Simon, but Radcliffe went even further to communicate the case to a broader professional audience. On April 1, 1867, before the Epidemiological Society, he used the study to draw critical lessons for proving the waterborne theory and for shaping the methods of outbreak investigation.[14] He reflected that "this outbreak furnishes the most complete, because least doubted and doubtful, illustration . . . of the propagation of cholera by means of the drinking water."[15] George Wilson, in his 1873 *Handbook of Hygiene* called it a "remarkable outbreak," and that Radcliffe had proved—following Snow in 1854—that cholera was a waterborne disease that followed the fecal-oral route.[16] Radcliffe's waterborne hypothesis, following Budd and John Snow, rested on the fundamental idea that cholera was caused by a specific, living agent able to be transmitted through water charged with the excreta of those suffering from the disease. We can compare Radcliffe's 1865 Theydon Bois study with Snow's Broad Street study in 1854. Radcliffe and Snow shared basic assumptions about the biological world and the nature of epidemic disease. The connection was not lost on Radcliffe, who concluded his report by reflecting that Snow's Broad Street study and his investigation at Theydon Bois "furnish invaluable data in estimating the probable effect of water contaminated with diarrheal

---

Upon drawing water, he found the unmistakable smell of carbolic acid. See Seaton, "Impure Water as a Cause of Typhoid Fever."

14   Radcliffe's Epidemiological Society address was covered in *The Lancet*. See "Medical Annotations," *Lancet* 2280 (May 11, 1867): 575–76.

15   Radcliffe, "On the Outbreak of Cholera at Theydon Bois," 85.

16   Wilson, *A Handbook of Hygiene*, 205.

discharges in determining explosions of cholera."[17] Comparison with Snow was a rhetorical nod before the members of the Epidemiological Society; by connecting his work to Snow, Radcliffe was both acknowledging an intellectual debt and attempting to validate the waterborne theory.

But more than rhetorical grandstanding, Radcliffe's investigation at Theydon Bois helped dictate preventative action. In late 1865 Simon issued a memo to local authorities recommending precautionary measures against the spread of cholera, diarrhea, and typhoid.[18] The memo warned that "sources of water-supply should be well examined. Those which are in any way tainted by animal or vegetable refuse, above all those into which there is any leakage or filtration from sewers, drains, cesspools, or foul ditches, ought no longer to be drunk from. Especially where the disease is cholera, diarrhoea, or typhoid fever, it is essential that no foul water be drunk." The memo extended Radcliffe's adherence to the exclusive waterborne theory, even if Simon in the mid-1860s was still waffling between it and Murchison's pythogenic theory. "In typhoid fever and cholera," Simon warned, "the evacuations should be regarded as capable of communicating an infectious quality to any night-soil with which they are mingled in privies, drains, or cesspools."[19] It was at least a nod to what Radcliffe had shown at Theydon Bois and a way for Simon to hedge etiological bets in making practical recommendations to local authorities who sought to prevent the spread of the disease.[20]

Epidemiological Methods during "The Final Catastrophe": Part Two—Urban London

Despite Simon's hopes in the 1865 memo, and only months after Radcliffe was experimenting with sewer drains in Essex, cholera struck London. Between July and early November of 1866, nearly four thousand Londoners were dead from cholera. It was an opportunity for Radcliffe to test his methods of outbreak investigation on a metropolitan scale. Radcliffe's 1866 metropolitan investigation of "the final catastrophe," to use Luckin's term,

---

17 Radcliffe, "On the Outbreak of Cholera at Theydon Bois," 98.

18 The 1865 circular was reprinted in the popular press as well. See "General Memorandum," 6.

19 "General Memorandum," 6.

20 Worboys, *Spreading Germs*, 113.

provides an interesting contrast to his investigation at Theydon Bois.[21] At Theydon Bois, Radcliffe confronted a rural, isolated outbreak, where he obtained detailed personal information about those dead and dying from the disease. He also had time and space to experiment. Less than a year later, in metropolitan London, Radcliffe was faced with a complex ecological web of people, sanitary systems, and vital statistics. Yet in both studies Radcliffe was inductive in his approach and set to prove the waterborne nature of the disease through carefully tracing the earliest cases of the outbreak. That Simon chose Radcliffe to lead the metropolitan investigation is telling of his reliance on Radcliffe's evolving methods of outbreak investigation.[22]

From the outset Radcliffe focused on the water supply of London, just as he had done at Theydon Bois. But he was also clear about his intellectual debt to Snow, from whom he borrowed "lessons derived from the outbreaks of 1848–49 and 1853–54," in linking cholera to a fecally infected water supply.[23] Examining the house drainage where the first cholera cases occurred, Radcliffe found that "the discharges of the patients first known to have been attacked with the epidemic, were cast, and they would pass rapidly along the line of sewers mentioned, over a distance of about 300 yards, into the river Lea."[24] Radcliffe employed an eclectic epidemiological set of practices; he collaborated with engineers, geologists, metropolitan MOsH, and statisticians. Even William Farr, who has been given the bulk of the credit for discovering the fault of the East London Water Company, noted that he referred "to his [Radcliffe's] report for a great many interesting details, and for an explanation or confutation of some of the fallacies set afloat."[25]

---

21   John Netten Radcliffe, "Report on Cholera in London."

22   Simon noted that "the East London epidemic was of such magnitude and concentration as peculiarly to require the vigilance of the department . . . so at various times Dr. Seaton, Dr. Buchanan, and Dr. Hunter were sent into the Eastern districts." Radcliffe alone, however, was responsible for conducting and writing up the department's report on the outbreak. See Simon, *Ninth Annual Report of the Medical Officer of the Privy Council*, 21.

23   Radcliffe, "Report on Cholera in London," 295. Radcliffe cited Snow's cholera research in pp. 295 and 305. On p. 304 he made direct reference to his 1865 Theydon Bois investigation.

24   Radcliffe, "Report on Cholera in London," 285.

25   Farr, "Report on the Cholera Epidemic of 1866," xii. Later in the report Farr described how Radcliffe was responsible for figuring out how the East London Water Company's water received the cholera discharges.

Farr was the first to suspect the East London Company's use of cholera-charged water. In a letter to Edward Frankland on August 4, 1866, Farr suggested, "My theory is, that is some strait they [the East London Company] supplied for some day or days their water from the *uncovered reservoirs* at Old Ford, contaminated in some way or other."[26] Farr's *Report on the Cholera Epidemic of 1866 in England* was an indictment of the East London Company and a complex analysis of the statistical distribution of cholera cases in the metropolis. Farr relied on Frankland for both water analysis—which was ultimately inconclusive—and for interrogation of the engineers and manual laborers at the company. He relied on Radcliffe for independent and "thoroughly impartial" epidemiological investigation, to trace individual cases of cholera and to determine how cholera discharges had made their way into the water supply. "Mr. Radcliffe," the *Lancet* noted, "has traced with the utmost minuteness the links in the chain of evidence inculpating the Water Company."[27] Radcliffe discovered what he believed was the index case, that key feature of Victorian outbreak investigation at the Medical Department. The case involved a laborer in a brush manufactory and his wife, who lived in the Bromley district of East London on Priory Street. A local physician reported that the couple had been seized with cholera on June 26, 1866, and died in rapid succession the next day. The couple were two of the first fourteen registered cholera deaths, and Radcliffe's epidemiological gaze narrowed on their movements throughout London. *The Lancet* was enamored with the minuteness of Radcliffe's tracing of the intimate links in the communication of cholera. It was a staple in the arsenal of outbreak investigation. The key to studying an outbreak of waterborne disease, Radcliffe believed, was to carefully follow the early cases, but it was also in spatially thinking through the epidemic that Radcliffe made his case.

Radcliffe, with help from geologist William Whitaker, created three epidemiological maps of the cholera deaths over the metropolis. The first was a large foldout of the distribution of cholera from June 27 to July 21, which marked cholera deaths, circled the two index cases in red, and overlaid the East London Water Company's lines and the metropolitan drainage system (figure 2.2). The second map compared the cholera field of 1866 to the earlier outbreaks of 1849 and 1854. The third map was a granular visualization of where the two index cases resided, a spatial attempt to show how the

---

26   "Mr. Radcliffe's Report on the London Cholera Epidemic," *Lancet* 2305 (November 2, 1867): 558.

27   Ibid.

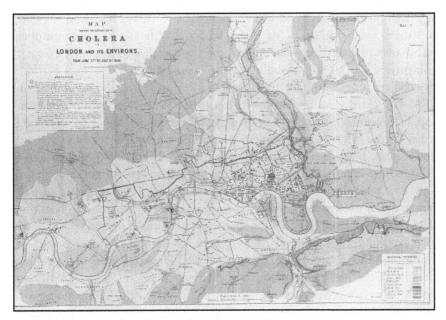

Figure 2.2 John Netten Radcliffe, map showing the distribution of cholera in London and its environs. Image courtesy of the Wellcome Library, London. CreativeCommons Attribution license CC BY 4.0.

outbreak began. Picturing the spatial dimensions of an epidemic was central to knowledge production in Victorian epidemiology.[28]

Radcliffe's cholera studies demonstrate the ways in which the waterborne theory of disease was put to the test in the 1860s.[29] Alexander Wynter Blyth, in his popular *Manual of Public Health,* argued in 1890 that Radcliffe's cholera studies in 1865 and 1866 were still "the most valuable which have ever

28 McLeod, "Our Sense of Snow." For a more recent account of how medical geographers have considered Snow's work, see Koch, *Disease Maps,* chapters 9 and 10.

29 Simon made this point clear in his *Ninth Annual Report,* summarizing Radcliffe's investigation, "that the person who contracts cholera in this country is *ipso facto* demonstrated with almost absolute certainty to have been exposed to excremental pollution; that what gave him cholera was (mediately or immediately) cholera-contagium discharged from another's bowels." Simon, *Ninth Annual Report of the Medical Officer,* 33.

appeared on the subject and will repay perusal."[30] The chief lesson for state medicine, Simon argued in his annual report, was the need for a continuous rather than intermittent water supply, and the overall accountability of water companies, which had "colossal power of life and death."[31]

Scholars have had a lot to say about the final visitation of cholera in 1865–66. Hardy and Luckin have shown that in the aftermath of the metropolitan outbreak there was a renewed political commitment to reforming urban health infrastructure, especially ensuring an efficient sewerage system, and a clean, filtered, continuous water supply.[32] Worboys has argued that it "allowed the experience to be packaged as a great success for sanitary science and state medicine."[33] The events surrounding the 1866 cholera outbreak represent, to use Luckin's phrase, the ascendance of "progressive" scientific methods of controlling epidemic disease; vital statistics teamed with water analysis and epidemiological fieldwork. It was a model often repeated in studies conducted by inspectors at the Medical Department in the last three decades of the nineteenth century. Radcliffe's studies at Theydon Bois and London provide a window into the evolving practice of epidemiology in Victorian Britain, particularly those "*avant garde* in the nascent profession of epidemiology," as Luckin suggests, who "gave unqualified support to the view that the outbreak of 1866 was decisively carried by water."[34] Eyler has argued that Farr's statistical work during the 1866 outbreak provided the crucial evidence in linking cholera and contaminated water, changing Farr's views to a more exclusivist position.[35] Hamlin, too, has shown that the outbreak led Frankland to abandon a strict Liebigian view about waterborne

---

30   Blyth, *A Manual of Public Health*, 512.

31   Simon, *Ninth Annual Report*, 28.

32   Luckin, "The Final Catastrophe"; Hardy, "Cholera, Quarantine, and the English Preventive System."

33   Worboys, *Spreading Germs*, 115.

34   Luckin, "The Final Catastrophe," 33. But there were still numerous critics. See, for example, the volatile debate that ensued at the Society of Medical Officers of Health meeting on March 21, 1868, between Henry Letheby, MOH for the City of London and Radcliffe. Henry Letheby, "On the Cholera Epidemic of 1866 Contrasted with Former Epidemics of the Disease, and an Examination of the Question Whether the Water Supply had any Connection with the Disease," read March 21, 1868, Wellcome Archives, London, Society of Medical Officer of Health Files, SA/SMO/G2/1/1.

35   Eyler, "The Changing Assessments," 229–30; Farr, *"Report on the Cholera Epidemic of 1866."*

diseases.[36] Radcliffe's efforts—and by extension epidemiological methods pioneered at the Medical Department—were critical to changing the views of both Farr and Frankland.[37] His involvement also deepens our understanding of how important rural epidemiological practices were in this period, as his 1866 investigation of the cholera outbreak in East London grew out of his study at Theydon Bois.

A "Close Aetiological Affinity": Local Investigations of Waterborne Typhoid in the 1860s

Radcliffe's cholera studies served as a springboard for a long career in professional epidemiology. He joined the Medical Department full time and began to provide vocal leadership for how to conduct outbreak investigation. In April 1868, for example, he gave a speech before the Epidemiological Society reflecting on his study of cholera in 1865–66. There Radcliffe compared epidemiology to meteorology, asserting that "to be fruitful of good . . . both must equally rest on accurate data collected in a wide area of observation, and over periods of time more or less extended."[38] He went on to lay out a six-point approach for studying outbreaks of waterborne disease:

1. What were the exact dates of the earliest recognized or ascertained cases of the disease, whether the cases proved fatal or not?
2. Did these cases occur among strangers or persons recently arrived in the place, or among residents who had not been recently away from it?
3. Had there been any unusual amount of bowel disorders, or other form of sickness, prevalent among the inhabitants prior to the occurrence of these cases?
4. What part of the town or village did the first cases occur, and what part or district suffered the most during the visitation?
5. What was the nearest place where the disease was known to exist at the time of the occurrence of the first cases, or to have existed shortly before such occurrence?
6. What precautionary measures have been taken by the authorities to avert, or to meet, the visitation?[39]

---

36 Hamlin, *A Science of Impurity*, 158–59; Hamlin, "Politics and Germ Theories in Victorian Britain," 116–17.
37 Contemporaries recognized Radcliffe's involvement. See, for example, MacNamara, *A History of Asiatic Cholera*, 317.
38 Radcliffe, "Report on the Recent Epidemic of Cholera," 232.
39 Radcliffe, "Report on the Recent Epidemic of Cholera," 233.

Radcliffe's point-by-point methodology provided a model for subsequent outbreak investigations. He became a leading voice for a new kind of epidemiology that flourished in the second half of the century. In 1875, for example, Radcliffe became the president of the society. But Radcliffe's methodology was applied to typhoid fever, not cholera.

British doctors in the period after 1866 coalesced around the view that there was a "close aetiological affinity . . . between the diffusion of cholera and the diffusion of typhoid fever."[40] The same truths hold for typhoid and cholera, Simon declared in his annual report for 1867: "excrement-sodden earth, excrement-reeking air, excrement-tainted water."[41] Leeds physician T. Clifford Allbutt, an early advocate of both experimental physiology and epidemiology, echoed as much in an 1870 article in the *British Medical Journal,* noting that "persons may drink fecal water for months or years, their cesspools may communicate with their wells, their drains may find a way into their water-pipes . . . but they do not suffer from enteric fever, unless they drink the specific poison of that disease."[42] In the period before the discovery of the typhoid bacillus, such an epistemological claim was at the center of the type of British epidemiology put into practice by inspectors at the Medical Department, who conducted local investigations of typhoid more than any other infectious disease. Typhoid served, the *Lancet* noted, as "a certain index of particular insanitary states."[43] It was a model disease, or as Lloyd Stevenson has called it, an "exemplary disease," for the health of a locality and for testing etiological hypotheses.[44] Remember, it was also a pressing public health problem, claiming the lives of 15,000 to 20,000 annually, and sickening over 150,000 each year.

---

40   Confidential memo sent by John Simon to the President of the Local Government Board, June 30, 1874, National Archives, Kew. MH 113/12, 5. Simon repeated the etiological connection between cholera and typhoid in Simon, *Twelfth Annual Report*, 31.

41   Simon, *Ninth Annual Report*, 33.

42   Allbutt, "On the Propagation of Enteric Fever," 308–9. The same conclusion was reached by the official report of the *Rivers Pollution Commission*, where in the *Sixth Report* they noted that "the existence of specific poisons capable of producing cholera and typhoid fever is attested by evidence so abundant and strong as to be practically irresistible. These poisons are contained in the discharges from the bowels of persons suffering from the disease." See Corfield, *The Treatment and Utilisation of Sewage*, 297.

43   "Typhoid Fever at Winterton," *Lancet* 2312 (December 21, 1867): 772.

44   Stevenson, "Exemplary Disease," 1.

A series of investigations of waterborne typhoid in the late 1860s, particularly because of the explosive and isolated nature of the outbreaks, were instructive for the evolving methods of outbreak investigation. These studies—by George Buchanan at Guildford and by Richard Thorne Thorne at Winterton and Terling—demonstrate a pattern developing at the Medical Department, one that in the 1870s and 1880s became routine, called the "*via exclusionis*, the favourite method in the department," Edward Ballard later noted.[45] MOH George Wilson, in his influential *Handbook of Hygiene and Sanitary Science*, called the late 1860s investigations of waterborne typhoid "examples of the painstaking and systematic way in which such inquiries should be conducted."[46] Local studies brought to the fore some of the as-yet-unanswered questions about the spread of the disease, such as how it spread differently in areas with shallow wells rather than those served by high-service reservoir public waterworks. And it was through local outbreak investigation that inspectors at the department began to use morbidity, as well as mortality rates, in their investigations of typhoid fever.

The small market town of Winterton, in north Lincolnshire, had rarely been free from typhoid from the mid-1850s. Among the local population of eighteen hundred, cases started to skyrocket in 1865 among middle- and upper-class homes in the west end of town. There, in one year, 100 of the 145 inhabitants contracted typhoid and 17 died. But in 1867 the disease took an abrupt turn, erupting in the east part of town among the laboring population, with 55 new cases and 6 deaths. The local officials wrote to John Simon for help. He sent Richard Thorne Thorne to investigate. Thorne was one of the most active researchers on typhoid in the 1860s and 1870s. He trained at St. Bartholomew's Hospital in the 1860s, qualified as a member of the Royal College of Surgeons in 1863, the Royal College of Physicians in 1865, and quickly began temporary work for Simon. He was hired full time in 1871 and worked tirelessly on outbreak investigation for two decades until he was promoted to chief medical officer in 1892.

Thorne began his investigation by consulting local union medical officer Mr. Bennett and interviewing the forty-nine people sick with typhoid. Knowing that the cases were localized to the east end of town, Thorne proceeded to field investigation, where he noted the "disgraceful state of the privies, cesspools, ashpits, and wells."[47] Only a few houses in east Winterton

45   Ballard, "Observations of Some of the Ways," 82–84.

46   Wilson, *Handbook of Hygiene and Sanitary Science,* 209.

47   Thorne, "Report on Epidemic Typhoid Fever at Winterton," 29.

had adopted water closets, with the majority being fitted with brick privies that had apertures, or openings, on the side or back for cleansing purposes. Walking house to house, Thorne found that at least half of the apertures were oozing excrement into gardens and penetrating into wells, using his own sensory experience to note that it was "producing the most offensive odour" and wafting under doors and into windows of houses.[48] The sanitary state was ripe for the excremental poisoning of shallow wells, but to prove his theory Thorne turned to granular case studies and visualization. In one example, he constructed a diagram of four cottages owned by Mr. Dale of Appelby (figure 2.3).

In front of cottage three, Thorne found an open, untrapped drain connected to the main sewer line that was full of holes and leaking. Eight feet away was the shallow well and pump, which included a waste pump that connected to the open drain line feeding to the main sewer. Because the drain was not emptying properly, sewage backed up to the pump. Thorne found other incriminating evidence of fecal pollution. The open ashpits near the privies, he learned through interviewing typhoid sufferers in the cottages, were home to the bowel discharges of typhoid patients. He found that the privies were so full of excrement that it nearly touched the seats, again sensorially noting that "the pestilential odour in the neighbourhood . . . would be almost impossible to describe."[49] Within a fourteen-foot range, Thorne concluded, there was an open leaking drain, an open ashpit, two pigsties, three privies, and one open cesspool, all situated one to three feet higher than a shallow well. Thorne examined the well's water with a microscope—he even tasted it—though he did not send a sample back to London for analysis. He found the water light brown in color, having a disagreeable taste and a large quantity of organic matter.

Thorne carefully interviewed the inhabitants of the cottages. Three people lived in Cottage One, two of whom were sick with typhoid. Cottage Two was free from typhoid, but only because it was empty. The previous inhabitants had been severely stricken, the father had died of typhoid, and the remaining family had relocated. In Cottage Three Thorne found Henry Driffell, a thirty-two-year-old bricklayer, "lying in a semi-comatose condition, on a mattress saturated with urine and fecal matter, to such an extent

---

48   Thorne, "Report on Epidemic Typhoid Fever at Winterton," 29. For a broader study of the senses in the Victorian period see the classic account of France, Corbin, *The Foul and the Fragrant*.

49   Thorne, "Report on Epidemic Typhoid Fever at Winterton," 31.

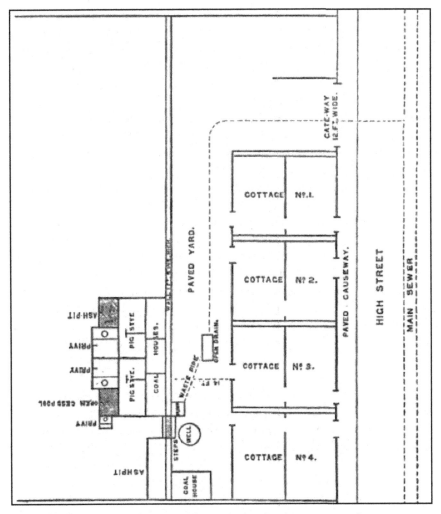

Figure 2.3 Diagram of the household spread of typhoid amongst rural cottagers. From Richard Thorne Thorne, "Report on Epidemic Typhoid Fever at Winterton," Tenth Annual Report of the Medical Officer of the Privy Council, 1868, 30. House of Commons Parliamentary Papers, Crown Copyright.

that the ammoniacal and fecal emanations were absolutely pungent."[50] In an adjacent room lay Driffell's wife in the same state. A parish nurse attended the Driffells, exhausted from watching the couple day and night and unable to move them or change their linens, since they did not have a spare set. Investigating Cottage Four Thorne found a family of four who were healthy and had been free of typhoid for many years. The key to their avoiding typhoid was that they never drank the well water on the premises—they found the taste disagreeable—instead obtaining it from a neighboring well. Thorne found the latter free of sewage contamination. He used the four-cottage case study to illuminate the sanitary standard in east Winterton. He was unable to determine the origination or index case of the outbreak, though it is interesting that he even sought to identify an index case, as typhoid had been endemic in the area for the past decade. Thorne was unwilling, in other words, to entertain the idea that the disease sprang up in Winterton *de novo*. *The Lancet* favorably reported on Thorne's Winterton study, praising the "honestly, comprehensiveness, and conscientious labour," which, they noted, were "characteristics of the reports which emanate from the Medical Department." Thorne had proved the excremental pollution of local shallow wells "clearly and conclusively," the article concluded, the study "is most instructive . . . a valuable contribution to the etiology of typhoid fever."[51] In 1868 the *Rivers Pollution Commission* made extensive use of Thorne's Winterton study, noting that his evidence was "so abundant and strong as to be practically irresistible."[52] William Whitaker, Britain's foremost expert on hydrogeology and a close colleague to the Medical Department, later noted in *Geology of London* that because of epidemiological studies such as Thorne's at Winterton, shallow wells had been proven to be "powerful factors in causing disease and death."[53]

While Thorne was in Winterton, his Medical Department colleague George Buchanan was investigating a sudden outbreak of typhoid close to London, in Guildford. With a population of around nine thousand,

---

50 Ibid.

51 "Typhoid Fever at Winterton," *Lancet* 2312 (December 21, 1867): 772. Thorne's Winterton study was even reported on in New Zealand and praised by local physicians as an instructive lesson. Vickerman, "The Sanitary State of Nelson," 2.

52 *Rivers Pollution Commission*, "Propagation of Typhoid Fever at Winterton," 183.

53 Whitaker, *The Geology of London*, 505.

Guildford, a mixed agricultural and manufacturing town home to the medieval Guildford Castle, had, like Winterton, rarely been free from typhoid.
But in late August and September 264 cases of typhoid rapidly occurred.
Examining the morbidity data (he was investigating while the outbreak
was occurring), Buchanan noticed that the outbreak struck both rich and
poor houses, but only those at the highest elevation in town, whose inhabitants were ten times more likely to get typhoid than those in low-lying
areas. Buchanan carefully examined the water supply of the town. Half of
Guildford received water from private wells, while the other half obtained
water from public waterworks. The public supply was fed by two wells sunk
twenty feet deep, one an old well that used a watermill and the other a new
well that raised water using a steam engine. On August 1, Buchanan learned,
the steam engine of the new well broke, and water was stored in a reservoir
used for the service of the high part of the town, where it sat until August
17. On that date only the high-lying areas of town received the stored water.
Buchanan sent several samples of the town's water to Miller in London.
While his tests were not conclusive, Miller found it probable that some
"excrementitious" contamination had occurred. With Guildford residents
still sick and dying of typhoid, Buchanan turned his attention to figuring out
how the new well had been contaminated, relying on the practical outbreak
investigation methods of case tracing and experimentation. He found that
the well was situated within ten feet of a main sewer line, in porous chalk
soil. When the pumping engine broke down, he learned from interviewing
workers that there was enough intense vibration to knock numerous bricks
loose in the adjacent sewer. Buchanan traced the sewer lines to show that the
pipes received the overflow of several cesspools in a poor part of town with
active typhoid cases. Buchanan was chuffed at his methodical sleuthing, noting that "a point in the natural history of typhoid appears to receive elucidation, if the deductions of this report as to causation are correct."[54] Buchanan's
suspicions of the contamination of the new well were later corroborated. The
local Poor Law medical officer, Mr. Taylor, later wrote to Buchanan to say
that after the outbreak, engineers working on the steam engine pump at the
waterworks noticed sewage-soaked soil.[55] They excavated and found that the
sewer line, full of holes and leaking sewage, had been constructed of old
unglazed tiles. "The ground was a quagmire of filth," Taylor wrote, "dark
coloured fetid slush had to be dug out and removed in baskets, making the

---

54   Buchanan, "On an Outbreak of Typhoid Fever at Guildford," 40.
55   For a background on poor law medical care, see Ritch, Sickness in the Workhouse.

men vomit who were employed in the work."[56] The entire episode had been, the *Lancet* noted, a "public calamity."[57]

Simon called Buchanan's study "peculiarly instructive."[58] Buchanan's investigative work had taught the local officials how to avoid typhoid in the future, and he had contributed "important matters towards the elucidation of the natural history and the etiology of the disease."[59] Taken together, Buchanan and Thorne in 1867 had demonstrated two very different ways in which fecally contaminated water could spread typhoid fever, in rural areas with shallow wells and rudimental drainage, and in suburban areas with deep wells and public works. The late 1860s marked the start of a flourishing period of epidemiology at the Medical Department. But not all outbreak investigations went smoothly. The swiftness and severity of some outbreaks, coupled with panicked local residents and stubborn local authorities, added up to the reality that outbreak investigation in this period was uneven and sometimes frustrating.

One illustrative case occurred in December 1867, when Simon received a letter from Colonel Shakespeare, a gentleman living in Witham, Essex, who complained that a sudden outbreak of typhoid was occurring in the village of Terling, and that the Board of Guardians of Witham, the administrative seat of Terling, was not supplying disinfectants. Thorne was sent to assist on the case, which erupted from a relatively unknown local outbreak into the national spotlight. Thorne arrived in Terling on December 21. Located on the banks of the River Ter, Terling boasted a modest nine hundred inhabitants, most of whom were impoverished agricultural laborers. The local outbreak had attracted national news, as about three hundred of the nine hundred residents were struck with clear-cut cases of typhoid in less than two months. Thorne was startled. Terling was a public health nightmare; when he arrived, about two hundred residents were already sick with the disease, and fresh cases were piling up daily. Entire families were attacked. He found houses where a father, a mother, or a child with mild diarrhea was nursing sick family members and neighbors. Due to a high rate of intermarriage, Thorne noted, everyone had someone either dying or dead. People were in a frenzy. Thorne even asked the vicar to stop the local custom of ringing the church bell every time someone died, because the town was "completely

---

56   Simon, *Tenth Annual Report*, 11.

57   "Typhoid at Guildford," *Lancet* 2306 (November 9, 1867): 587.

58   Simon, *Tenth Annual Report*, 10.

59   "Typhoid at Guildford," *Lancet* 2306 (November 9, 1867): 587.

panic-stricken," and the constant bells were having a "moral effect."[60] "Women with tears flowing down their cheeks called from their cottage doors for help," Thorne reported, and "no class of persons was exempt."[61] The *Medical Times and Gazette* on January 11 urged all residents to leave at once if they were able.[62]

Thorne began his investigation just as he did at Winterton, by consulting local officials, interviewing sufferers, examining the mortality and morbidity data, and closely inspecting the sanitary state of the local water supply, sewerage, housing, and local geological features. "All the nuisances which are generally associated with outbreaks of typhoid fever exist in great and unusual abundance," he lamented, but there was one peculiarity to the outbreak.[63] Examining the mortality returns, Thorne noticed that age and sex were determinate factors; of 145 cases where he was able to obtain the age of the victim, Thorne found that 79 were children under 14, and of the remaining 66, 50 were women. Thorne presumed this could be accounted for in the fact that men and boys over fourteen years of age spent most of their time laboring in the fields, and drank mostly beer, rather than well water, which Thorne inductively presumed was contaminated.

And like his colleagues at the department, Thorne was determined to locate an index case, made easier in Terling than in Winterton because the area had been free of typhoid for three months before the epidemic. Thorne turned to house-to-house inspection and interviewing local residents, which led him to the gardener's daughter at the dairy of Lord Rayleigh's dairy, who owned most of the agricultural land and cottages in Terling. The woman's case had commenced on November 13, a few weeks after returning from Somersetshire, where Thorne found active cases of typhoid. From there Thorne attempted to prove how the index case had spread so quickly and explosively throughout the village, which had only wells and no systematic sewerage works. The residents at the dairy drew their drinking water from the adjacent River Ter but insisted that they always boiled the water. It is interesting to note that Thorne considered it a possibility that "milk supplied from this dairy, could, after having been diluted with the river water,

---

60 Thorne, "Reports on an Epidemic of Typhoid Fever at Terling," 44.
61 Ibid.
62 "The Fever at Terling," *Medical Times and Gazette* 36 (January 11, 1868): 36
63 Hamlin has argued that the category of "nuisances" in this period was malleable. See Hamlin, "Public Sphere to Public Health." See also Hanley, "Parliament, Physicians, and Nuisances."

have caused the general outbreak."[64] Milk was only seriously considered a vehicle for the transmission of typhoid after 1870, as we will see in chapter 3. Although Thorne quickly dismissed the milk-borne hypothesis, it is likely, considering the demographic profile, that milk was a factor in communicating the disease. Without the kind of theoretical backing of the milk-borne hypothesis, Thorne moved to a waterborne theory. The cases had exploded so suddenly in Terling that even though Thorne had found the index case, he found it difficult to trace the communication of the outbreak throughout the village.

Much as he had done at Winterton, Thorne turned to granular case studies and visualization to prove the contamination of the local surface wells. Crucial to his methodology was the spatial element of mapping the wells, sewer drains, cottage cesspools, and geological formations. Thorne's visual strategies were coupled with interviewing and inspection. One important case study featured a diagram of a group of cottages called "Old Workhouse Row," in a populous part of the village where typhoid prevailed (figure 2.4). During the summer of 1867 the well the cottagers used dried up, and they were forced to use a neighboring one called Middleditch's Well. On November 26, Thorne found from interviewing residents that the cottagers' well had refilled, and they began to reuse it for drinking purposes. The first case of typhoid occurred ten days later, which Thorne noted matched the incubation period for typhoid. The same pattern was true of the two cottages north of Main Road.

Thorne believed he had unraveled a new fact in the etiology of typhoid: that the rise in groundwater corresponded to a rise in typhoid. Part of what was known as Pettenkofer's "ground water theory," was informed by his Munich colleague Professor Buhl, who argued that mortality rates from typhoid rose when groundwater levels were low and declined when water levels rose. Thorne found the opposite had occurred at Terling. With his suspicions awakened, Thorne was vocal that the Witham Board of Guardians "had entirely neglected its duty."[65] George Wilson, MOH for North Warwickshire, echoed as much in 1876, noting that rural MOsH often faced a "do nothing policy" by local authorities.[66] But Thorne pushed on, going before the board on December 23, imploring them to disinfect and clean out derelict cesspools and other accumulations of filth around cottages, to

---

64   Thorne, "Reports on an Epidemic of Typhoid Fever at Terling," 45.

65   Thorne, "Reports on an Epidemic of Typhoid Fever at Terling," 51.

66   Wilson, "Sanitary Work in Rural Districts," 158.

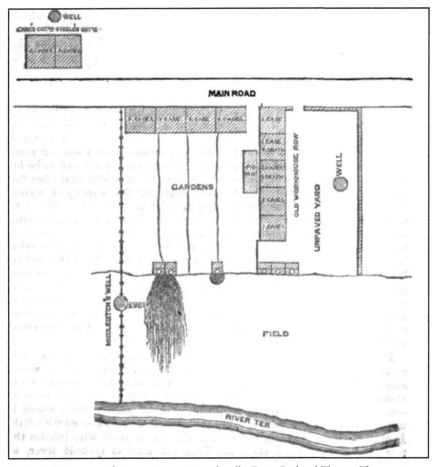

Figure 2.4 Diagram of sewage-contaminated wells. From Richard Thorne Thorne, "Reports on an Epidemic of Typhoid Fever at Terling." Annual Report of the Medical Officer of the Privy Council for 1865. Parliamentary Papers (London: Eyre and Spottiswoode, 1867), 46. House of Commons Parliamentary Papers, Crown Copyright.

provide a pure water supply, and to reduce overcrowding. The board argued that it was the local Terling vestry's duty under the Sanitary Act of 1866 to act, and Thorne and the board "did not quite agree."[67] The confusion about which political arm responsible was so great that Thorne returned to London

---

67   *First Report of the Royal Sanitary Commission*, Testimony of J. H. Blood, June 17, 1869, 210.

to seek advice from Simon. Simon advised Thorne to return to Terling, which he did, speaking before the board again on January 13, 1868, to say that they had "seriously neglected" his recommendations; walking around the village he found cesspools still "full to the brim."[68] "It is hardly possible to speak in sufficiently strong terms of the culpable neglect shown by that authority," Thorne lamented, "when the villagers were dying around them."[69]

Back in London again Thorne convinced Simon to make a formal complaint to Tom Taylor, secretary of the Local Government Act Office. Simon made the case that under the forty-ninth section of the Sanitary Act, the Home Office could force the Terling officials to enact sanitary improvements and enforce the nuisance laws. On February 5, Simon and Taylor petitioned the Home Office in a formal letter to intervene at Terling. Taylor called it "a most frightful epidemic. In the proportion of the number of deaths to the number of the population, it was the worst epidemic . . . that has been known in modern times in England."[70] The Home Office sent Thorne and Taylor back to Terling to speak before the Witham Board of Guardians, which they did on February 10, and with the ratepayers of Terling, whom they met on February 12. Taylor wrote to the secretary of state on February 17 with a full report. The Home Office responded, issuing several orders to resolve the matter. First, instead of the Witham Board, the local police were to oversee the nuisance removal per Thorne's recommendations and to pay for disinfectants, to the sum of £60.[71] Second, the Terling vestry had to oversee the construction of digging new wells. In concert with Lord Rayleigh, the vestry complied, and all of the cesspools at the local cottages (78 out of 164 in the village) were cleaned out, rebuilt with cement, and covered.[72]

The Terling outbreak cast a grave light "upon indolent nuisance authorities throughout the country."[73] Thorne was not the only one with an inter-

68   Thorne, "Reports on an Epidemic of Typhoid Fever at Terling," 51.
69   Thorne, "Reports on an Epidemic of Typhoid Fever at Terling," 54.
70   *First Report of the Royal Sanitary Commission,* Testimony of Tom Taylor, May 10, 1869, 78.
71   *First Report of the Royal Sanitary Commission,* Testimony of Tom Taylor, April 26, 1869, 12.
72   The measures were delayed for months, however, as local officials could not find enough able-bodied men to cleanse the cesspools, and the new well came up dry. "The Fever at Terling," *Medical Times and Gazette* 1 (February 8, 1868): 152
73   "The Epidemic of Fever at Terling," *Builder* 26 (February 15, 1868): 106.

est in Terling, as the rural outbreak attracted national attention. *The Builder* called it "a valuable addition to sanitary science," and the medical press in London issued weekly updates, which, like Thorne, castigated the "apathy of the local officials."[74] The popular press rallied around Thorne too. *Punch* went as far as to publish extensive sections from Thorne's report as a warning against idealizing the countryside, jokingly calling Terling "A village in Arcadia."[75] With Terling in the spotlight, local officials slowly started to implement sanitary improvements. During the proceedings of the *Royal Sanitary Commission* in 1869, J. Howell Blood, clerk to the local board, confidently stated that because of the outbreak and Thorne's recommendations, "Terling is now really a most extraordinary example of a country place . . . a model village."[76]

Thorne was not the only investigator at Terling. Although it is unclear whether he collaborated with Thorne, Alfred Haviland, who in 1873 became MOH for Northamptonshire, also studied the outbreak. Haviland at the time was undertaking an extensive nationwide study of the relationship between weather, geology, and disease. In the last three decades of the century Haviland became a renowned medical geographer, offering a Geography of Disease course at St. Thomas's Hospital. He published two landmark books on the topic, in 1875 and later in 1892, but material that would later serve as a basis for the books was first published in 1868. Haviland embodied the burgeoning epidemiological conviction of the second half of the nineteenth century that the nation's health needed to be studied spatially. His mapping of the geographical distribution of cancer, heart disease, and tuberculosis was pioneering for the late Victorian period and echoed work done by the Medical Department; it made him an epidemiological ally, even if he was not a metropolitan elite or a government insider.[77] Haviland's report, published in the *Medical Times and Gazette* on January 11, 1868, bore a striking similarity to Thorne's, although he only mentioned that "a gentleman has

---

74   "The Epidemic of Fever at Terling," *Builder* 26 (February 15, 1868), 105; "Typhoid at Terling," *Lancet* 94 (February 8, 1868): 204; "The Fever at Terling," *Medical Times and Gazette* 36 (February 22, 1868): 209.

75   "A Village in Arcadia," *Punch* 54 (February 22, 1868): 87. Interestingly, *Punch* noted that the disease at Terling was "King Typhus," suggesting the persistent confusion between typhoid and typhus well into the 1860s, and despite Thorne's very clear language.

76   *First Report of the Royal Sanitary Commission*, Testimony of J. H. Blood, June 17, 1869, 210.

77   On Haviland, see Arnold-Forster, "Mapmaking and Mapthinking."

been sent down by the Medical Department of the Privy Council to investigate the matter."[78] Like Thorne, Haviland narrowed in on Lord Rayleigh's
dairy farm as the *fons et origo mali* of the outbreak, and Haviland, too, was
hesitant to push for milk-borne transmission. Haviland's conclusions were
much in line with those of Thorne: that the outbreak began at the dairy farm
and spread via the contamination of shallow surface wells. In 1872 Haviland
delivered the first of numerous lectures on the geographical distribution of
disease at St. Thomas's Hospital, two of which were on typhoid. He extensively cited the reports of the Medical Department, showing a growing sym-
metry between the local work of the department and broader arguments
about the spread of disease throughout the country.

Simon called the outbreaks at Witham, Guildford, and Terling, in his
typically rhetorical and lyrical tone, the "filthiest chapter in the history of
our pestilences."[79] Combined, the studies of 1867 left "no possible doubt as
to the relation being that of cause and effect" between typhoid and its waterborne route of transmission, as the *Lancet* noted.[80] Haviland was clear that
there were no finer studies of typhoid than the Medical Department's late
1860s investigations, which went to prove, "in the simple words, 'poisoned
air and water' . . . the better classes suffer from the inhalation of mephitic air
within their houses . . . and the poorer classes . . . fall victims to the poison
by drinking the water of superficial wells having direct or indirect communication with sewage."[81] By 1870 sewer air and water were understood to be
the key media by which typhoid was spread.

In addition to showing the class dimensions of typhoid, local studies
were revealing, as *Punch* wryly noted, the unhealthiness of many rural locations throughout England and Wales. Fueled by a growing antiurbanism in
Victorian Britain, as Luckin has shown, the growing consensus coming out
of outbreak investigation was quite grim.[82] But the Medical Department's
investigations were doing more than just amassing anecdotal evidence of
the sanitary state of the nation. Instead, local—especially rural—outbreaks
were critical testing grounds for the epidemiological methods of outbreak
investigation and the epidemiological gaze. In sparsely populated areas it was

78   Haviland, "Special Report on the Epidemic at Terling," 40–41.

79   Simon, *Tenth Report of the Medical Officer of the Privy Council*, 9.

80   "Public Companies and the Public Health," *Lancet* 2344 (August 1, 1868):
      150.

81   Haviland, "The Geographical Distribution," 232.

82   Luckin, "Revisiting the Idea of Degeneration."

easier for inspectors to interview a greater number of those involved in an outbreak. And it was easier to find an index case, trace the spread of the disease, construct maps and diagrams, and carefully inspect the sanitary arrangements and cajole local authorities into action. Local investigations by the Medical Department's inspectors were also beginning to reveal the inadequacy of mortality records in gauging the health of a local community. Thorne's Terling outbreak showed as much. So, too, did Radcliffe's investigation of Stamford.

In late 1869 Radcliffe traveled to Stamford, an ancient market town in the county of Lincoln, which had "a high local reputation for healthiness."[83] From 1868 to 1869, however, typhoid cases flooded the local hospital, creating so much worry that local officials contacted Simon and pleaded for help. Radcliffe was put on assignment and first conducted a sanitary survey of the area; he investigated the local geology, the housing conditions, the methods of waste disposal, the water supply, and the distribution of typhoid in the area. Of 152 cases, only eight deaths occurred. It was enough, however, for Radcliffe to suspect excremental contamination.

He consulted local physicians and the district MOH. He also carried out house-to-house inspections where typhoid had attacked, interviewing local residents about their personal habits and recent travel, always on the search for an index case. Radcliffe sent samples of local water to London, which were analyzed by his colleagues Miller and Burdon Sanderson. With the local death certificates in hand, and with his own house-to-house visitations, he constructed a spot map of Stamford that showed the incidence of typhoid for the entire year from September 1868 to 1869. On the map (figure 2.5), he marked a circle at each house where there had been either a typhoid death or typhoid sickness. He also added to the map the location of cesspools, wells, and the nature of the soils—sand, gravel, clay, or oolite. "It is no exaggeration," he noted in a private memo to Simon, "to say that the inhabitants . . . drink water which is polluted with their own stools."[84] Radcliffe's inves-

---

83 John Netten Radcliffe, "Typhoid Fever at Stamford," confidential draft to John Simon, February 6, 1870, National Archives, England. MH 113/2, 2. There was a general feeling among Britons around midcentury that rural districts were healthier than their urban counterparts. By the 1870s this cultural notion was gradually being replaced by sentiment that rural areas were unhealthy and backward in their sanitary practices. See Fergus, "Excremental Pollution."

84 Radcliffe, "Typhoid Fever at Stamford," National Archives, England, MH 113/2 12.

tigation confirmed the contamination of the local water supply as the cause of the typhoid outbreak.

Radcliffe's Stamford study represented a turn both toward mapping morbidity and mortality and calculating house attack rate. He marked houses infected with typhoid where individuals were either sick or had died of the disease. This practice was common to epidemiological investigations in the last two decades of the century. In doing so Radcliffe was not only challenging the popular perception that Stamford was a healthy town but also the broader use of mortality rates as indexes of healthiness. Radcliffe argued, "The healthiness of localities with low death-rates cannot be judged by the death rate alone, but has to be estimated by the absence or prevalence of certain causes of death, and certain forms of sickness, particularly fever and diarrheal diseases."[85] Death rates alone, Radcliffe claimed, were a "fallacious index" of healthiness. Early use of morbidity statistics came out of epidemiological necessity to fieldworkers such as Radcliffe. "The damage to a community from sickness not ending in death," he noted, "cannot yet be stated with any near approach to accuracy, and its magnitude is too commonly overlooked or lightly estimated."[86] In 1876 Radcliffe was charged with examining the working conditions of the new Public Health Act of 1875, which made compulsory MOsH posts. In a confidential memo Radcliffe noted that although sickness records were of the "highest value" to outbreak investigation, such data was only available to local MOsH via pauper-sickness returns compiled for Poor Law medical officers.[87] These sickness records, he lamented, were often marred by ineffective reporting; such as not including patients' names, addresses, or causes of sickness, information that was critical to the methods of outbreak investigation by the mid-1870s.[88] The notification of infectious diseases could clarify this matter but was not compulsory until 1889. Local investigations were demonstrating a multitude of problems and not just in sanitary arrangements and in the use of vital statistics. Sometimes it was a simple matter of nosology, and the clinical diagnosis of typhoid remained a nagging problem of outbreak investigation throughout the late Victorian period. Conducting an investigation of waterborne typhoid in Bradford and

---

85   Radcliffe, "Typhoid Fever at Stamford," 3.

86   Radcliffe, "Typhoid Fever at Stamford," 4.

87   On Poor Law medical officers, see Price, *Medical Negligence*.

88   John Netten Radcliffe, "Report on Certain Questions Relating to Medical Officers of Health of Combined Sanitary Districts," May 18, 1876, National Archives, Kew, MH/113/6.

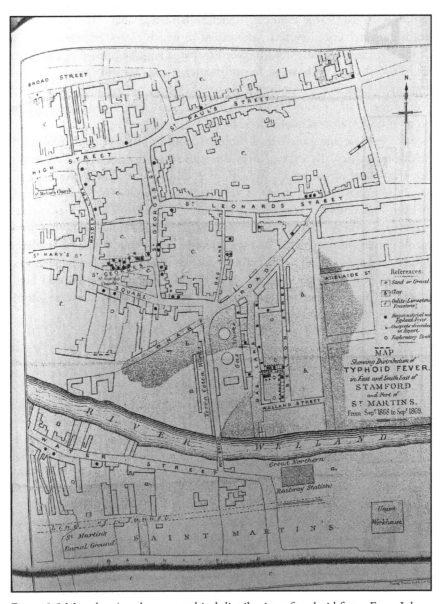

Figure 2.5 Map showing the geographical distribution of typhoid fever. From John Netten Radcliffe's "Typhoid Fever at Stamford." National Archives, England. MH 113/2, 12. Crown Copyright.

Yorkshire in 1871, for example, Radcliffe lamented that "The registers of death indicate very imperfectly the extent to which *enteric fever* is prevalent in the borough . . . but, still, the word *typhus* is largely adopted as a generic term, and the less understood forms of enteric fever are still commonly designated as "simple" or "continued" fever, or "febris." A considerable proportion of the deaths registered as from "typhus" and "continued" fever, I have no doubt, were instances of enteric fever."[89]

Such clinical and nosological problems could obfuscate epidemiological fieldwork, particularly in rural areas where the inspectors believed they could not trust local physicians.[90] T. Clifford Allbutt, for example, lamented in the *BMJ* in 1870 that "it is not yet clearly understood by the profession at large that enteric fever is a specific fever."[91] Horace Swete, a part-time inspector for the Medical Department offered the same conclusion, that rural medical men think typhoid "springs directly from a cold."[92] Cornelius Fox, MOH for Essex, declared that country doctors often replied to the question, "Where did the patient catch the fever?" with "nowhere; he (or she) bred it, sir."[93] There was lasting confusion until the widespread use of the serum antigen Widal Test in the 1890s.

---

89 John Netten Radcliffe, "Report on Certain Defects in the Sanitary Administration of Bradford (Yorkshire), and on the Recent Prevalence in the Borough of Enteric Fever and other Diarrhoeal Diseases," May 1871, National Archives, Kew, MH 113/10. By 1880 this was not such a problem. See Cayley, "On Some Points," 4.

90 But it was not just rural physicians. The 1900 Examination for a Diploma in Public Health, which most British epidemiologists were obtaining by that time, still asked students to "compare and contrast Typhus and Typhoid Fevers from an etiological view." See Examination Papers for Diploma in Public Health, 1900 in Wellcome Archives, London, MS 6807/17–23.

91 Allbutt, "On the Propagation of Enteric Fever," 308–9.

92 Horace Swete, "Report to the Local Government Board on an Inquiry into the Sanitary Condition of the Haverfordwest Rural Sanitary District (Pembrokeshire), with special reference to the frequent Prevalence of Enteric Fever," National Archives, Kew, Medical Department Files, MH 113/16.

93 Fox, "Is Enteric Fever Ever Spontaneously Generated?," 376.

John Simon, William Budd, and the Politics of Filth

By the late 1860s Simon was using local studies of typhoid to make vocal political arguments. Before the Royal Sanitary Commission of 1869, for example, he sought to persuade officials that the typhoid outbreaks of 1867 were "remarkable instances" that shed important light on the need for local sanitary improvements in sewerage, water supply, and housing. After 1872, when Simon and the Medical Department were administratively shuffled to the Local Government Board, he became even more outspoken. As noted in the introduction, Simon's landmark 1874 report *Filth Diseases* argued that typhoid was a preventable disease wreaking havoc on the country. As Radcliffe, Buchanan, and Thorne had shown through routine outbreak investigation, typhoid was amounting to an "incalculable amount of physical suffering and disablement . . . sorrows and anxieties . . . permanent darkening of life destitution and pauperism."[94]

Using the reports of his inspectorate to draw out general sanitary lessons, Simon generalized that the filth diseases—typhoid and cholera, but also diarrhea and dysentery—were caused by "uncleanliness" and the "fatal influence . . . of filth." All across the nation, Simon lamented, "gross and scandalous and very often, I repeat, truly bestial" states of filth prevail.[95] Simon's rhetorical stance narrowed in on two "gigantic evils" that marred public health, the disposal of excreta through public sewage, faulty house drains, or bog privies, causing "nuisance by its effluvia and soakage," and the movement of those suffering from disease and their ability "to scatter abroad the seeds of their infection."[96] Only preventive, compulsory sanitary legislation, he argued, could bring about "the rudiments of sanitary civilisation."[97] Simon was calling for a rethinking of filth, "that awful entity," Hamlin has wryly noted, "at which Victorians loved to shudder"[98] Whereas "it had long been an accepted doctrine that filth was in some way related to the production of disease," Simon focused on "the chief morbific agencies in Filth."[99]

Simon was thus engaging in a decades-long debate in British public health about the causal relationship between filth and infectious disease, one

---

94 Simon, *Filth Diseases*, 5.
95 Simon, *Filth Diseases*, 5, 18.
96 Simon, *Filth Diseases*, 7, 8, 17.
97 Simon, *Filth Diseases*, 18.
98 Hamlin, *Public Health and Social Justice*, 4.
99 Simon, *Filth Diseases*, 8.

whose agenda was set in the 1820s and 1830s by Thomas Southwood Smith and later popularized by Edwin Chadwick, as Michael Brown and John Pickstone have shown.[100] Simon's redefinition of filth was a savvy attempt at merging the long-standing idea that filth contributed to the production of disease with newer epidemiological evidence about the specific ways that fecally contamined water spread disease. Fetid air, like that arising from a cesspool, Simon argued, might be harmful to breathe and cause discomfort or headache, but it was only when the *morbific ferments,* or *contagia,* specific living organisms, were present that infectious disease arose. The ferments of disease, Simon urged, might even be odorless, reversing Chadwick's dictum that "all smell is disease," and upending Southwood Smith's classic formulation of infectious diseases arising from "local influences," of which, as Kerr has noted, the "fever dens" or "fever nests" were "a powerful literary trope."[101] That did not mean that fetid smells should be ignored, Simon argued, but that air and water were the "respective media of diffusion" only when charged with the specific excreta of those suffering from typhoid or cholera.[102] Studying and intercepting the "media of diffusion," namely air, water, and milk, Simon argued, could prevent the spread of the filth diseases, which made him a kind of English advocate of what David Barnes has called the "sanitary-bacteriological synthesis" of the late nineteenth century.[103] Simon's contemporary Benjamin Ward Richardson called Simon and the department's inspectors "scientific epidemiologsts" as opposed to "sanitarians," who had "untenable theories as to origins of disease."[104]

Simon's 1874 report demonstrated a turn toward Budd's exclusivist waterborne theory, which he argued was "rapidly growing more positive and precise."[105] He was not alone. Thomas Watson, in his widely read 1871 *Lectures on Medicine* endorsed Budd's views. So, too, did William Aitken, whose *Science and Practice of Medicine*—one of the standard works in British medicine at home and across the empire—firmly stood by Budd's idea that

---

100 Brown, "From Foetid Air to Filth"; John Pickstone, "Dearth, Dirt, and Fever."

101 Kerr, *Contagion, Isolation, and Biopolitics,* 46. Simon cited the experience in London in 1858 of the Great Stink, where, despite massive pollution and stinking of the Thames in London, rates of infectious disease were down that year in London.

102 Simon, *Filth Diseases,* 10.

103 Barnes, *The Great Stink of Paris,* 135.

104 Richardson, "The Present Position and Prospects," 127.

105 Thorne, *On the Progress of Preventive Medicine,* 25.

typhoid was chiefly spread via the fecal-oral route of transmission.[106] "As facts have accumulated," Simon suggested, the fecal-oral theory "has gradually been changing into conviction."[107] The third edition of Aitken's *Science and Practice of Medicine,* for example, noted that "the Privy Council have now made the principle [Budd's] of this method an integral part of their general memorandum."[108] In other words, what Gull two years earlier had called a "good working theory," Simon, at the center of the epidemiological practice of outbreak investigation, was calling a conviction. Although Budd had "constantly and very powerfully" argued for an exclusive waterborne theory of typhoid for over fifteen years, Simon, especially before 1874, had hedged etiological views between Budd and Murchison.[109] After the growing body of outbreak investigation, especially of waterborne typhoid, Simon had adjusted his stance. In giving primacy to local investigations of typhoid, Simon in *Filth Diseases* was also giving primacy to the power of outbreak investigation and an epidemiological way of knowing. In his 1873 *Typhoid Fever* Budd laid out a nine-point deductive theory of typhoid fever that followed from two assumptions: that typhoid is a contagious disease and that the intestinal discharges of those sick with the disease contain the essential "poison" that produces the disease in others. Budd's theory, paraphrased, was that typhoid rates will be higher in areas where human excreta contaminates the soil and air of an area;typhoid "will show little or no contagious power" in areas not thus contaminated; the tendency of typhoid to run in families is more apparent in country districts, where houses share a common privy. The phenomenon is less likely where houses have a water closet, and even less so in urban districts with public works;typhoid is distributed differently in urban versus rural districts. In the country the disease tends to occur in a "thickly clustered manner," as the intestinal discharges are thrown in the air and soil near dwellings without sewers or public water supply. In cities the disease appears more scattered, as the intestinal discharges are conveyed longer distances by sewers;the sewer falsely appears to be the source of the disease, when in fact it only contains the most virulent part of the disease: the intestinal discharges of the sick. The source of the disease, therefore, is the infected person, and the sewer is simply the medium;the contagious nature of the disease is more obvious in rural areas, whereas in the city it will seem

---

106 Aitken, *The Science and Practice of Medicine,* 410–14.
107 Simon, *Filth Diseases,* 14–15.
108 Aitken, *The Science and Practice of Medicine,* 414.
109 Simon, *Filth Diseases,* 14.

"masked and obscure";in the country typhoid will be epidemic and thickly clustered, where in the city it will be endemic and scattered;separating the sick from the healthy will not stop the spread of the disease unless the intestinal discharges are not allowed to spread; andthe severest outbreaks of typhoid will be in large institutions such as schools and barracks.

Budd, in his most important and widely read treatise on typhoid, laid out not just a theory but a practical methodology for studying and preventing the disease.[110] Of particular importance was his geography-minded interest in the distribution of the disease in urban versus rural areas. He was not alone in this pursuit. From the early 1860s Simon had questioned why typhoid was unequally distributed throughout England and Wales. So, too, had some early epidemiological thinkers. Haviland. For example, in his 1872 lectures at St. Thomas's Hospital, examined typhoid mortality rates for the entire country in the 1860s. He confidently stated that typhoid was "essentially a fever of the *country*, more than of the *town*."[111] Local studies at the Medical Department in that same decade demonstrated that typhoid was prevalent in urban, suburban, and rural districts, but stemming from local studies of typhoid in the 1860s, special attention was placed on rural outbreaks. By the 1880s and 1890s, as chapter 4 shows, it was becoming increasingly clear that the health of urban Britons was very much entwined with the sanitary faults of rural dwellers.

Much of the history of epidemiology has focused on work done in urban spaces, such as the shoe-leather practices of Snow and the statistical innovations of Farr studying cholera in London.[112] Budd's early epidemiological studies of typhoid fever in North Tawton, as well as the Danish physician Peter Panum's epidemiological work on measles in the isolated Faeroe Islands bear testimony to rural practices in the history of epidemiology around mid-century.[113] Yet, scholars have not seriously engaged with the epistemic differences between urban and rural practice, particularly in the second half of the

---

110 Budd included an appendix with simple rules for preventing the spread of typhoid.

111 Haviland, "The Geographical Distribution," 148.

112 Vinten-Johansen, et al., *Cholera, Chloroform, and the Science of Medicine*; Pelling, *Cholera, Fever, and English Medicine;* Eyler, *Victorian Social Medicine.*

113 Winslow's *The Conquest of Epidemic Disease,* chapter 13. Even so, Budd's cholera studies, for which he is perhaps better remembered, were largely conducted in Bristol.

nineteenth century. Armchair debates in urban spaces, Worboys contends, have been given priority over field practices in rural ones.

Historians have tended to favor urban-centered stories in examining Victorian epidemiology, largely as the result of an overemphasis on the cultural impact of cholera, or what Hamlin has recently called a "cholera forcing."[114] Gerry Kearns has argued that Victorian public health officials were uniquely aware of an urban-rural gap (what he calls an "urban penalty") that showed a marked increase of infectious disease in cities.[115] Comparative mortality statistics confirmed the rhetoric of an urban penalty. Consider, for example, Farr's concept of the "healthy district."[116] As Kearns has shown, cholera was uniquely understood as a foreign and urban disease, bred from concentrations of filth and immorality, where "particularly the poor and unskilled . . . bore the brunt of the urban penalty."[117] The urban pattern seemed to hold true for some infectious diseases. Franklin Parsons, an inspector at the Medical Department writing in 1899, for example, noted that while diphtheria, formerly understood as a "disease of rural districts and rare in towns, is now much more fatal in the large towns."[118] Such appeared to be the pattern for diarrhea and scarlet fever, Parsons added, but not typhoid. He noted that typhoid "is now not much more prevalent in the great towns than in the country districts."[119] From the 1870s it was a common belief that typhoid was a particular problem for rural areas, reversing the urban penalty and the common logic of filth diseases.[120] Contemporary epidemiologists, while acknowledging the urban penalty, were suggesting an equally operable rural penalty for typhoid fever. Budd went a step further and suggested that the reason why typhoid had long been considered noncontagious was because most medical authorities, like his chief rival Murchison, lived in cities, and experienced scattered outbreaks of the disease. Investigating rural

---

114 Hamlin, "Cholera Forcing."

115 Kearns, "Biology, Class, and the Urban Penalty," 18.

116 Late Victorian statistically minded epidemiologists such as H. Franklin Parsons were still hammering on about urban and rural mortality differences. In his Inaugural Address to the Epidemiological Society of London in 1899, Parsons brilliantly demonstrated Kearns's concept of the "urban penalty." Parsons, "On the Comparative Mortality of English Districts."

117 Kearns, "Biology, Class, and the Urban Penalty," 15.

118 Parsons, "On the Comparative Mortality of English Districts," 3.

119 Ibid.

120 Sedgwick, Taylor, and MacNutt, "Is Typhoid Fever a 'Rural' Disease?"

outbreaks, as Budd and the inspectorate of the Medical Department demonstrated, made it easier to recognize the contagious nature of the disease, specifically its spread via media.[121] Summarizing eight years of country practice, R. Bruce Low, MOH in Yorkshire and later inspector at the Medical Department, repeated as much, noting that rural outbreaks were "free from the ordinary sources of error which surround similar investigation in large towns or populous centres."[122] And yet, Low lamented in 1880 that most country practitioners still believed that typhoid arose *de novo*, long after most urban practitioners had abandoned the idea, particularly the vanguard of epidemiologists at the Medical Department.[123]

Part of what made typhoid a model disease of Victorian public health was that it struck both rich and poor, urban dweller and country cottager. Some geography-minded MOsH, such as Haviland and Low, were keen to see the wide-ranging implications of the distribution of the disease, and so, too, were some general practitioners such as Budd. But it was principally at the Medical Department where this view was put into practice, and many rural MOsH and urban hospital physicians continued to support Murchison's flexible model of spontaneous generation and typhoid poisons fermenting in the environment. Looking back on the last twenty years of the Medical Department in 1886, then chief medical officer George Buchanan said that it had long been the goal of the department to examine the "prevalences, appearances, and outbreaks of disease in many places, and at different times," so as to answer etiological questions.[124] Simon had orchestrated a national epidemiological gaze. His strategy in *Filth Diseases* and Budd's in *Typhoid Fever* were similar: to lay out an exclusive theory of typhoid as a self-propagating disease through evidence gleaned by local epidemiological investigation. Budd's was a sober, calculated account, a blow-by-blow account of his theory as to the spread of typhoid, and an emphatic denial of the spontaneous origin of the disease. Simon's *Filth Diseases* differed in its rhetorical

---

121 Budd's magnum opus on typhoid was defended by John Tyndall, who had made typhoid a point of controversy in 1871 during the prayer-gauge debate. Just two years later, in 1873 following the publication of *Typhoid Fever*, Tyndall, in the *Times*, called Budd's work "remarkable, its logic is so strong, and it conclusions are so momentous." See Tyndall, "Typhoid Fever," 7.

122 Low, "The Origin of Enteric Fever," 733–36.

123 Low, "The Origin of Enteric Fever," 735.

124 George Buchanan, "Memorandum as to the Duties of the Board's Medical Department as at Present Constituted (1886)," National Archives, Kew, NA/ MH78/1.

strategy in discussing filth, a word only used twice in Budd's book, and one very directly aimed at Murchison. Repeated again and again in Simon's report was an emotional, sensorial view of typhoid that the disease was spread by "an invariable source in that which of Filth is the filthiest" and by "successive inoculations from man to man, by instrumentality of the molecules of excrement which man's filthiness lets mingle in his air and food and drink."[125]

Simon and Budd's works of 1873 and 1874, respectively, suggest several important conclusions. A particular kind of epidemiology, predicated on outbreak investigation, was crucial to a general transition in etiological theory, where the mediums of infectious disease—water, milk, shellfish, flies, and later human carriers—were the foci of scientific research and preventive public health. As Simon argued in an 1879 article "Contagion" in Quain's *Dictionary of Medicine*, the focus on disease media was essential to the ascendency of the theory of indirection contagion.[126] The pattern was set by the mid-1870s, and, as the *Times* reported, the Medical Department's investigations "throw much light upon the particular conditions under which enteric fever is developed and propagated both in towns and in rural districts."[127] The Local Government Board was also incorporating the department's findings into official warnings to local sanitary authorities. An 1874 memo, for example, warned that during summer droughts local communities should be especially vigilant not to let inhabitants turn to excrement-polluted water sources.[128] An 1878 memo, likewise, advised local authorities that in cases of typhoid, "evacuations should be regarded as capable of communicating an infectious quality to any night-soil with which they are mingled in privies, drains, or cesspools."[129] Nearly half of all department investigations from the 1870s to the 1890s were local outbreaks of typhoid, and most of these were traced to contaminated water supplies. The vast majority were sudden,

125 Simon, *Filth Diseases*, 14.

126 Simon, "An Essay on Contagion," 923.

127 "Enteric Fever," *Times*, April 17, 1873, 4.

128 John Lambert, "Water Supply," June 29, 1874, National Archives, Kew, MH113/6.

129 Edward Seaton, "General Memorandum on the Proceedings which are Advisable in Places Attacked or Threatened by Epidemic Disease," National Archives, London, MH/113/6.

virulent outbreaks in rural areas, but there were exceptions, such as large-scale outbreaks at Maidstone and Malvern in the late 1890s.[130]

Filth Diseases was also important because it was Simon's bureaucratic swan song. He resigned in 1876 amidst growing tension between himself and the civil servants at the Local Government Board. Simon and the department's role had long been advisory. But after the move to the LGB, Simon began to demand more legislative power. He wanted three key changes: more access to James Stansfeld, president of the Local Government Board, instead of first going to the secretaries; for the department to report directly to local authorities on sanitary matters rather than all correspondence passing through the secretaries; and for the chief medical officer to alone oversee outbreak investigation. In other words, Simon wanted more power and independence. State medicine, according to Simon, had surrendered "medical influence to the traditions of a Circumlocution Office."[131] Officials at the Local Government Board were furious. In a series of private memos to Simon in 1873, Stansfeld, John Lambert, and George Fleming categorically refused his requests.[132] Simon's tenure has been seen as a political failure "unfortunate for public health," and one of the few key pieces of sanitary legislation passed on his watch was the compulsory appointments of MOsH via the Public Health Act of 1872.[133] Even in *Filth Diseases* Simon lacked the coherent vision to tackle the vast array of political challenges needed to successfully implement his version of preventive, or state medicine, which he argued in a private memo to the president of the Local Government Board, was "the primary aim" of the department.[134] He also lacked the personality and communication routes to convey this to Parliament. His rhetorical, even indiscriminate use of the term "filth" was meant to shock and dismay, a strategy that might work on medical practitioners and the public but not on Whitehall civil servants. Even though his agenda was to redefine filth, he seemed inexorably tied to Chadwickian-era debates. Narrowly defined by acts of Parliament, Simon's career was lackluster and his voice overshadowed by Victorian bureaucracy, at least in the opinion of most historians. But this opinion misses a crucial

130 The Malvern outbreak is fascinating and understudied. See Wellcome Library, GC/63/4.
131 Seaton, "Evolution of Sanitary Administration," 1637.
132 National Archives, Kew, MH/78/44.
133 Hamlin, "State Medicine in Great Britain," 148.
134 Memo from Simon to Stansfeld, "Staff of the Medical Department," National Archives, London, MH78/44.

point, and we might see it another way. Simon's lasting contributions were twofold. First, he prioritized a specific type of epidemiological knowledge production. Field-based, local investigations of infectious disease were key to making arguments about public health reform. Second, he provided a model of preventive medicine by developing the system of a centralized, watchful eye over the health of the nation (the Medical Department) that was coupled with on-the-ground sanitary support staff (MOsH). Simon uniquely nurtured the burgeoning science of epidemiology (he was less successful in nurturing pathology or chemistry at the department) as the key science of state medicine. The health of the nation, Simon had firmly established, had to be overseen by epidemiological expertise. He left the department in the hands of his inspectors—Seaton, Buchanan, Thorne, and Power—who continued, if still stifled by the bureaucracy of the Local Government Board, to press for the primacy of epidemiological knowledge in guiding preventive health. In the process, during what most historians consider the Medical Department's least influential period, the inspectorate worked out the major pathways by which typhoid was spread. In other words, the years 1860–1900 were anything but a failure. Simon, no doubt in part helped by Budd, had established the view that typhoid was a model disease. The 1870s were critical in shaping the direction of British epidemiology, and nowhere was this more apparent than at the Medical Department.

"*Via Exclusionis*": Richard Thorne Thorne's Epidemiology at Caterham in 1879

One last example typifies the fruition of epidemiological methods at the department in tackling waterborne typhoid before the discovery of the typhoid bacillus. In early February 1879 Thorne descended into one of the wells of the Caterham Waterworks Company. It was there, he believed, that he could find the source of a violent outbreak of typhoid. Caterham, a sparsely populated London suburb in the Rural Sanitary District of Godstone, and its more populous neighbor Redhill, in the Urban Sanitary District of Reigate, had been attacked by an explosive outbreak of typhoid; upwards of 350 individuals were struck within a six-week period. Caterham had largely been free of typhoid the preceding twelve months; now it was faced with a public health crisis. Such sudden, fulminating outbreaks, according to Thorne's colleague and prolific public health writer Edward Cox

Seaton, "attracted so much notice that no wonder the impression they created in this country has been deep and lasting."[135]

Thorne had descended into the Caterham well because he believed it was there that the outbreak had commenced. He was looking for the index case, what the Epidemiological Society of London described in 1863 as "tracing with scrupulous minuteness the history of the first cases."[136] It was by using basic statistical methods and case tracing, long established at the department, that Thorne had come to suspect the Caterham Waterworks Company. Early in the outbreak, Thorne found that of the forty-seven persons attacked from January 19 to February 2, forty-five received water from that source alone. He interviewed Dr. James Adam, medical superintendent at the Caterham Asylum, and Dr. James Magill, of the Caterham Barracks, and found that among the two thousand patients at the former institution, and five hundred soldiers at the latter—both of which were supplied by their own wells—no cases of typhoid fever had arisen. Moreover, Thorne found that in the neighboring town of Redhill, typhoid cases were exclusive to those houses supplied with water from the Caterham Waterworks Company. With a "very strong presumption that it had been caused by the use of the Caterham Company's water," Thorne narrowed the investigation.[137]

In late 1878 the Caterham Waterworks Company began constructing an adit from the well in question to a new bore being sunk. A number of men were employed in this work, some on the surface and others below. Enquiring into the health of these workers, Thorne interviewed one, identified as "J. K.," aged thirty-two, a "loading man" who had been suffering from a case of typhoid fever preceding the outbreak in early January 1879.[138] While down in the well, J. K. confessed that he regularly used the loading buckets, meant for raising the excavated chalk to the surface, for his frequent diarrhoeal dejections—at least two or three times per shift—despite the complaints of his fellow workmen on the surface. With this knowledge in hand, Thorne conducted a simple experiment in the well. He found that every time a bucket was hoisted up the rope to be emptied, it oscillated to and fro, coming into violent contact with the walls of the well.[139] About ten days after J. K.'s fecal mishaps in the well, Thorne deduced from the statistical

135 Seaton, *Infectious Diseases and Their Prevention*, 96.
136 Babington, "Objects of the Epidemiological Society," 7.
137 Thorne, "On an Extensive Epidemic of Enteric Fever at Red Hill," 81.
138 Thorne, "On an Extensive Epidemic of Enteric Fever at Red Hill," 85–86.
139 Ballard, "Observations on Some of the Ways," 82–84.

distribution of the typhoid fever cases and contemporary knowledge about the incubation period of the disease—about a fortnight—the epidemic had become widespread across Caterham and Redhill, both of which received water from the Caterham Waterworks Company.[140] Typhoid cases, Thorne found, were largely limited to those who received water from the fecally polluted Caterham Waterworks Company. Such was "one of the most striking instances" Thorne later noted, showing "how great was the potency for mischief of even minute portions of the specifically diseased evacuations of enteric fever patients."[141]

Thorne's public health practices at Caterham were emblematic of epidemiological investigations inspectors at the Medical Department conducted between 1860 and 1880.[142] Such practices were observational and experimental; when, on February 5, 1879, for example, Thorne arrived in the Caterham and Redhill area—he left the day after the department received word of the outbreak from a local physician—he examined the local water supply, the milk supply, the house drainage, and the sewerage. He consulted local medical practitioners, especially E. L. Jacob, MOH for the combined sanitary districts of Surrey, and William Whitaker on the soil composition of the area. Thorne tabulated the mortality statistics of the outbreak and inquired from house to house about the particulars of every case of suspected or confirmed typhoid, which led him to the abovementioned index case of J. K.[143] Thorne and the late Victorian practitioners of epidemiology, as Anne Hardy has shown, championed careful case tracing, simple sanitary experimentation, and the marshalling of evidence predicated on statistical inference.[144] Thorne's investigation spanned urban and rural physical environments—and the administrative categories of Urban and Rural Sanitary Districts—it also included basic experimentation, quantitative statistical analysis, and qualitative case tracing and interviewing. Though it was

140 William Cayley, Physician to the Middlesex Hospital and the London Fever Hospital, noted in his 1880 Croonian Lectures before the Royal College of Physicians of London, that although variable, it was "well established" that the incubation period for the disease was "about fourteen days." See Cayley, "Some Points in the Pathology," 431.
141 Thorne, *On the Progressive of Preventive Medicine*, 29.
142 Hardy, "Methods of Outbreak Investigation," 199–206.
143 Both the rich and the poor had been struck down by the disease, and inhabitants in Lower Caterham had been affected as had those living in Upper Caterham, which included the old village.
144 Hardy, "On the Cusp."

population centered, individuals, especially the search for the index case, were also the focus of Thorne's study. By 1879 these had become hallmarks of Victorian epidemiology.

Placed into the twenty-year context of investigations of waterborne typhoid at the Medical Department, Thorne's 1879 Caterham investigation was characteristic—it even later served as a model—of epidemiological practice at the department in an age when epidemiology, rather than the incipient practices and rhetoric of bacteriology, dominated British public health. Yet, in one critical way Thorne's Caterham study diverged from many of the investigations conducted through the department: no bacteriologist or chemist was involved in the investigation. Thorne did not send a sample of Caterham water to be analyzed by one of the department's bacteriological or chemical analysts, a common, though inconclusive practice for field epidemiologists from the 1860s.[145] By refusing to seek chemical or bacteriological confirmation of his etiological hypothesis, Thorne was actively constructing the rhetorical claim that epidemiological knowledge alone best informed practical decisions in preventive public health.

Thorne's 1879 investigation reveals the way in which epidemiology, at perhaps its height in Britain before the discovery of the typhoid bacillus, was, to borrow a phrase from Vassiliki Betty Smocovitis, "part of a culturally embedded belief system" that Victorians used to understand the spread of disease.[146] That Thorne did not appropriate chemical or bacteriological science, a practice others at the department often did, albeit "uninfluentially," as Hamlin as shown, makes him emblematic of a practitioner who embodied the fullest expression of the scientific authority of epidemiology.[147] Thorne's practices at Caterham, as well as the process by which his findings were communicated, represent a vision of epidemiological authority that was widespread in the period. What makes this an especially interesting case, furthermore, is that it was conducted and communicated at a time before the widespread acceptance of bacteriology, explored in chapter 4.

Addressing the Epidemiological Society in 1878, a year before his Caterham investigation, Thorne admitted that he had "little acquaintance with the laboratory," and that he relied "for most of his data on experience

---

145 Thorne did refer in his 1879 report to the influence of John Burdon Sanderson's research on the "intimate pathology of contagion." See Sanderson, "Intimate Pathology of Contagion," *Twelfth Annual Report*.

146 Smocovitis, *Unifying Biology*, 86.

147 Hamlin, *A Science of Impurity*, 270.

gained in what I may perhaps term the field-work of epidemiology."[148] No doubt he was following his old mentor, Simon, who had recently left the department. Before the *Royal Sanitary Commission* of 1869, Simon reported that the department typically sent water for analysis to Miller at King's College but that such tests rarely provided the proof needed to condemn a local authority. "A chemical analysis perhaps would sometimes be an imperfect addition" to outbreak investigation, Simon noted.[149] As was the case earlier at Winterton, Guildford, and Terling, it was epidemiological investigation that provided sufficient evidence that wells were contaminated by privies, cesspools, and sewers. "Sometimes too much" emphasis is put on water analysis, Simon concluded, "the real test of the poisonousness of the water has been in the killing of people, and not in what the chemists have been able to demonstrate."[150] Simon echoed this view into the mid-1870s. In *Filth Diseases* he maintained that "till chemistry shall have learnt to identify the morbific ferments themselves, its competence to declare them absent in any given case must evidently be judged incomplete, and waters which chemical analysis would probably not condemn may certainly be carrying in them very fatal seeds of infection."[151] Such a programmatic dismissal of laboratory science both reflected a shared disciplinary awareness among British epidemiologists and reified the role of field over laboratory work in the generation of scientific knowledge about disease. In this way we can more fully understand the epidemiological practices Thorne employed at Caterham in the course of his 1879 investigation in the longer history of outbreak investigation stretching back to the early 1860s. Yet, as we will see in chapters 4 and 5, departmental apathy to laboratory studies began to change in the last two decades of the nineteenth century.

That Thorne descended into the Caterham well and conducted an experiment with water buckets used for diarrhoeal dejections was tantamount to fulfilling the duties of what Radcliffe, called a "day labourer" or "journeyman worker," in Victorian epidemiology.[152] Thorne's practices of case tracing to find and interview the index case, J. K., were constitutive performances of the epidemiological gaze that both guided practice and provided a corporeal

148 Thorne, "Remarks on the Origin of Infection," 234.
149 *First Report of the Royal Sanitary Commission*, testimony of John Simon, May 31, 1869, 108.
150 Ibid.
151 Simon, *Filth Diseases*,11.
152 Radcliffe, "On the Recent Progress of Epidemiology," 459.

and gestural basis for how such practices were communicated to larger audiences.[153] But how was Thorne's study communicated, and how was the epistemic claim made that Thorne "has perfectly succeeded in proving his case," as Ernest Hart, the sagacious medical reformer and editor of the *British Medical Journal*, noted in 1879?[154] In part, Thorne himself provided the agency for rationalizing the epidemiological findings; his colleagues—at the department and in the wider community of epidemiologists and medical writers—also justified the conclusions and public health outcomes that followed the Caterham study.

Thorne's report was published in the *Ninth Annual Report of Medical Officer of the Local Government Board* and also separately as a pamphlet. In his commentary, Buchanan, then chief medical officer, noted that Thorne's investigation at Caterham had offered "conclusive proof of the manner of its distribution . . . from this one case [J. K.] the deep water was specifically contaminated, and fever was spread over a large district."[155] The legitimacy of Thorne's study, judged Buchanan, lay in Thorne's ability to convince contemporaries that he had discovered the index case. Not only was such a finding integral to making epidemiological knowledge in this period, it was also predicated on the performative reality of descending into a well, conducting experiments, and interviewing individuals. The contemporary medical press joined in the praise. *The Medical Times and Gazette* found it "difficult to escape from accepting the conclusion that the Caterham works were infected by this workman."[156] "The conditions of this huge and involuntary experiment," the article noted, "seem to have been as nearly perfect as may be, and the indictment against the implicated water-supply appears at least fair and justifiable."[157] This referred to the discernible outcome of Thorne's Caterham investigation, namely public health action by the Caterham local authorities. Thorne was able—through persuasion that rested on a foundation of his epidemiological methods of outbreak investigation—to convince the local Sanitary Authorities to issue public notices that the Caterham water

---

153 Wintroub, "Taking a Bow," 779.

154 Hart, "The Recent Epidemic of Enteric Fever in the Caterham Valley," 668–70.

155 George Buchanan, *Ninth Annual Report of the Local Government Board, 1879–80. Supplement Containing the Report of the Medical Officer for 1879*, viii.

156 "The Late Epidemic of Enteric Fever at Caterham and Redhill," *Medical Times and Gazette* 1 (Saturday May 10, 1879): 507.

157 Ibid.

had been "accidentally contaminated."[158] Residents were recommended not to use the company's water until further notice, or, if necessary, to boil water before use. Thorne successfully prompted the Caterham Waterworks Company to pump a large portion of their water to waste for three weeks, at an economic loss, and thoroughly to cleanse, scour, and disinfect the walls of the wells, adits, reservoirs, and surrounding soil with chloride of lime and permanganate of potash. Thorne noted, with more than a little smugness, that "the Company acted with considerable energy and prompitude in adopting all measures which were found possible to do away with the results of the accidental contamination to which their water had been subjected."[159] It is worth reflecting on the complex and delicate relationship between Thorne's epidemiological field practices, the communication of his methods and results, and the political outcome of his recommendations. As an inspector for the Medical Department, Thorne could only make recommendations to local authorities; that the Caterham authorities, as well as the local water company, fully complied with Thorne was the product of an agreement with Thorne's epidemiological methods, which rested on the performative nature of Thorne's experiments, interviews, and statistical tabulations. At Terling a decade earlier he looked to Simon and the Home Office for help. At Caterham he was confidently on his own. The local authorities at Caterham and Redhill responded favorably to Thorne in spite of (or perhaps because) he relied exclusively on an epidemiological way of knowing to convince contemporaries of the necessary and sufficient cause of the local outbreak.[160] In this way, Thorne's epidemiological gaze at Caterham embodies what Steven Shapin has recently called the "practices of securing and maintaining credibility."[161] Thorne's study sheds light on earlier frustrations with local authorities in the 1860s and early 1870s.

Much of the contemporary approbation of Thorne's 1879 study focused on his methodology, which, as we have seen, was dependent on routine epidemiological practice that even Thorne himself had been doing for over a decade. *The Practitioner* was direct in praising Thorne's epidemiological methods, stating that his investigation exhibited "in a perspicuous and

---

158 Thorne, "On an Extensive Epidemic of Enteric Fever at Red Hill," 90.

159 Thorne, "On an Extensive Epidemic of Enteric Fever at Red Hill," 91.

160 Thorne's 1879 study in this way fulfils Richard Doll's criteria of an epidemiological study that provided, at least according to Thorne's 1879 contemporaries, proof beyond reasonable doubt. See Doll, "Proof of Causality."

161 Shapin, *Never Pure*, 9.

intelligible manner the method of inquiry which is usually adopted by the Medical Inspectors of the Board, and which has hitherto been attended with results which leave little to be desired."[162] Later that year Edward Ballard, Thorne's colleague and close friend at the Medical Department, addressed the Section of Medicine at the Annual Meeting of the British Medical Association held in Cork and echoed remarks published in *the Practitioner* and *Medical Times and Gazette*. Ballard called Thorne's epidemiological methodology at Caterham the "*via exclusionis*, the favourite method in the department, and indeed the only one applicable to such difficult inquiries."[163] It was, put another way, quoting an early twentieth-century description, "the Sherlockian method in epidemiology," which typified the deductive basis of epidemiological practice in the late Victorian period. To his contemporaries, Thorne's success rested on a sound methodology, one that Radcliffe pronounced in 1875 as signaling "the gold of scientific epidemiology."[164] Such professional back-patting of Thorne suggests important ways in which epidemiological methods were standardized in this period. It is clear that the activities of infectious disease investigation conducted through the Medical Department were crucial to such standardization of practice.

Also crucial were the performative ways that local studies were made known to wider medical, scientific, and public audiences. Even outside his cadre of like-minded public health workers at the Medical Department, where we might expect praise, Thorne's Caterham investigation garnered a great deal of interest and acclaim.[165] This was due to the complex ways that Thorne projected epidemiology to larger audiences. In May 1879, for example, he was requested to present a paper at the *Annual Conference on National Water Supply, Sewage and Health*, held in London by the Royal Society of

---

162 Brunton, "Enteric Fever," 473.

163 Ballard, "Observations on Some of the Ways," 82–84.

164 "The Sherlockian Method in Epidemiology," 639; Radcliffe, "On the Recent Progress of Epidemiology in England," 464.

165 "Typhoid Fever Spread by Water," *Bristol Mercury and Daily Post*, 1897, 3; Tyndall, "Cholera and Disinfection," 6. Edward Klein, presenting evidence before the *Royal Commission to Inquire Into the Water Supply of the Metropolis* in 1893–94, argued that Thorne's typhoid study at Caterham was "perfectly sufficient to establish the proposition that water fouled with cholera dejecta or typhoid dejecta may produce infection, the one with cholera, the other with typhoid fever." Edward Klein, minutes of evidence, *Royal Commission to Inquire Into the Water Supply of the Metropolis*, 417.

Arts, a special conference convened at the request of the Prince of Wales, who as we saw in chapter 1 was no stranger to the filth disease.[166] Thorne summarized his Caterham findings by noting that "in short there can be no doubt that the pollution of this water, as the result of the man's [J. K.'s] disease, and the epidemic in question, were related to each other as cause and effect; indeed the several essential incidents recorded are linked together in point of date, with a precision characteristic of the results which might have been expected to have followed a scientific inoculation."[167] Presenting before a large and prestigious audience, Thorne was at pains to defend epidemiological ways of knowing, particularly the authority of proving cause and effect. The eminent sanitary engineer Baldwin Latham was supportive of Thorne's claims, noting in the minutes of the meeting that Thorne's was "a very valuable paper . . . the lessons to be drawn from it would be of great use in the future."[168] Thus, Thorne's 1879 Caterham study was both emblematic of epidemiological practices and one that many practitioners recognized as indicative of the power of the epidemiological gaze.

In the lively discussion that followed his presentation at the *Annual Conference on National Water Supply, Sewage and Health,* Thorne was asked about the chemical state of the Caterham water. His response was that he had "specially avoided having the water analysed," as "you might have taken 100 samples and never found any evidence of specifically diseased matter in it; but in the one hundred and first you might have discovered it."[169] Such indifference to the chemical analysis of water was common, as Hamlin has shown.[170] W. F. Bynum has claimed that "Britain remained a relative bacteriological backwater through the last third of the century, and clinical and epidemiological features of what were often called the 'acute specific fevers' were just as important as the French, German and British laboratory evidence."[171] Thorne's 1879 study—both his projection and self-fashioning of the investigation, as well as its reception by contemporaries (including local political

---

166 "Conference on National Water Supply, Sewerage and Health," *Journal of the Society of Arts* 28 (June 20, 1879): 662.

167 Thorne, "The Recent Outbreak of Enteric Fever," 118.

168 Thorne, "The Recent Outbreak of Enteric Fever at Caterham and Redhill," 174.

169 Thorne, "The Recent Outbreak of Enteric Fever at Caterham and Redhill," 173.

170 Hamlin, *A Science of Impurity,* chapter 8.

171 Bynum, "The Evolution of Germs," 54.

authorities and scientific colleagues)—is suggestive confirmatory evidence of such a "bacteriological backwater," at least before 1880. By examining the projection and reception of epidemiology—in other words, how Thorne and others defended, constructed, and maintained epidemiological ways of knowing—we are better able to see the larger significance of his study and understand the reasons why the Caterham local authorities placed trust and authority in Thorne's recommendations. Without the often-inconclusive practices of chemical or bacteriological analysis, Thorne could, through performance, command public health recommendations. To Thorne, a quintessential Victorian epidemiologist, ignoring bacteriology and chemistry was a deliberate strategy.

The public health lessons that contemporaries gleaned from Thorne's Caterham study were fourfold: (1) even a minute quantity of the germ or poison of typhoid fever, under favorable conditions when introduced into a water supply, could lead to an extensive outbreak; (2) mild or "perambulatory" cases of typhoid fever represented a special public health danger by reason of their intensely poisonous diarrhea; (3) all sources of excremental pollution near water sources should be extensively investigated; and (4) no persons suffering from diarrheal complaints should work in the construction or storage of water.[172] To contemporaries, Thorne's 1879 investigation was one of a series of confirmations of the developing waterborne hypothesis; into the early twentieth century it remained a classic study in Victorian epidemiology.[173] Late Victorian epidemiological investigations of typhoid fever reinforced the cultural assumptions that typhoid was bred of filth, and, as Hamlin has argued, that the protection of water supplies and the revamping of sewerage systems in rural and provincial areas was behind advancements made in numerous metropolitan locales.[174] The image of Thorne, who only a few years later became the administrative leader of British state medicine, climbing into a well in 1879 forms more than just an interesting anecdote; it was both routine epidemiological fieldwork as well as a powerful performance that Thorne used to convince local authorities to act on his otherwise powerless recommendations. Such performances by Victorian epidemiologists accompanied experimentation, interviewing, case tracing, mapmaking, and statistical tabulation, which we must also treat as performative. Field performances were accompanied by rhetorical strategies of self-promotion

---

172 Brunton, "Enteric Fever," 480.
173 Sedgwick, *Principles of Sanitary Science*, 191–200.
174 Hamlin, "Muddling in Bumbledom."

by Victorian epidemiologists. Through his epidemiological methods, Thorne had also placed his finger on one of the more controversial aspects of state medicine that continued into the twentieth century; the index case, J. K., whose perambulatory case of typhoid fever enabled him to continue working in the Caterham well while being highly infectious, was the late Victorian precursor to the infamous Typhoid Mary, although the latter was recognized as a healthy carrier.[175] To Thorne and his contemporaries around 1879 the perambulatory problem loomed larger than the identification of the typhoid germ or poison. And while this was a product of the belief in the epidemiological practices Thorne employed at Caterham, in the next two decades, American, French, and German bacteriologists began to discover some of the specific microbes responsible for the major infectious diseases.

Conclusion

By 1880 the waterborne theory had come to fruition.[176] Edward Ballard, who had himself conducted countless investigations of waterborne typhoid for the department, presented in the *BMJ* the most definitive account on the waterborne theory of the spread of disease. Ballard proclaimed that it was an epidemiological "creed" that the "enteric fever contagium . . . has an ancestry; and, however long and widely and through whatever media it may have traveled about prior to finding a lodgment suitable for its development in a human system, it or its ancestor at one time issued with excremental matter from some individual affected with the disease." [177] It was a summary of the waterborne theory advocated by John Snow and William Budd in the 1850s, advanced by epidemiologists such as Radcliffe and Thorne in the 1860s and 1870s, and to Ballard now a "doctrine," a "salutary rule of practice, inasmuch as it is calculated to foster a minuteness of investigation which has, at any rate, the chance of being fruitful."[178] Ballard's article, not

175 Leavitt, *Typhoid Mary*. See also Mendelsohn, "A Bacteriological Approach," 185–88.
176 Hudson, "The Germ-Theory of Enteric Fever"; Thomson, "Typhoid Fever"; Murphy, "The Etiology of Enteric Fever"; Collie, "The Etiology of Enteric Fever"; Kerr, "Enteric Fever, Diarrhoea, Diphtheria, and Scarlatina"; Hudson, "Facts Illustrative of the Spread of Enteric Fever."
177 Ballard, "Observations of Some of the Ways," 82–84.
178 Ballard, "Observations of Some of the Ways," 82.

unlike Thorne's Caterham study, was a disciplinary crowing for the particular kind of outbreak investigation becoming central to British epidemiology in the late Victorian period. In an 1886 memo to the Local Government Board, Buchanan echoed these views, saying that the etiological connection between typhoid and excremental pollution shown at the department was one of the single biggest factors in improving the sanitary conditions of the nation in the last twenty years, reducing the mortality rates of typhoid by one third.[179]

Epidemiological investigations, such as those explored in this chapter, were crucial for several reasons: they solidified the waterborne hypothesis, made clear the extensive need for sanitary reform (especially in remediating the water supply in urban and rural areas), and established epidemiology as a state-supported science worthy of parliamentary and public attention. Water supply was often the first thing epidemiologists investigated during an outbreak of typhoid fever in the second half of the nineteenth century. As the protection of water supplies in urban areas increasingly came under municipal regulation, rural areas often lagged behind in overall sanitary hygiene. This was true also of waste disposal and sewerage.

The focus on water, once coupled with the exclusivist theoretical perspective shared by a cadre of British epidemiologists, also led to the fear that anything that came into contact with fecally polluted water might be a medium of disease as well. Such was the case with milk beginning in the 1870s, explored in the next chapter. By the mid-1890s sewage-contaminated shellfish and ice cream were understood as disease media; H. T. Bulstrode, inspector at the Medical Department, conducted the first wide-ranging epidemiological study of the threat of oysters in spreading typhoid. A year later Arthur Newsholme, as MOH for Brighton, produced a similar epidemiological study on sewage-contaminated shellfish. Foodborne studies, which proliferated in the 1890s and early twentieth century, were a logical extension of the waterborne hypothesis. Such investigations also added, as Morabia and Hardy have shown, another layer onto already difficult epidemiological studies.[180]

Delivering the famous Chadwick Lectures at the University of London in 1910, Edward Cox Seaton, well-known MOH for Surrey, reflected on a lifetime of epidemiological practice by rhetorically asking his audience the very

---

179 George Buchanan, "Memorandum as to the Duties of the Board's Medical Department as at Present Constituted (1886)," National Archives, Kew, NA/ MH78/1.

180 Morabia and Hardy, "The Pioneering Use of a Questionnaire."

same question we started this chapter with: "Looking back from our present standpoint, may we not well ask whether Gull's assertion was very far wrong even thirty or forty years ago? Sir William emphasized the fact that the waterborne view was 'a good working hypothesis,' and so it undoubtedly proved to be in the after years, both home and abroad." But, Seaton added, "the subject we have to consider is much wider . . . in order to discuss this fairly, it is essential to reduce the water-carriage factor to its proper proportions."[181] Seaton had a privileged view throughout the second half of the nineteenth century; his father, Edward Cator Seaton, was first in line to replace Simon as chief medical officer. By the early twentieth century, as Seaton's comments indicate, British epidemiologists were too reliant on the waterborne theory. It was a telling admission. Was water becoming another sewer gas, another scapegoat in inconclusive investigations?

As we will see in the next chapter, however, epidemiologists, especially Radcliffe and Ballard, used the waterborne hypothesis to discover the ways that vehicles other than water could also spread disease. The most important medium was milk, the subject of chapter 3. While the epistemological claim that milk could spread disease was dependent upon the waterborne claim, and part of the same typhoid culture that dominated epidemiological networks, studying milk and investigating dairy farms brought epidemiologists into contact (and sometimes into conflict) with a wide range of competing cultural and scientific visions for public health. To many Victorian reformers, milk was nature's most perfect food, and animals were rarely the domain of epidemiologists at this time. In other words, investigating milk-borne outbreaks presented new challenges to epidemiologists that expanded and at times frustrated the professional claims of the burgeoning science.

---

181 Seaton, *Infectious Diseases and Their Prevention*, 98.

Chapter Three

Nature's Not-So-Perfect Food

The Epidemiology of Milk-Borne Typhoid

In the summer of 1873 London was again the center of a public spectacle over the filth disease. It began with England's fever expert. On July 22 three of Charles Murchison's children—the two oldest and the baby—came down with well-marked cases of typhoid. They were sent on July 25 to recover at the family's Cumbrian summer home in Westmorland, far away from the fetid air of London. But days later, on July 31, three more Murchison children came down with the disease, sending the house into a panic. With his children "hovering between life and death," Murchison set out to answer why his house had been attacked.[1] He was one of Europe's leading authorities on typhoid and had been physician at the London Fever Hospital for fifteen years. A month earlier, in June, he had finished a second edition of the magisterial *Continued Fevers of Great Britain,* judging that a revised work was needed because of increased "public as well as professional interest in the subject."[2] England was just recovering, after all, from the Prince of Wales's near-death experience from typhoid, as we saw in chapter 1.

---

1   Charles Murchison to *the Times,* August 8, 1873. Royal College of Physicians, London (RCP). Charles Murchison Papers, MS 710, book labeled "News Papers Cuttings, The Milk Epidemic of 1873."

2   Murchison, *Continued Fevers* (1873), iv.

What Murchison did not suspect was that soon typhoid would demand all of his personal attention. Typhoid, Murchison had long held, was not contagious, although as he concluded in the 1873 edition, in rare instances it might be communicable. So he went peering around his house's drains and water closets. But his house on Wimpole Street, in the St. Marylebone parish of London, was in scrupulous order, "the most perfect sanitary condition." He had consulted none other than the engineering expert Robert Rawlinson.[3] Convinced that it was not the usual domestic sanitary suspects at fault, Murchison turned to his neighbors, who were doctors in the popular West End. What he found was astonishing: on Wimpole Street and Harley Street, at Cavendish, Grosvenor, and Portman Squares, "the hidden foe has struck at some of the best known among his medical opponents."[4] Although Murchison knew better, public discourse held that typhoid was supposed to be the "disease of dirt," as the *Daily Telegraph* noted. So why had it struck the children of London's best doctors? Even from the first edition of *Continued Fevers, with* evidence gleaned from statistical analysis of patients at the London Fever Hospital, Murchison had argued that typhoid had a proclivity for the well-to-do, and especially children. But in two decades of studying the disease, he had never found a link between typhoid and the children of doctors. In fact, evidence from the London Fever Hospital suggested that doctors and nurses in the metropolis were notably free of the disease.[5] So why, "like a cunning besieger," as the *Telegraph* hyperbolized, had "the disease which latest struck down the Prince of Wales . . . found its secret road into these fortalices of medical security"?[6]

With no official assistance—why would such an authority as Murchison need assistance?—Murchison started an investigation. After consulting neighbors, he was confident their homes were also in proper sanitary order. It was not water. Or sewer gas. Through a deductive process of elimination, one

---

3   Unpublished letter from Charles Murchison to the *Times*. RCP, Murchison Papers MS 710.

4   *Daily Telegraph*, August 14, 1873, RCP, Murchison Papers, MS 710, book labeled "News Papers Cuttings, The Milk Epidemic of 1873."

5   Alexander Collie, medical officer to the Homerton Fever Hospital, who argued against Murchison's pythogenic theory in favor of the spread of the disease by direct personal contact, nonetheless found, like Murchison, that nurses at his institution were rarely struck with typhoid. See, Collie, "The Etiology of Enteric Fever," 84–87.

6   *Daily Telegraph*, August 14, 1873, RCP, Murchison Papers, MS 710, book labeled "News Papers Cuttings, The Milk Epidemic of 1873."

common to Victorian epidemiological practices of outbreak investigation, he found one common factor in the cases. In forty out of forty-three families that he visited, all close friends whose children were suffering from typhoid, received milk from one source: the Dairy Reform Company (DRC). Since the outbreak was a public calamity that was garnering national attention, it rapidly became a public relations nightmare for the DRC, a supposed pinnacle of progressive milk operations. Coupled with the near death of the Prince of Wales in 1871, typhoid was earning its reputation as "a national disgrace" in more ways than one, as Alfred Haviland had quipped in 1872.

The "Marylebone Milk Crisis," or "Marylebone Milk Panic," as it came to be known, was not the first outbreak of typhoid to be traced to a contaminated milk supply. And Murchison was not the first to suspect milk as a vehicle for typhoid. Edward Ballard, MOH for Islington and later inspector at the Medical Department, first brought widespread professional attention to the milk-borne theory in 1870. But the Marylebone episode was critical for raising the profile of milk's link to typhoid to an unprecedented level; it was the most public case of milk-borne typhoid in the second half of the nineteenth century. That it happened in London, which increased its visibility, and struck the houses of England's elite doctors, no doubt contributed to the popularization of the outbreak and the heightened anxiety over milk. But the Marylebone Milk Crisis also produced a model epidemiological investigation, one that combined a private inquiry by Murchison, William Jenner, and Ernest Hart, the efforts of Marylebone's MOH Charles Whitmore, St. George's MOH William Henry Corfield, Buckinghamshire MOH G. W. Childs, and the Medical Department's John Netten Radcliffe and William Henry Power. Taken together, the milk-borne investigations of typhoid at Islington and Marylebone were landmark studies in the history of public health. The two examples form the central part of this chapter.

Linking typhoid to milk was an important scientific discovery in the history of the disease, but equally important were the ways in which milk-borne investigations served to bolster epidemiological expertise. English epidemiologists were forced to ask new types of questions, acquire new forms of knowledge, and devise new types of public health practices. Milk-based investigations expanded the explanatory framework of epidemiology, giving the burgeoning science the space to make more extensive claims about its role in state medicine. But studying milk also frustrated epidemiological practice. Studies of typhoid prior to 1870 had shown that epidemiological knowledge was critical in understanding and improving water supply, drainage, domestic plumbing arrangements, and excrement disposal. After 1870 typhoid was on a national stage, and as epidemiologists were unraveling its etiology, the milk-borne hypothesis raised new questions about epidemiological, chemical, and veterinary expertise; about the culpability of milk sellers, dairymen, and farmers; and about the imaginary geopolitical lines between urban, suburban, and rural food pathways.

In advocating for the milk-borne hypothesis epidemiologists had to contend with a new set of causal theories about the spread of disease. Fear of the zoonotic transfer of epidemics, highlighted by the 1865 cattle plague led many English scientists, particularly veterinarians, to suggest that milk-borne typhoid was the product of diseased cows: or, as the Croydon chemist and surgeon Alfred Smee argued, what cows ate, like sewage grass. Coupled with this potential etiological confusion was a politically charged discourse against food adulteration that began around midcentury, one that highlighted milk as a vital nutritional product—nature's perfect food—especially for the burgeoning middle classes. Milk was the beverage *par excellence* of liberal subjectivity, and reformers sought to protect it from adulteration. The milk industry was changing around the 1870s, responding to growing trends in the industrialization of food production that saw disparate traditions of rural and urban cowkeeping being replaced by large-scale, aggregate rural dairies and suburban milk shops that mixed, bottled, and distributed milk throughout urban centers.

Epidemiological studies of milk-borne typhoid fever, in other words, collided with already contentious debates about food safety and agricultural productivity. Before 1870 the two biggest fears among the English middle classes—the principal consumers of milk—were that adulterated milk not only deprived children of the nutritional qualities needed to grow and flourish into productive citizens but also robbed honest tradesmen. After 1870, as a result of epidemiological studies of milk-borne typhoid, the public discourse on milk had to contend with a grave new worry: that milk, infused with typhoid excreta, often spread infectious disease. This chapter begins by exploring an investigation of milk-borne typhoid by Michael Taylor in 1858 in the northern English town of Penrith. Little remarked on at the time, by the 1870s Taylor's study was seen as an important contributor to the milk-borne hypothesis. The chapter then moves to consider the burgeoning interest in milk and disease that resulted from the 1865 cattle plague. From there I examine two precedent-setting studies of milk-borne typhoid, by Edward Ballard in Islington in 1870 and the 1873 Marylebone Milk Crisis. The chapter ends by considering the way in which milk-borne studies of the early 1870s became models of epidemiological inquiry and were enshrined in English epidemiological history and the broader history of British public health.

Michael Taylor and the Origins of the "Milk Hypothesis"

In a relatively brief and unprecedented article in the *Edinburgh Medical Journal* in 1858, Scottish-born physician Michael Waistell Taylor proposed that milk could be a vehicle for the spread of fever. Taylor was a rural physician and antiquarian in Penrith, located in the Lake District of northwest England, but his humble position belied his Edinburgh University training and professional contacts. He worked with renowned botanist John Hutton Balfour and was one of the earliest presidents of the Hunterian Medical Society. Taylor had even helped establish a regional branch of the British Medical Association.[7] If we consider Budd's argument that the communication of typhoid was more easily studied in rural areas and isolated outbreaks, it is not surprising that a country practitioner first recognized the milk-borne route of transmission.

Titled "On the Communication of the Infection of Fever by Ingesta," Taylor's article described a violent outbreak of what he called "epidemic typhus" in Penrith and the surrounding countryside that peaked in the autumn of 1857.[8] Taylor knew the area well and was attending most of the cases, so he easily traced the source of the outbreak to a fifteen-year-old girl, E. O., who had been working as a servant in Liverpool for three months. E. O. became so sick from fever that her friends brought her back to her parents' home in Penrith, which had been free from disease for some years. She remained feverish for two weeks in Penrith but convalesced and recovered. Two of her siblings caught the disease but also lived. Taylor had found the index case but had yet to explain how the disease spread throughout the community. He was struck by the demographic profile of the outbreak. The earliest cases had been children who received milk from one dairy farm, a small-scale operation run by E. O.'s own parents. Taylor went to the farm

---

7   "Obituary for Michael Waistell Taylor," *British Medical Journal* 1667 (December 10, 1892), 1315.

8   Late nineteenth-century medical writers acknowledged that Taylor was actually describing an outbreak of typhoid and that "epidemic typhus" was a Scottish term used for the disease. But W. H. Hamer in 1921 believed Taylor was studying typhus, not typhoid. Hamer, "A Bird's Eye View."

and examined the sanitary conditions and interviewed E. O. and her family. He found that the mother had nursed E. O. and her two siblings back to health, in addition to her daily duties milking cows. Once she was supposedly well enough to work again, E. O. distributed milk to houses in town. Taylor adduced a number of case studies; sick families who only came into contact with E. O.'s family via the milk, and others, living next to the small dairy, who were free of fever and took no milk. He argued that the facts of the case were "strong in favour of the argument of the milk having been the medium by which the infectious agent was conveyed."[9]

Taylor's etiological views were multifactorial, but he drew on the analogous research of Snow and Budd, citing them both, in thinking about milk as a medium, nidus, or conveyor—he used all three terms. The poison of fever, Taylor argued, was ingested, not inhaled. His chain of evidence focused on showing that the earliest cases of fever had not come into contact with dangerous miasmas but only milk from one source. He could find no other explanation and believed that "it was during the process of milking, while the thin warm stream was flowing, or whilst standing exposed to this atmosphere of fever-miasms, that the warm freshly drawn fluid absorbed the fever-virus, and afterwards communicated the disease to those who drank it."[10]

Taylor's article "received but little publicity" in the medical press despite his own efforts.[11] He boldly ended the piece by saying that the milk-borne hypothesis was "a new one in the etiology of fever."[12] But Taylor's case was mostly built on inference and weak causal connection. The earliest cases had milk in common, but Taylor had not proved how the milk became infected, then only weakly and without citing evidence. Anything but tepid, Taylor jumped at another chance to demonstrate the milk-borne hypothesis in 1868, this time arguing that scarlet fever could also be spread via milk.[13] But that article also failed to find much of an audience. Before 1870, it seems, English sanitary thinking was not fertile enough to sustain the milk-borne

---

9   Taylor, "On the Communication of the Infection of Fever," 996.

10   Ibid.

11   Thorne, *On the Progress of Preventive Medicine*, 26. Taylor published a later article on typhoid in 1872, one he had read before the Cumberland and Westmoreland Branch of the British Medical Association. See Taylor, "Notes of a Recent Epidemic of Typhoid Fever."

12   Taylor, "On the Communication of the Infection of Fever," 1004.

13   Taylor, "On the Transmission of the Infection of Fevers," 623–25. See also Wilson, "The Historical Riddle," 321.

hypothesis. Recall from chapter 2 that at Terling, all signs had pointed to milk-borne transmission, and Thorne had even narrowed in on one particular dairy. But he quickly dismissed the idea, unable to frame a broader argument about the role of milk and unable to direct his investigation along a milk-borne route of transmission.

Taylor was later vindicated, albeit anachronistically, by later epidemiologists who were trying, through a bit of epidemiological hagiography, to bolster their own milk-borne investigations and further their own epidemiological expertise—not to mention construct their own version of epidemiology history. Arthur Newsholme's *The Last Thirty Years in Public Health,* for example, called Taylor's Penrith investigation "a great event in public health history."[14] Harold Swithinbank and George Newman, who cowrote the definitive *Bacteriology of Milk* in 1903, lauded Taylor's work as "the opening page in a chapter of public health, which has proved to be one not only of exceptional interest, but of vital importance."[15] W. H. Hamer, looking back with a "bird's eye view" of typhoid research in 1921, called Taylor's "the original milk outbreak."[16] But if Taylor's study had opened a new page, as Swithinbank and Newman pronounced, it was a slow-turning book for over a decade.

Competing Conceptions of Milk and the 1865 Cattle Plague

That the milk-borne hypothesis was not widely recognized until the 1870s was not because of a lack of interest in the safety or purity of milk. Scientific interest in milk before the mid-nineteenth century took three forms: chemical studies that sought to understand the constituents of milk and what made it a nutritious article of diet, agricultural studies that sought to improve animal husbandry and commodify the production of milk, and medical studies that sought to situate milk in debates about the effectiveness of wet nursing.[17] Milk was also widely recognized from the eighteenth century as an essential part of *materia medica,* typically arranged as a demulcent or emollient, used to treat a wide range of inflammatory conditions and fevers up through the nineteenth century.[18]

---

14   Newsholme, *The Last Thirty Years,* 37.
15   Swithinbank and Newman, *The Bacteriology of Milk,* 261.
16   Hamer, "A Bird's Eye View," 60.
17   Orland, "Enlightened Milk," 195.
18   Orland, "Enlightened Milk," 146–47.

Early food reformer and London doctor H. Hodson Rugg epitomized the Victorian, idealist attitude toward milk in 1850 when he noted that "milk appears to be that which was intended by nature should constitute to man in general, and children in particular, an agreeable and nutritious food . . . it is thus a most perfect diet."[19] But it was clear that milk rarely made its way to households in a perfect state. The 1850s saw a public frenzy over milk adulteration, created in large part by analytical studies of milk adulteration by microscopist Arthur Hill Hassall, who worked in connection with Thomas Wakley's Analytical Sanitary Commission of the *Lancet*.[20] It was widely known that milk was adulterated with water, but contemporary reports claimed unscrupulous dairymen used flour, chalk, or, as one popular urban legend held, even sheep's brains to bolster profits. Charles Cameron, MOH for Dublin, lamented in 1868, for example, that "milk is rarely obtained in a state of absolute purity in towns."[21]

The consumption of raw cow's milk varied throughout the nineteenth century, but generally speaking women and children, especially those in rural agricultural areas, drank larger quantities than men. The class-based dimensions were not lost on contemporary medical observers. George Ross, MOH for St. Giles, in his annual report for 1869 noted that "I have hardly ever known a child in a poor family supplied with the quantity of milk which experience has shown to be necessary for its due nourishment and growth."[22] In urban areas, particularly by the mid-nineteenth century, as Peter Atkins has shown, the consumption of cow's milk was largely confined to the middling and wealthy classes due to its increased cost, as urban cowsheds had been relocated to more sparsely populated areas and milk had to be transported, unrefrigerated, via railroads.[23]

By the mid-1850s the urban cowshed had become vilified as a dangerous urban space in need of reform. The dissolution of urban cowsheds was a product of the growing vigilance of veterinary inspectors and MOsH. Such inspection was permissible under the older Nuisance Removal Acts, but rigorous sanitary supervision often depended, as veterinary reformer John Gamgee noted, upon both progressive local authorities and an active

---

19   Rugg, *Observations on London Milk*, 1.

20   Charnley, "Arguing over Adulteration," 129–33.

21   Cameron, *Lectures on the Preservation of Health*, 99.

22   Ross, *Report on the Sanitary Conditions of the St. Giles District*, 13.

23   Atkins, *Liquid Materialities*.

MOH.[24] Numerous scholars have shown that there was increased attention to the health of cows, and by extension, the health of their meat and milk, as a result of the 1865 outbreak of rinderpest, or cattle plague. Worboys and Romano, for example, have demonstrated the ways in which the 1865 cattle plague was a vital testing ground for early variations of the germ theory. The widespread public nature of the 1865 outbreak facilitated an increased network of communication between medical authorities and veterinarians, intensifying mid-Victorian fears of zoonotic and epizootic diseases.[25]

Kier Waddington and Chris Otter have also shown that the 1865 cattle plague was critical in turning veterinary and public health attention to the reality that the consumption of milk and meat from diseased cows was harmful to human health.[26] There were important precedents even before 1865. Edward Ballard, MOH for Islington and active member of the Metropolitan Association of Medical Officers of Health (MAMOsH), led a committee on the dangers of diseased animal products as early as the late 1850s and early 1860s. The committee included John Burdon Sanderson and John Syer Bristowe, and also worked closely with Gamgee.[27] On April 18, 1863, Gamgee was invited to the monthly MAMOsH meeting to give a speech titled "The Diseases of Animals in relation to Public Health and Prosperity," where he laid out an extensive argument for the contagiousness of cattle diseases such as pleuro-pneumonia, foot and mouth disease, rinderpest, and the harmful effects of diseased milk and meat. Metropolitan MOsH were sympathetic to Gamgee's views, noting that "the Association also has reason to believe that much disease is produced in the human subject by the consumption of meat of diseased animals."[28] Although the management of cattle diseases was not in the direct purview of MOsH, "It could not fail to have considerable interest for them, as illustrating general epidemic laws, and practically as affecting the milk supply and the management of cow-houses

24 Gamgee, *The Cattle Plague and Diseased Meat*, 8. On Gamgee see Fisher, "Professor Gamgee and the Farmers"; Hall, "John Gamgee and the Edinburgh New Veterinary College."

25 Worboys, *Spreading Germs*, chapter 2; Romano, "The Cattle Plague of 1865."

26 Waddington, *Bovine Scourge;* Otter, "The Vital City."

27 Gamgee had a particular interest in zoonotics and especially the dangerous state of diseased meat. See Woods, *A Manufactured Plague*, 6–19.

28 John Gamgee, The Diseases of Animals in Relation to Public Health and Prosperity," read April 18, 1863, Society of Medical Officers of Health Collection, Wellcome Archives, London, England, SA/SMO/G2/1.

within the Metropolis."[29] Later legislation such as the Contagious Diseases (Animals) Act, passed in 1869, and the Public Health Act of 1875 bolstered the inspection and supervision of dairies, slaughterhouses, and butchers, but problems remained throughout the second half of the nineteenth century.[30]

But medical attention had been drawn to the idea that milk could spread infectious disease. Gamgee's hand-gesturing was making ground, at least among urban MOsH like Ballard and Henry Letheby, who noted that pleuro-pneumonia and aphtha "are contagious, and they give to the milk properties which cannot fail to be injurious to those who make use of it."[31] An outbreak of foot and mouth disease in 1869 was an opportunity for Simon at the Medical Department, and for epidemiological expertise, to join the fray.[32] Simon put Thorne on the task. Working with James Simonds at the Veterinary Department, Thorne conducted a sanitary survey of areas where the epizootic was widespread, particularly in Suffolk. In some towns, such as Beccles and Bungay, where foot and mouth disease struck nearly all stock, Thorne found an increased number of children sick with "soreness and vesicular eruption about the mouth."[33] He concluded that in some (but not all) cases milk from diseased cows could infect humans. But investigating dairies and dairymen was charting new epidemiological ground at the department, and Thorne was aggravated by the lack of compliance from dairy farmers, a foreshadowing of many later studies of milk-borne typhoid in the 1870s and 1880s. He lamented:

> The difficulties encountered in making this inquiry have been very much increased by the careful reticence observed by farmers and dairymen whenever questioned as to the quality of the milk supplied by them at given dates, and the almost invariable impossibility of tracing the milk of any special cow, to any particular person or persons.[34]

---

29   Secretary Report for 1865–1866, *Annual Report of the Society of Medical Officers of Health,* Wellcome Archives, London, England, SA/SMO/G2/1, 4.

30   See, for example, George Buchanan's private remarks about the inadequacies of the acts in 1889, National Archives, Kew, MH 113/26.

31   Letheby, "Cows in Cow-Houses, and their Milk,"185; McBridge, "Report on Cases of Contagion," 536–37.

32   Woods, *A Manufactured Plague.*

33   Thorne, "Effects produced on the Human Subject," *Twelfth Annual Report,* 295.

34   Thorne, "Effects produced on the Human Subject," 298.

By 1870, within public health and veterinary circles, it was becoming provisionally accepted that, at least under certain circumstances, "milk is an extremely dangerous agent for the spread of contagion," as Lawson Tait noted in the *BMJ*. Up until that time, however, the *modus operandi* was narrowed to sick cows. But given the widespread attention to epizootics and the media frenzy over milk adulteration in the 1860s, the stage was set for at least inferring that milk, when diluted, could spread typhoid. Lawson Tait suspected as much. In an 1870 *BMJ* article he warned that

> if we bethink ourselves of any instances of disease which might in certain instances be communicated by milk, typhoid fever stands out with fearful probability. Enteric fever is nowhere more common nor more fatal than in country farm-houses, where means for the removal of the dejections are not sufficiently well adapted for security, and much too convenient for safety.[35]

It was a prophetic statement, as Edward Ballard, MOH for Islington, was at that very moment investigating an outbreak of milk-borne typhoid.

Edward Ballard's "Model" Milk-Borne Investigation at Islington

What happened in the fall of 1870 was unprecedented. "Suddenly and without premonition," between July and September cases of typhoid fever exploded in one Islington neighborhood, causing 168 people in sixty-seven houses to get sick and twenty-six to die. Edward Ballard, MOH for one of London's largest metropolitan districts for fifteen years, stepped in to investigate. "The occurrence of a serious outbreak of typhoid fever in a district supposed to be under sanitary surveillance," Ballard howled, " is . . . an opprobrium to sanitary administration." It was a "remarkable" outbreak, one that left Ballard "staggered." He was one of the most vigilant MOsH in London, and initially blamed himself, wondering, "What was it? Was the fault mine? Had I failed to warn the local authority where warning was my duty?"[36]

Ballard was a prototypical early professional epidemiologist in Victorian England. Born in 1820 to a middling family in the north London suburb of Islington, he apprenticed with a workhouse medical officer before entering

---

35   Tait, "The Influence of Milk," 344.
36   Ballard, *On a Localised Outbreak of Typhoid Fever*, 5.

University College London. He received an MD in 1844, and spent his early professional years dividing his time as physician among the St. Pancras Royal General Dispensary, St. George's Hospital, and at University College London. His 1845 treatise titled *Elements of Materia Medica and Therapeutics* showed a propensity for botanical classification, and two publications on nutrition and digestion, titled *On Pain After Food* (1854) and *On Artificial Digestion as a Remedy in Dyspepsia, Apepsia, and their Results* (1856) provide insight into Ballard's aspiring interests.[37] Inducted as a fellow of the Royal Medical and Chirurgical Society of London in 1848 and the Royal College of Physicians in 1853, Ballard was an early member of the New Sydenham Society and the ESL. His career in public health began in 1856 when he was appointed the first MOH of Islington, a post he held for sixteen years until John Simon offered him a position as inspector at the Medical Department in 1871, where he spent the last twenty-five years of his life.[38]

Throughout his sixteen-year period as MOH, Ballard was involved in a wide range of sanitary activities typical of urban MOsH. He investigated outbreaks of scarlet fever, smallpox, diphtheria, cholera, typhoid fever, and epidemic diarrhea. As MOH he became interested in the health effects of trade nuisances—chiefly factory pollution and urban cowkeeping—a subject he studied for over thirty years. Ballard's interests ran the gamut of what today we would call the ecology of urban-industrial health. Islington's Holloway Cattle Market and the factories of Belle Isle—glue making, soap boiling, pottery, and varnish factories—kept Ballard busy. He was a sanitary reformer and keen advocate of the professionalization of the metropolitan MOsH. He was a founding member, for example, of a Committee on Trade Nuisances for the metropolitan group and served as a witness before the Royal Commission on Rinderpest in 1866, acting as a close ally to Gamgee. As MOH, Ballard proved uniquely proficient in the use of vital statistics (he was close with William Farr) and epidemiological mapping during the 1866 cholera epidemic—he once called John Snow "my old friend." Simon went so far as to say that Ballard was "among the foremost representatives of

---

37 In the mid-1850s he also supervised a comprehensive clinical study of post-mortem observations through the London Medical Society. See Ballard, *What to Observe at the Bed-Side*.

38 On public health in Islington before Ballard, see Kearns, "Cholera, Nuisances, and Environmental Management."

English sanitary knowledge and practice."[39] During his distinguished career at the Medical Department, from 1871 until his death in 1897, Ballard made important contributions to understanding waterborne disease, industrial health, and infant mortality. But his most important epidemiological investigation was carried out in 1870.[40]

At the outset of the investigation Ballard was struck by the unique features of the outbreak. It was limited to a quarter-mile radius. The 168 cases were middle- and upper-class residents of Islington, "not of the class among whom fevers are most commonly observed, but were persons in very comfortable positions in society, attended by private medical men, and residing in some of the best houses in the parish."[41] The streets were wide, the houses well drained. Consulting with local physicians and conducting a house-to-house sanitary inspection of the area, Ballard came up with four hypotheses that could account for the outbreak: (1) an alteration of the railway had cut into several old sewers and drains and produced typhoid miasmas, (2) a local "dung-shoot" (or dung heap) induced the epidemic, (3) local sanitary and domestic drainage was at fault, or (4) a single source of milk had been polluted.[42] While the first three hypotheses, either alone or in combination, would have been acceptable and logical conclusions for most Victorian observers—and would have fit into Budd or Murchison's etiological framework—Ballard started the investigation with a broad understanding of typhoid causation. His multifactorial views were in line with most MOsH, and he considered air and water to be the vehicles of typhoid. But he was already leaning toward a living germ theory of disease. On November 19, 1870, for example, he read a paper at the meeting of the Association of Medical Officers of Health titled "On the Practical Aspect of the Previous Sewage Contamination Question," in which he sided with the view that the most important danger to public

---

39   "Obituary for Edward Ballard," *British Medical Journal* 1883 (January 30, 1897): 281–82. Edward Ballard, "Observations on Some of the Ways," 82.

40   Ballard's industry at the Medical Department was evident from his first set of duties, which was to inspect local vaccination practices in Warrington. Ballard found the local physician in charge of vaccination incompetent, using dirty instruments and causing much mischief, including several cases of erysipelas. See Edward Ballard to John Simon, November 28, 1871, and two letters on November 30, 1871, National Archives, Kew, MH 25/22, Medical Department, LGB, Miscellaneous Files.

41   Ballard, *Report on the Sanitary Condition*, 8.

42   Ballard, "On a Localised Outbreak of Typhoid Fever in Islington," *Medical Times Gazette* 2 (1870): 612.

health was the contamination of water by specific morbid discharges from the bowels of people suffering from epidemic diseases, which contained living agents of typhoid and cholera.[43]

Ballard was unconvinced of the first three hypotheses, because they were unable to explain why on some streets typhoid picked out certain houses and within certain houses picked out only certain family members. And though he admitted that at first he was skeptical of "what appeared a rather far-fetched theory," the overwhelming qualitative and quantitative evidence pointed to milk.[44] His method was, as the *British and Foreign Medico-Chirurgical Review* applauded, a thorough process of scientific deduction "by the process of exclusion."[45] It was the method in place at the Medical Department, as we have seen in previous chapters. But Ballard's use of vital statistics, for example, his calculating case-fatality rates, was pushing methodological boundaries of outbreak investigation. He was using vital statistics not only to identify a public health problem but to combine statistical methods with outbreak investigation on the ground. He found that in no cases where two families occupied the same house did typhoid occur except where both families used the same milk. Attacks within families followed consumption practices, even by sex; adult females, who habitually drank more milk than males, made up 69 percent of those attacked. The preference of the disease for females perplexed Ballard, as he noted, "I am not aware that under ordinary circumstances typhoid shows any such decided preference for the female sex."[46] But the skewed gender distribution also assisted in narrowing the cause of the outbreak to the milk from one dairy. It is possible that Ballard had read Taylor's 1858 article, but he did not cite it in any of his publications in 1870. Curiously, though, Ballard ended his annual report to the vestry of Islington noting that "I have long suspected the possibility of the propagation of Typhoid Fever by milk in this way, the water added to

---

43   Ballard, "On the Practical Aspect of the Previous Sewage Contamination Question," read at the November 19, 1870 meeting of the Association of Medical Officers of Health. See Wellcome Archives, London, England, SA/SMO/G2/1/1.

44   Ballard, *On a Localised Outbreak,* 12.

45   "Typhoid Fever in Islington," *British and Foreign Medico-Chirurgical Review* 48 (July to October 1871): 25–26.

46   Ballard, *Report on the Sanitary Condition,* 9. The gendered distribution was observed by Murchison.

it being contaminated."[47] Up to this point Ballard's investigation was not unlike Taylor's, in methodology or scope. Both pointed to milk as the probable cause of the outbreak based on correlation and the statistical grouping of cases. What distinguished Ballard's study, and in fact what made it stand out to contemporaries, was that Ballard was adamant in his quest to provide proof that the milk consumed had been contaminated with the specific excreta of typhoid patients. He tenaciously ruled out mere coincidence.

Visiting the dairy, Ballard found that the owner of the farm and seven others, family and employees, had died of typhoid preceding the Islington outbreak. He had been fortunate to get the assistance of local medical practitioners, but even more critical was that the father of the deceased owner provided Ballard with a customer list, which Ballard called essential to "unravelling the mystery of the outbreak."[48] The dairyman's list, when compared to Ballard's compiled list of those sick or dead from typhoid, told the story. The dairy in question supplied milk to 142 out of 2,000 families in the quarter-mile radius of where the outbreak occurred. Out of those 142 families 70 were struck with typhoid, a relative risk of 50 percent. Of the 70 families invaded there were 175 cases, with 30 deaths, a case fatality of 17 percent. The statistical evidence was striking: "The fever was confined to persons who had consumed milk from one particular dairy . . . in particular streets, rows of houses &c., the typhoid poison picked out as it were the customers of the dairy, leaving the others free from the attack.[49] With the milk-borne theory fully solidified in his mind, Ballard then had to surmise how the milk became infected—what he called the "origin of the case."

Moving away from statistical analysis, Ballard turned to interviewing, environmental inspection, and spatial thinking. He drew a visual diagram similar to what Thorne had done at Winterton and Terling, explored in the previous chapter. The diagram (figure 3.1) helped Ballard visualize the spatial conditions of the farm and the source of the outbreak. But the diagram was antecedent to quantitative case tracing, interviewing, and environmental inspection. Although clean and tidy, with healthy-looking cows, there was danger lurking under the surface at the dairy. Ballard narrowed his investigation to a wooden underground water tank, "I." It was rotten in one corner "P," and with the aid of a candle Ballard found that it connected to a series of rat burrows, marked as dotted lines on the map. He then started

47   Ballard, *Report on the Sanitary Condition*, 18.
48   Ballard, *On a Localised Outbreak*, 14.
49   Ballard, *Report on the Sanitary Condition*, 8–9.

digging around the tank in the direction of the rat burrow, where he found that it freely connected to three old drains, including one from the water closet "F." The rat burrows also linked up with the main drainage of the farm, "B," which led to the sewer pipe "D." Through simple experimentation of flushing the closet and filling the tank, Ballard found that the rat burrows were the link between excreta and water. But the discovery had not solved the entire mystery of the outbreak. The water in question was only used for dairy purposes—feeding animals and washing equipment. The first cases had originated at the farm, and so, following the sanitary problems, had probably compromised the water supply, loading it with the typhoid discharges of the owner. Once in the water supply, milk could be contaminated in two ways: the milk was either deliberately adulterated with water, or the milk pails were accidentally polluted when they were washed with fecally contaminated water. Ballard lamented that he was now getting into probabilities.[50] The dairy employees swore that they did not water down the milk, but several customers, upon Ballard's inquiry, had complained that it had been done. Because of his extensive experience as MOH, Ballard knew the watering of milk was "all but universal among milk sellers in London."[51] Nefarious practices of milk adulteration were not the sole problem, however, and Ballard condemned a much wider set of cultural attitudes toward milk production and milk selling, arguing the following:

> That it is in the nature of a fraud upon the purchasers must be generally allowed, but it is one which the public seem to unite in condoning. . . . If the public choose to be parties to the arrangement by which an indefinite amount of dilution, according as may be convenient to the seller or necessary for his trade interests, shall be permitted, provided that the price of the article sold be not varied, no one can interfere with the tacit contract. But it is my place to proclaim the risk which the public run in thus submitting to the habitual adulteration of so common an article of food as milk, and especially to raise my voice against a practice the danger of which the poorer classes of the community cannot guard against, even if they should be aware of its extent. We take a great deal of trouble to secure the purity of the water in dwelling houses, and to guard against its contamination from house-drain emanations, and from the emanations from cesspools; but with all our care a wholesale

---

50 Ballard argued that milk was infected from typhoid-laced water, but others were adamant that milk that came into contact with sewer gases could likewise become infective.

51 Ballard, *Report on the Sanitary Condition*, 10.

poisoning may take place because the article received into houses and used as *milk* is diluted with water mixed with the contagium of typhoid fever.[52]

Ballard was initially careful not to place too much emphasis on what he first thought was mere coincidence. What started as skeptical suspicion, however, increasingly became vehement indictment, combining an attack on dishonest milk sellers who routinely adulterated their milk for profit, on the public for demanding cheap milk, and on local authorities for not regulating the milk trade. It was the kind of practical methodology in epidemiology that Simon was developing at the Medical Department, and the type of powerful public engagement that aligned with Simon's vision of state medicine.

Ballard's epidemiological study of milk-borne typhoid in Islington was careful, methodological, and precise; it represents Victorian practices of outbreak investigation in the period. But part of what made it so important is the way in which Ballard publicized his findings and showcased his expertise. The performative aspects of Ballard's epidemiology dovetail with Thorne's Caterham study later in the decade, which was explored in the previous chapter. Reporting to the Islington vestry, Ballard minimized the blow-by-blow account of his investigation, noting that "many of the details of this very remarkable outbreak of a fatal disease will possess little interest for the non-professional reader." To the local authorities Ballard focused on the facts and only those "of the highest practical importance."[53] The vestry report did not contain the diagram (figure 3.1) but instead warned of the practical dangers of milk adulteration. It was accompanied by a lengthy section that included chemical figures produced by analytical chemist Alfred Wanklyn, who had conducted an investigation of all the milk sold in Islington as a result of Ballard's epidemiological study.[54] "In Islington alone," Wanklyn's report concluded that "dairymen receive many thousand pounds annually for water." Not one dairy, Wanklyn found, sold pure milk, which Ballard said was "hideous to contemplate" given his finding that adulterated milk could spread typhoid.[55]

Ballard's interests were far greater than the local sanitary politics of Islington. On November 19, 1870, he read an extended version of his study

52   Ballard, *Report on the Sanitary Condition*, 11.
53   Ballard, *Report on the Sanitary Condition*, 7.
54   For more on Victorian debates over milk analysis, and Wanklyn's mercurial career, see Steere-Williams, "A Conflict of Analysis."
55   Ballard, *Report on the Sanitary Condition*, 14.

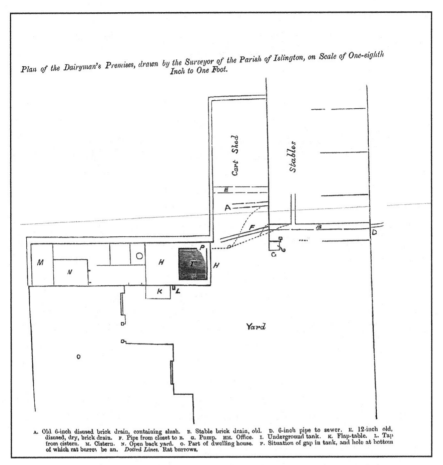

Plan of the Dairyman's Premises, drawn by the Surveyor of the Parish of Islington, on Scale of One-eighth Inch to One Foot.

Cart Shed

Stables

E

A

F

P

M

N

H

I

H

K L

C

Yard

o

A. Old 6-inch disused brick drain, containing slush. B. Stable brick drain, old. D. 6-inch pipe to sewer. E. 12-inch old, disused, dry, brick drain. F. Pipe from closet to B. G. Pump. HH. Office. I. Underground tank. K. Flap-table. L. Tap from cistern. M. Cistern. N. Open back yard. O. Part of dwelling house. P. Situation of gap in tank, and hole at bottom of which rat burrow be an. *Dotted Lines*, Rat burrows.

Figure 3.1 Diagram of local dairyman's premises. From Edward Ballard, On a Localised Outbreak of Typhoid Fever in Islington, Traced to the Use of Impure Milk (London: J&A Churchill, 1871). Image courtesy of the Wellcome Library, London. Creative Commons Attribution only license CC BY. 4.0

to the Metropolitan Association of Medical Officers of Health. "It was listened to with marked attention," Robert Druitt, president of the Association and late MOH to St. George's Hanover Square, noted, "and followed by an unanimous burst of approval." So impressed were his MOH colleagues that the association printed a pamphlet of Ballard's presentation and circulated it to all members of the association, which included MOsH, doctors, chemists, and lawyers. They especially praised his methodology, his "untiring industry in collecting the minutest facts," and "in linking together the chain of evidence," which led "him to the irresistible conclusion" that milk had been the vehicle "of a most terrible and fatal disease."[56]

The medical profession heaped on even more praise. Reviewing the pamphlet in the *Lancet,* James Wakley said that "the pamphlet is one to be read carefully, and to be possessed by every medical man, not only as a model of careful investigation in etiology, but as a history of one of the most remarkable outbreaks of typhoid on record."[57] Similar commendation followed in the mainstream medical press, and the medical profession in Europe and North America took notice. Almost overnight Ballard's name and the Islington study became yoked to the milk-borne theory of typhoid. Charles Cameron, MOH for the City of Dublin, communicated Ballard's study throughout Ireland, and James Russell did the same in Scotland. Using Ballard as a model, both Cameron and Russell conducted a series of important milk-borne investigations in the 1870s and 1880s. In his *Half-Yearly Report on Public Health* for 1871 Cameron, for example, began with a lengthy discussion of Ballard's Islington study, concluding that "Dr. Ballard has undoubtedly proved that typhoid fever was largely spread through the medium of milk, and it is impossible not to believe with him that the contagium was introduced into the milk by water which had been contaminated with sewage."[58] In other words, Ballard had powerful champions backing his work and bolstering the epidemiological gaze toward dairies and milk. His study received praise in Budd's *Typhoid Fever* (1873), which warned that "I have no doubt that this mode of infection is much more common than it is generally supposed to be."[59] And in real ways the lessons gleaned from Ballard's 1870 Islington study entered public health practice. The updated fourth edition of E. A. Parkes's widely popular handbook, *A Manual of Practical Hygiene* (intended for MOsH and army medical officers), noted that Ballard's Islington investigation was "exhaustive" analysis that "decidedly" traced the epidemic to watered milk.[60]

In the last three decades of the century, Ballard's Islington study became public health lore. In 1890, preparing his self-congratulatory public health

56   Ballard, *On a Localised Outbreak,* 3.
57   "On a Localised Outbreak of Typhoid Fever in Islington During the Months of July and August, 1870," *Lancet* 1 (1871): 120.
58   Cameron, "Half-Yearly Report," 478; Cameron, *A Manual of Hygiene.*
59   Budd, *Typhoid Fever,* 103.
60   Parkes, *A Manual of Practical Hygiene,* 246.

history, *English Sanitary Institutions*, John Simon called Ballard's work "a new line of epidemiological accuracy."[61] Writing Ballard's obituary for the Royal Society of London in 1897, William Henry Power, another close colleague at the Medical Department, powerfully noted that the Islington study "necessarily served as a model to later investigators."[62] And Ballard's name continued to be written into British epidemiological history into the twentieth century. In an address titled "Milk and its Relation to Health and Disease," delivered before the Wimbledon Medical Society in November 1901, University College Hospital physician George Vivian Poore was clear that the entire history of research into the relation between milk and disease started with Ballard's Islington study. Poore went as far as to excuse himself to the audience: "I am perfectly well aware that everybody in this room is acquainted with this historic instance." Poore noted that because of Ballard's work at Islington, it "was no longer a 'view' held by this man or that man, but it was a fact." "Indeed," Poore declared, it was "an epoch-making investigation by a man with a scientific and logical mind. He knew what care was necessary to prove his case, and he definitely proved it."[63] Curiously enough, as British epidemiology changed in the first half of the twentieth century, Ballard's name was written out of the history of the field. The afterlife of Ballard's Islington study, in other words, proved to be just as interesting and important as the work itself, which provided a framework investigation of milk-borne disease.

While Taylor in 1858 had suggested that milk might act as a vehicle in spreading disease, Ballard's was the first to trace more carefully how milk might become infected with typhoid excreta and cause an outbreak. Ballard was also more convincing and had a greater professional platform to broadcast his views. That his investigation was "successful" by contemporary logic rested on Ballard's cajoling of multiple audiences. He had gained the trust of local Islington medical practitioners through his diligence as MOH. He had obtained a list of the customers of the dairy by gently accusing milk as the vehicle that spread the disease. And he stressed different aspects of the study to different audiences—reports of milk analysis to the local vestry versus the

---

61   John Simon, perhaps notes for his *English Sanitary Institutions*, Royal College of Surgeons of England untitled manuscript, John Simon Collection, Sir John Simon PRCS, 67.h.5 Letters & Papers re: College affairs.

62   Power, "Obituary Notice for Edward Ballard," *Proceedings of the Royal Society of London* 62 (1898): iii–v.

63   Poore, "Milk and Its Relation," 178.

spatial diagram to his MOH colleagues. It all amounted to a landmark investigation and an indicative case study that embodied the emerging belief in epidemiological expertise in Victorian England.

In some ways Ballard was lucky during the Islington study. Later investigators in the 1870s and 1880s often struggled to find the source of milk-borne outbreaks. Often dairy farmers were obstinate about giving away private information regarding customers and letting public officials dig about their farms. The confined nature of the outbreak meant that it was easy for Ballard to trace it to one local dairy. In many later cases a complex mix of farms throughout the country supplied urban areas. Ballard's study became the standard, in other words, even if it could not always be replicated. The Medical Department, where Ballard went to work as an inspector from 1871, led the way in epidemiological research on milk-borne outbreaks. It was no surprise that Ballard was often the first called to investigate a suspected outbreak related to milk. In 1872 he traced an outbreak of typhoid in Armley (near Leeds) to a milk source, and again in 1873 he did the same in Moseley and Balsall Heath.[64] In the next several years Thorne, Power, Buchanan, and Radcliffe all studied outbreaks of milk-borne typhoid. Whenever the demographic profile of an outbreak skewed toward the wealthier inhabitants of an area, and especially where women and children were unequally struck, the department's inspectors suspected a milk-borne route of transmission. By the mid-1870s the milk-borne theory was so fully ingrained into the everyday activities of Victorian epidemiology that nearly every outbreak investigation of typhoid at least considered the possibility that contaminated milk had been the cause. The dairyman and the so-called perfect food had come under the epidemiological gaze.

Milk Adulteration Reframed

Ballard's Islington study stirred up more than epidemiological interest. It provided fuel for antiadulteration reformers. If milk could spread disease as a result of unscrupulous trade practices, the likes of Gamgee and Hassall thought, then perhaps national and local authorities would be more willing

---

64   NA, MH 113/11, "Dr. Ballard's Report upon an Outbreak of Enteric Fever at Armley, in the Borough of Leeds," and "Dr. Ballard's Report upon an Outbreak of Enteric Fever at Moseley and Balsall Heath, near Birmingham." See also Robinson, "The Cause of the Contagion," 451–52.

to entertain progressive reform. Gamgee, using Ballard's Islington investigation, argued as early as December of 1870 that

> the simple dilution of milk has been regarded by many as the worst form of deterioration injuring the milk consumer. But when it is considered that impure water, used in washing milk-pails, or diluting the milk, transfers from the cesspool to the breakfast cup, or infant feeding bottle, the germs of enteric fever . . . it is high time that, as practical men, we should consider the whole subject, and devise a remedy at once efficacious, and of possible or probable application.[65]

His solution was a complete surveillance of dairy matters: a watchful eye on the transportation of milk from country to town, an intervention at dairy farms, and chemical scrutiny over milk composition. Gamgee was not alone. The first edition of the food reformist periodical the *Milk Journal*, in January 1871, for example, contained a lengthy article summarizing Ballard's epidemiological evidence linking milk and typhoid. The opening issue also contained an article by Ballard, titled "On Some Sanitary Aspects of Cowkeeping, and the Trade in Milk in London," where he argued that the flawed and unsanitary system of cowkeeping in the metropolis unavoidably led to public health dangers, from diseased cows to germ-laden milk.[66] Ballard's clarion call for epidemiology was growing louder and was far from a conservative warning, particularly considering that *the Milk Journal's* readership was mostly dairy farmers. Ballard demonized and even threatened dairymen who adulterated their milk, urging that

> from this time forth, the water supply upon the premises of a dairyman will be jealously scrutinized by public authorities. Let us hope, too, that another session of Parliament will not slip away, without imposing upon milk adulterators, such a punishment as the gravity of their delinquency warrants. From henceforth no one can plead ignorance—no one ought to be permitted to plead the "custom of the trade."[67]

---

65   Gamgee, "Country Versus Town Milk," 38–39, 67–68.

66   Ballard, "On Some Sanitary Aspects of Cowkeeping," 6–8.

67   Ballard, "On Some Sanitary Aspects of Cowkeeping," 8. This was in spite of the widespread recognition that the "ordinary dairy farmer knows nothing of the meaning of purity as applied to water, or of hygienic regulation of his farm and his dairy." See "The Regulation of the Sale of Milk," *Sanitary Record* 3 (September 18, 1875): 199–200.

Ballard's voice, alongside Hassall and Gamgee, was quickly becoming the standard in antiadulteration circles. In the absence of compulsory antiadulteration legislation, which was not passed until the 1880s and 1890s, epidemiological and analytical evidence was pushing a reformist agenda. But eliminating milk-borne epidemics had to be considered in light of what was already known about the communication of typhoid, and Ballard was one of the first to present a broader, protoecological vision for understanding the disease and its prevention. As early as 1872 in an investigation of milk-borne typhoid in Leeds, Ballard argued this position, saying that

> the Adulteration of Food Act of last Session enables local authorities to deal with persons who add water to milk; but if a dairyman's own drinking water is permitted by local authorities to be a fluid little better than sewage, is it not rather a reflection on those authorities than an aggravation of his commercial fraud that he, only meaning to dilute his milk, ignorantly supplies infection to his customers?[68]

The onus was on local sanitation authorities to control and maintain sewerage, water, and now milk supplies. Ballard's vision thus meshed with Gamgee's, and both reformers saw a marriage between chemical and epidemiological expertise. After 1870 analytical chemists like Wanklyn and the broader organization, the Society of Public Analysts, found their own professional platform in milk analysis. In 1875 these posts became compulsory to all local authorities, although often the duties of analyst fell on already overworked MOsH. However, scientific inaccuracy, political jockeying, and professional controversy—what I have called "conflicts of analysis"—mired the science of milk analysis in the second half of the nineteenth century.[69]

As we have seen, Taylor's 1858 study of milk-borne typhoid received little notice. Ballard's 1870 investigation at Islington earned widespread professional notice and praise. But it was not until three years later, in the fall of 1873, that the milk-borne hypothesis entered a broader public discourse. It came as a result of a notorious outbreak of typhoid among London's wealthy, West End elite. It was known as the "Marylebone Milk Crisis."

---

68 "Dr. Ballard's Report upon an Outbreak of Enteric Fever at Armley, in the Borough of Leeds," 11, NA, MH 113/11.

69 Steere-Williams, "A Conflict of Analysis."

The Marylebone Milk Crisis of 1873

On Saturday, April 18, 1874, Sir Thomas Watson, physician-in-ordinary to Queen Victoria, delivered a private address before a group of London elites gathered at Charles Murchison's home on Wimpole Street. Watson's speech, of "great eloquence and force," was a recognition of Murchison's dogged sagacity the previous summer in tracing a virulent outbreak of typhoid fever in Marylebone to milk distributed by the Dairy Reform Company. Watson presented Murchison with a testimonial, signed by a hundred residents—doctors, colonels, lords, and baronesses—and with a pair of candlesticks and a timepiece, the latter bearing the inscription, "Presented to Charles Murchison, M.D., F.R.S., L.L.D., on April 18, 1874, in admiration of his sagacity in detecting, and his courage in exposing, the cause of the outbreak of Enteric Fever in the Western Districts of London in 1873."[70] Though flattered by the event, Murchison must have been miffed that his friends engraved the watch with "enteric" rather than "pythogenic" fever, a fitting reminder that theoretical knowledge on typhoid was giving way to Budd's ideas.

The Marylebone Milk Crisis, or as Ernest Hart later called it, "The Great Marylebone Epidemic of 1873," began and ended at Murchison's home. Recall from the introduction of this chapter that Murchison had found no fault with the sanitary arrangements of his Wimpole Street home to account for five of his children being struck with typhoid. So, on August 4, 1873, he turned to his neighboring friends, including William Jenner and Ernest Hart, where in house after house he found the same pattern. The children and some servants were sick with typhoid, but the owners were spared. Like his own, the homes of his medical colleagues were without sanitary fault. Within hours of making house calls in Marylebone, Murchison narrowed his search to the milk from the Dairy Reform Company (DRC), whose central office at 29 Orchard Street was a mere ten-minute stroll from his house. Nearly all of the victims purchased milk from this particular source. Murchison was familiar enough with the mounting evidence that milk could spread typhoid after Ballard's 1870 Islington study and never strayed from

---

70 "The Murchison Address and Testimonial," *British Medical Journal* 695 (April 25, 1874): 555. The testimonial was originally written on October 10 by John Murray, five days before his death. See Murchison Papers, RCP MS 710, titled "Original Proof of Testimonial Written by Dr. Murray Five Days Before His Death on October 15th."

a milk-borne hypothesis during the 1873 outbreak. And while he continued to gather facts to support his suspicions, on the afternoon of August 4, Murchison turned to John Whitmore, the MOH for the parish of St. Marylebone.

Whitmore held the post of Marylebone's MOH from the early 1860s until ill health forced him to retire in 1879. He was seventy when he died in 1880. Originally trained as an apothecary-surgeon, Whitmore obtained an MD at the University of St. Andrews before settling in London as MOH, succeeding Dundas Thomson. He was an active but not especially vocal MOH, taking on additional responsibilities as analytical chemist and gas inspector in the early 1870s. Murchison had used simple case tracing and statistical comparison to suggest the culpability of the DRC's milk. The initial evidence was convincing enough for Whitmore. On the same day that Murchison came to him, August 4, Whitmore went to the dairy to speak with the manager. Later that day Whitmore wrote a letter to the Dairy Reform Company. His communiqué was tepid but nonetheless suggestive. Whitmore, not directly accusing the DRC, called it a "remarkable coincidence" that children and servants sick with typhoid had all drank DRC milk. Following Murchison's plea, Whitmore suggested that it was his "duty" as MOH for the parish to insist that the DRC take "serious consideration the necessity of your at once ceasing to supply the public with milk obtained from your present sources."[71] A response came the following day from the hand of the DRC's secretary and manager, D. S. D. Maconochie. He assured Whitmore that the company had "made a very full investigation" into all the London districts that received DRC milk and found no complaints other than in Marylebone. They were the best dairy company in London, Maconochie argued, "so I cannot believe the cases of typhoid fever . . . can really be traceable in any way to the produce which we send to our customers."[72] But Maconochie's tone was defensive. Whitmore's allegation—if it even was one—might hurt their business. Besides, Maconochie grilled Whitmore, had he even analyzed the water of the houses in question? Were there cases other than among those who drank DRC milk?

Whitmore was no stranger to the milk supply of Marylebone, but his mild response to the DRC was no doubt shaped by a recent professional disaster. In the summer of 1873 Whitmore had undertaken a special investigation of

71   "The Dairy Reform Company and the Typhoid Outbreak in London," *British Medical Journal* 663 (13 September 1873): 336.

72   Ibid.

the quality of milk sold in Marylebone. Having just been dually appointed public analyst under the Public Health Act of 1872, it was his first foray into food analysis. He had chosen milk as his initial subject of study, "because this article constitutes the sole nutriment of Infants, and to a very large extent the diet of young children, and because, also, their vigorous and healthy growth must in a great degree depend upon its purity."[73] He produced the special report in June 1873 to the Marylebone vestry, just as cases of typhoid started to appear in his parish. Out of 62 samples of milk, Whitmore found that 22 were genuine, 15 deteriorated, and 25 adulterated.[74] Whitmore was confident that he was fulfilling his new duties with diligence and care, even ending his report by declaring that "if at a future period Milk is brought to me that is found to be adulterated, it will be my duty to recommend the Vestry to prosecute the Vendor of it."[75] The report quickly made its way to the medical press, and soon it blew up in the rather naïve Whitmore's face. *The Pharmaceutical Journal* noted that Whitmore had "insufficient familiarity with the details of analytical work."[76] Whitmore's "absurd and confused" report, they noted, was exactly why MOsH should not be serving double duty as public analysts. *The BMJ* likewise lambasted Whitmore, calling on the authority of Wanklyn to show that Whitmore was "quite at sea" in his methods of milk analysis and probably not fit for office.[77] Whitmore had mistakenly argued that the percentage of water in a sample of milk alone dictated whether it was adulterated, which Wanklyn showed was erroneous in his manual *Milk Analysis*, completed in November 1873.[78]

It had been a blow to his ego and accounts for Whitmore's initially cautious approach to the DRC. The confrontation with the DRC did not go well initially for Whitmore. He had learned from Maconochie's first letter that the DRC's board of directors was meeting that afternoon and requested that he attend. But instead of questioning the DRC, Whitmore was the one under fire. Had he ever analyzed DRC milk? (he had) Was it ever found to be adulterated? (It had not.) Did he analyze the water supplied to houses

73   Whitmore, *Report of the Medical Officer*, 3–4.

74   "The Adulteration of Food in Marylebone," *Food, Water, & Air* 1 (November 1871): 91.

75   Whitmore, *Annual Report*.

76   "The Adulteration Act," *Pharmaceutical Journal* 32 (June 7, 1873): 979.

77   "Detection of Adulteration of Milk," *British Medical Journal* 647 (May 24, 1873): 594.

78   Wanklyn, *Milk Analysis*.

with typhoid? (He had not.) It was not the meeting Whitmore had expected. One of the DRC's directors, William Hope, noted that Whitmore was "disillusioned," likely Murchison's puppet, and that even Whitmore himself did not believe that the DRC's milk was the problem.[79] Hope admitted that at least he, unlike the other two directors, entertained the idea that DRC milk might be at fault. He convinced his partners to draft a letter to all of the farms that supplied the company with milk and to inquire about the health of their employees. They also let Whitmore inspect the Orchard Street operations and interview the employees. Finding no problems, the directors considered the whole matter a "false alarm." Even Whitmore seemed to agree in part. He reported to the Marylebone vestry that the August 5 meeting had "satisfied me that there was nothing in the condition of the premises to account for the outbreak, nor did it appear possible that the milk could be contaminated either by the milk carriers or any other persons employed by the company at the dairy."[80] But the meeting had not ruled out the DRC milk, and the board had not proved that the milk was not contaminated before it came into their possession in London.

Whitmore continued with what saw as the due diligence of an MOH. He wrote to the London medical journals asking that any cases of typhoid be brought to his attention, and he drew up a circular asking the same of every doctor in the parish. He was staggered by the response, receiving 200 answers, bringing the number of families struck to 90 and individuals attacked to 320. Whitmore found the cases "are of the most interesting kind and tend to prove incontestably that they owed their origin to the infected milk."[81] It was becoming clear to Whitmore that the outbreak was beyond his control, so he made three decisive moves on August 7. The first was to inform the Marylebone vestry of the widespread nature of the outbreak and the strong likelihood that it was due to DRC milk. The second was to visit John Simon's office at the Medical Department, where he pleaded that he might "have the assistance of some gentleman from his department," not "because I felt personally incompetent to the task, but because it was apparent that the origin of the outbreak was to be sought for in places far away from the Parish

---

79   Hope, "The Dairy Reform Company," 337.

80   John Whitmore, *Report of the Medical Officer of Health, on the Recent Epidemic of Typhoid or Enteric Fever, St. Marylebone*, September 23, 1873, Parkes Pamphlet Collection, Wellcome Library, Box 89, Volume 53.

81   Whitmore, *Report of the Medical Officer of Health*, 6.

of St. Marylebone, beyond which I could exercise no power of authority."[82] Simon at first balked at the request, believing Whitmore capable of inquiring and not wanting to meddle with the business of an MOH. But he agreed and put John Netten Radcliffe on the case. Whitmore's third decision on August 7 was to write again to the DRC, presenting the mounting evidence against their milk "in terms as strong as I felt justified in using . . . warning them that, by neglecting to do so, they would be alone responsible for the ill consequences that might thereby ensue."[83] Maconochie doubled down, saying Whitmore's "hypothesis" was a "slur on our good name."[84] The DRC would gladly stop the sale of their milk, Maconochie added, if the vestry compensated them for "the loss and injury they may sustain in loss of profit and reputation."[85] It was a bad look for the DRC, and Murchison and the medical press later took the statement to show that the company's interest in profit was secondary to their commitment to the public's health.

The following day, on August 8, the DRC received a letter from Simon at the Medical Department stating that John Netten Radcliffe was beginning an investigation that should be fully assisted. Bringing in Radcliffe, a government official and expert on waterborne disease and leading English epidemiologist, must have worried the DRC, as they responded with their own hired guns: William Corfield, MOH for St. George's parish, and J. Chalmers Morton, a noted agriculturalist and one of Edward Frankland's longtime assistants with the Rivers Pollution Commission. Morton was also the editor of the *Agricultural Gazette* and a prominent member of the Royal Agricultural College. But although the DRC might have hoped the expertise of Morton and Corfield could be pitted against Whitmore and Radcliffe, things worked out quite differently. Early in the morning of Saturday, August 9, Radcliffe met with Whitmore and Murchison to get up to speed on the details of the outbreak, and at 10:00 a.m. Radcliffe and Whitmore proceeded to the DRC's office where Corfield, Morton, Hope, and Maconochie were waiting. It was anything but dramatic or contentious, despite the escalating tension between Whitmore and Maconochie. Radcliffe noted that although the DRC was "unconvinced" that their milk was at fault, they "offered every

82   Whitmore, *Report of the Medical Officer of Health*, 3.

83   Whitmore, *Report of the Medical Officer of Health*, 2.

84   "The Dairy Reform Company and the Typhoid Outbreak in London," *British Medical Journal* 663 (13 September 1873): 336.

85   Whitmore, *Report of the Medical Officer of Health*, 2.

facility for pursuing the investigation."[86] Though he said little of Morton, Radcliffe was pleased that Corfield was there and that he "had the advantage of his co-operation."[87] It came as no surprise that Corfield had been an occasional inspector at the Medical Department, and he and Radcliffe served as joint secretaries of the Epidemiological Society of London from 1870 to 1872. At the DRC meeting, Corfield and Radcliffe agreed that all eight of the DRC farms should be inspected. The DRC consented, drawing up a list and a map for their investigation, which would begin Monday morning.

In the meantime, Radcliffe spent the rest of the day Saturday and all of Sunday conducting his own outbreak investigation of Marylebone. Whitmore and Murchison had done as much, but Radcliffe inquired personally into a number of cases and inspected the house drainage, water supply, and sewerage of the area. He wanted to make sure all signs pointed to the DRC, and without much difficulty he, too, settled on the evidence implicating the milk. In about 24 hours Radcliffe had inspected and interviewed 28 households where typhoid was present; 26 of them received DRC milk. As Murchison had already shown, Radcliffe corroborated that cases were limited to children or adults who frequently consumed milk. Typhoid, Radcliffe found in the limited time he had studying the outbreak in Marylebone on August 9 and 10, "picked out as it were the houses supplied from the particular dairy . . . the disease picked out the members who drank the suspected milk, and those only."[88] The area where the disease raged was supplied by two water companies, the West Middlesex and the Grand Junction, and Radcliffe found nothing suggestive of fecal contamination.

On Monday morning, August 11, Radcliffe, Whitmore, Corfield, and Morton set off to investigate the eight farms in Oxfordshire. The group, akin to a "royal commission," that favorite arm of Victorian inquiry, agreed to examine five sanitary factors at each farm: the drainage and nature of the soil, the quality and quantity of water supply, the health of the cows, the health of the occupants and laborers, and the methods of milking. Even before the field investigations began, Radcliffe, typical of epidemiologists at the time, was already trying to narrow the search to an index case of sorts: the farm that supplied the contaminated milk. He had pulled mortality returns from the GRO for the first and second quarters of 1873, which showed that

---

86 Radcliffe, "Preliminary Report," 132.
87 Ibid.
88 Radcliffe, "Preliminary Report," 133.

three of the eight farms were in subdistricts rife with typhoid, indicative of a broadening methodological scope of outbreak investigation.

The group visited the first six farms on August 12, and all proved in sanitary order and above suspicion that typhoid-laced excreta had found its way into the milk supply. That evening, however, consulting with M. H. Humphreys, a local surgeon in Thame (where the two remaining farms were located), the group uncovered new evidence: the owner of Chilton Grove Farm, Mr. Jessop, had died under suspicious circumstances. From the second week of May, Jessop had been sick, ailing under a fever and profuse bloody diarrhea. Humphreys diagnosed him with "latent" typhoid fever and told Mrs. Jessop to place all of her husband's diarrheal dejections into the ash heap, instead of the privy, to prevent the dangerous accumulation of typhoid gas. Although he seemed to be convalescing the first week of June, Jessop collapsed and died on June 8. Humphreys listed the official cause of death as "heart disease" but later admitted that he should have listed "typhoid fever" instead. It was a "grave suspicion," and even before they went to inspect the farm the following day, Corfield, on the evening of June 12, sent a telegraph message to the DRC in London advising them to stop the distribution of milk from that particular farm.

They spent the entire day inspecting Chilton Grove Farm, a forty-cow operation situated in a valley between the villages of Brill and Chilton. The group first questioned the district MOH, G. W. Child, and tabulated the cases of typhoid that had occurred between June and August 1873 in the surrounding area. There were nine workers employed by the farm who came from the villages of Brill and Chilton, both of which were infected with typhoid preceding the Marylebone outbreak. Led by Radcliffe and Corfield, the investigators next carefully surveyed the farm for defects in drainage, water supply, and sewerage, which proved to be numerous. The whole place was "incommodious," "old," and "ramshackle."[89] The water supply, from an old eleven-foot-deep well on the premises located between the bedroom and the piggery (figure 3.2), was "manifestly polluted," Radcliffe noted, "so manifestly as to prevent its being used for ordinary drinking purposes."[90] Because of the increasing "distastefulness" of the well, the Jessop family drew their drinking water from a nearby spring. But they still used the well water for dairy operations. It was rather easy for Corfield and Radcliffe, experienced

---

89 Radcliffe and Power, "Report on an Outbreak of Enteric Fever in Marylebone," 122

90 Radcliffe, "Preliminary Report, 133.

in the investigation of waterborne outbreaks, to figure out how the well water had become contaminated. Soakage from the privy was initially thought to be the culprit, as it was situated some fifty feet above the well. But upon making a series of excavations from the well to the privy drain, they found no leaks. Radcliffe and Corfield then excavated on the south side of the well, along the farmyard wall, and found a leak in the well—once pumped free of water—and soakage all along the wall. In their diagram of Chilton Grove Farm (figure 3.3), the excavation sites are marked by dotted lines. It was now obvious why the water had tasted poorly and how the well had been contaminated. The well was in a recessed valley, and about twenty-five feet above it was the piggery, dung heap, and ash heap on the southeast side of the property. Discovering the leak in the well, which pointed directly at the ash heap and piggery, was an aha moment for Radcliffe. It all made sense: "by an unhappy and altogether unforeseen chance, and in carrying out precautions to obviate any possibility of mischief the matters from which mischief was most apt to arise were deposited in perhaps the only spot on the farm premises where they would certainly find their way into the water used for dairy *purposes.*"[91]

Though they had discovered exactly how the well water was contaminated with the discharges of Mr. Jessop, they still had not proved how excreta-laced water was mixed with the milk sent to London. And Radcliffe and Corfield never did. They knew from interviewing laborers on the farm that the well water was used for dairy purposes—cleaning churns and utensils—but none admitted deliberate adulteration. The group never sorted out the precise method of infection. Radcliffe argued, however, that did not matter, as such solutions "will probably prove insuperable," and "does not in the least militate against the evidence of infection." The stakes of preventive action were too high, Radcliffe warned, and "probability" must "not wait upon a minute etiological elaboration."[92] Corfield had already telegraphed the DRC to warn them to discard the Chilton Grove Farm milk—which they promptly disinfected and threw away. Radcliffe, too, on August 13, sent a telegram to Murchison in London, which simply and confidently noted "source

---

91   Radcliffe and Power, "Report on and Outbreak of Enteric Fever in Marylebone," 125. Italics in original. Radcliffe had sent water for analysis to Dupre in London, who found that sewage contamination was all but certain.
92   Radcliffe and Power, "Report on and Outbreak of Enteric Fever in Marylebone," 126–27. Their argument still being made a decade later. See Hart, "The Influence of Milk," 492.

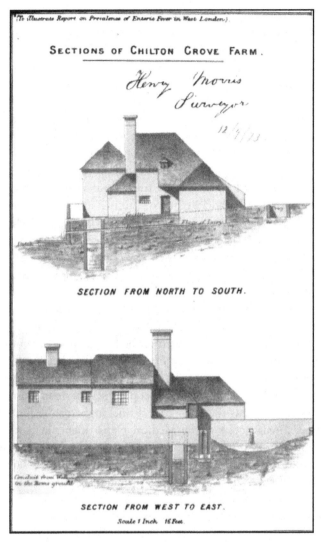

Figure 3.2 Diagram of Chilton Grove Farm. From John Netten Radcliffe and W. H. Power, "Report on an Outbreak of Enteric Fever in Marylebone and the Adjoining Parts of London," in Annual Report of the Medical Officer of the Local Government Board for 1872. Parliamentary Papers (London: Eyre and Spottiswoode, 1873). House of Commons Parliamentary Papers, Crown Copyright.

dis-covered and stopped."[93] Corfield called the whole matter an "accident that . . . could not have been foreseen."[94] Mrs. Jessop, now running the farm, was also compliant; she insisted that the milk should not be distributed and immediately ceased to use the leaky well.

To Radcliffe, Corfield, and Whitmore—who returned to London on August 13—the entire ordeal was an exemplary model of collaborative outbreak investigation.[95] Whitmore had learned of the suspected milk on August 4. The Medical Department began its inquiry four days later. By August 12 the mischief was discovered, and the distribution of the milk was stopped. "It will rarely happen that the source of an outbreak of the kind under consideration will be so readily traced and rapidly followed out as in the present instance," Radcliffe noted. From Radcliffe's perspective both the DRC and the farm owners were compliant with his investigation, and a potential rival, Corfield, was actually on his side. The two used statistical evidence and induction to narrow their gaze onto the milk. They utilized evolving methods of outbreak investigation such as interviewing and case tracing to discover an index case and employed environmental and spatial knowledge to dissect the Chilton Grove Farm. The diagram (figure 3.2) was consistent with the methods of outbreak investigation at the department, but the additional inclusion of a sketch of the farm (figure 3.3) provided yet another visual tool in outbreak investigation and the rhetorical communication of epidemiological arguments. Whereas most epidemiological studies took place in a limited geographical scope, the Marylebone investigation began in London and was traced to a rural Buckinghamshire farm, marking it an unprecedented success at the Medical Department, in particular, and in English epidemiology in general. Less than a year later, J. C. Morton and the Rivers Pollution Commission noted that it was a grave "illustration of the way in which the water supply to a country place may affect the health of town populations."[96] But the success, gauged by Radcliffe's epidemiological criteria, was mitigated by the reality that the investigation was post facto, and the outbreak was probably over before the discovery of the problems at

---

93   Telegram from Radcliffe to Murchison, August 13, 1873, RCP, Murchison, Personal Papers, MS 710.

94   Corfield, "Typhoid Fever in Marylebone," 7.

95   Radcliffe returned to Chilton Grove Farm on August 19 to ensure that the milk was not being sent for purchase and that the well was disused. Both were in order.

96   *Rivers Pollution Commission*, 415.

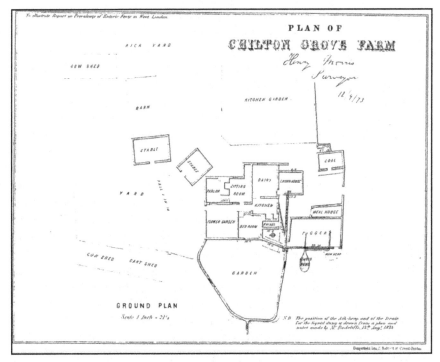

Figure 3.3. Sketch of Chilton Grove Farm. From John Netten Radcliffe and
W.H. Power, "Report on an Outbreak of Enteric Fever in Marylebone and the
Adjoining Parts of London," in Annual Report of the Medical Officer of the
Local Government Board for 1872. Parliamentary Papers (London: Eyre and
Spottiswoode, 1873). House of Commons Parliamentary Papers, Crown Copyright.

Chilton Grove Farm. This point was not lost on Radcliffe, who lamented
that the state of rural sanitary arrangements and misguided sanitary legislation would lead to more milk crises.

Radcliffe spent August 14 and 15 preparing a preliminary report for the
Medical Department, but he knew a complete inquiry was needed back
in Marylebone. Simon provided Radcliffe's colleague W. H. Power to help
with what was a several-month-long study. In their final report, included in
Simon's famous *Filth-Diseases and Their Prevention* supplemental report for
1874, Radcliffe and Power began with quantitative evidence of the milk-
borne route of the outbreak. Of the 244 cases, 218 (nine-tenths) were in
households that obtained milk from the DRC. Through intricate case

tracing and interviewing, the case became even more striking, and they found numerous examples like the following:

> The mistress and the kitchenmaid were the only persons in a family who habitually drank uncooked milk: they both had enteric fever. Two children in the same family who did not take milk in this form escaped. A physician, in the habit of taking nightly half a pint or more of cold milk, "as it came from the dairy," was the only person in his household who did so, he alone had enteric fever.[97]

Anecdotal, individualized examples were crucial for cementing the epidemiological chain of evidence; however, remember that they were marshalled after the Chilton Grove Farm had been shown to be the culprit. The diagram and illustration, likewise, only appeared in the final report as confirmatory and persuasive tools to prove the source of the outbreak.

While Radcliffe and Power were investigating granular facts surrounding the outbreak into August and September, and as cases dwindled and the distribution of milk from Chilton Grove stopped, the Marylebone Milk Crisis raged in the press. Continuing his own line of inquiry, Murchison teamed up with England's other fever expert, William Jenner, his Marylebone neighbor and longtime London Fever Hospital colleague. Together the two wrote to the DRC on August 11 warning them to stop the sale of their milk lest it extend the outbreak.[98] They also enlisted the help of another influential colleague and Marylebone resident Ernest Hart, whose children, like Murchison's, had sickened with typhoid. Though he later took to the pen, Hart, the editor of the *British Medical Journal*, first took to foot, visiting the DRC office on Orchard Street. But just like he had with Whitmore, Murchison, and Jenner, Hope dismissed Hart as well, insisting that it was "mere coincidences" that those who were sick had been supplied with DRC milk. Radcliffe had reported that Hope was "unconvinced" early on about the milk-borne hypothesis, but at least he was open to the epidemiological investigation. To Murchison, Jenner, and Hart, the DRC was flat-out combative. Hope was so perturbed by Hart's visit on August 11 that he brought him to the mixing and bottling operation of the Orchard Street office, took up a tumbler full of milk, and drank it to prove that it was harmless. The

---

97 Radcliffe and Power, "Report on and Outbreak of Enteric Fever in Marylebone," 116.

98 Murchison, "The Dairy Reform Company," 7.

performance left Hart unimpressed, and he left the office not wanting to argue further with "a gentleman who regarded it as an act of heroism to drink the milk which was being supplied to his customers."[99]

The case against the DRC quickly heated up following Corfield's public pronouncement in the *Times* on August 14 that the milk-borne theory was correct and the Chilton Grove Farm, through an "accident," was to blame. Hart, who had tried in vain to persuade Hope in private, turned to the pages of the *British Medical Journal*, listing a series of individual cases he obtained from Murchison, in which DRC milk drinkers alone were attacked with typhoid. The outbreak was, Hart noted, "something in the nature of a vital experiment, such as physiologists would employ to test a case."[100] Hart shamed the DRC for not stopping the sale of their milk sooner, when Whitmore and Murchison warned them on August 4. "It is impossible to tell how much damage has been done," he noted gravely. Hart's article was followed by a full rundown of the investigation by Corfield, who praised Radcliffe's skill in leading the epidemiological investigation of the DRC farms. Throughout the report, Corfield's tone against the DRC was measured. The outbreak was a "lamentable accident," which "will tend in the end to the ensuring of much greater safety than at present exists in the matter of the milk-supply of the metropolis. It is impossible to say at present what dairy might not be the cause of a similar outbreak."[101] A follow-up article by Hart, on August 23, repeated as much, saying that the Marylebone outbreak provided "a remarkable stimulus" to sanitary science.[102]

The whole matter might have been put to rest had it not been for an attempt by the DRC's manager, Maconochie, to save face. In a "manifesto" in the *Times* on August 26, Maconochie started with an admission of guilt.[103] It was "painful and humiliating in the extreme" that the DRC's milk was to blame.[104] He was right in part. That the DRC was embroiled in the biggest dairy-related scandal to date in England was somewhat ironic. Founded in 1867, the company began as a new enterprise whose chief aim was to correct the rampantly adulterated and inconsistent supply of milk to

99   Hart, "The Dairy Reform Company," 338.
100   Hart, "The Outbreak of Typhoid Fever," 206.
101   Cofield, "The Source of Infection," 208.
102   "The Outbreak of Typhoid Fever in London," *British Medical Journal* 660 (August 23, 1873): 230.
103   "Sanitary Science and the Milk Panic," *Engineer* 36 (August 29, 1873): 137.
104   Maconochie, "The Late Typhoid Epidemic," 8.

the metropolis—particularly to the upper classes. In an advertisement for the DRC in the first edition of the *Milk Journal*—the same edition that featured Ballard's Islington study and came out publicly in favor of the milk-borne theory—the company proudly publicized that "this Company established four years ago for the sale of Pure Milk and Cream, has met with such continued and hearty support from the Public, that its deliveries now cover a very large portion of London."[105] The advertisement noted that the company was committed to seven principles: unadulterated produce, imperial measures, moderate prices, regularity of delivery, punctuality and correctness of accounts, immediate investigation of all complaints, and weekly payments (and for small quantities, cash on delivery). In February 1871, shortly after Ballard's Islington investigation linked milk to typhoid, the company filed to conduct their business under the limited liability law, which provided a kind of shareholder immunity, so that if indicted, investors could not lose personal assets.[106] The DRC widely advertised that "the means the Directors possess of preventing Adulteration of the Produce . . . are complete and absolute," and we "will continue in the future as in the past to give that personal attention to the business which has made its success."[107] By 1873, in other words, the DRC was fully aware of the dangers of adulterated milk, and had striven to prevent fecal pollution in their supply. They even hired a chemist to analyze the milk coming from the eight farms twice a day. It was always rich and free from suspicion, they argued.

Maconochie's *Times* article insisted that what happened at Chilton Grove was an anomaly. The DRC was recommitted to the purity of its milk. Maconochie announced a new plan of continuous medical, veterinary, and chemical inspection. Each week London doctors would visit each farm. District MOsH would inquire about the health of workers. Veterinary surgeons would inspect the cows. More analytical chemists would be hired. It was a lacteal version of Benjamin Ward Richardson's *Hygeia*, sanitary surveillance *par excellence*.[108] But sprinkled in Maconochie's *Times* article was a not-so-masked animosity at the whole ordeal. "Some persons," Maconochie

---

105 "The Dairy Reform Company," *Milk Journal* 1 (1871): 6.

106 Dairy Reform Company, "Memorandum of Association of the Dairy Reform Company, Limited," Board of Trade, BT/1/591/5277, National Archives, Kew.

107 "The Dairy Reform Company," *Milk Journal* 3 (1871): 30.

108 Richardson, *Hygeia*. Cassedy, "Hygeia." Such sanitary supervision on dairy farms would not come to pass until the very late nineteenth century. But some notable early examples of dairy farms that voluntarily reformed before

noted, "have not yet been able to bring themselves to consider the evidence against the milk as conclusive." He never cited the names of these mysterious medical observers but noted how some thought the outbreak was due to sewer gases. Children after all, he observed, were physically closer to sewer drains and often ran with their mouths open. Others, Maconochie maintained, thought the contaminated Thames water was to blame or that typhoid was imported from Belgium, Munich, or Vienna. Moreover, Maconochie grasped at hypothetical lines of spurious defense—that Murchison had sat on the information for too long, Whitmore had been uninformed, and Radcliffe was mum as to details of the case. In other words, it was not their fault.

The following day, a leading *Times* writer characterized Maconochie's excuses as "a farrago of nonsense which is scarcely worth the trouble of serious refutation." Maconochie's attempt was pathetic, the article noted, and if the DRC was the top dairy in London, with scientific backing and prestige, they could not have been ignorant of the milk-borne hypothesis. To reinforce this point, the *Times* cited earlier investigations like Ballard's at Islington, which "have obtained a very wide publicity."[109] Because they were now dragged into what was amounting to a public scandal, Whitmore and Murchison responded in the *Times*, defending their actions and the timing of their warnings. The whole matter especially irked Murchison, who became increasingly vocal and aggressive against the DRC, who, he argued, was not only lying about the early advice he and Whitmore had given but had put profit before lives.[110] Maconochie, frustrated by what he had started, wailed in the *Times* on September 3, "What is it that Dr. Murchison wants? . . . Why, therefore, is he attacking us now, when all danger is over?" Murchison's attack, which was really just a rejoinder, had amounted to an accusation of "manslaughter of an aggravated character," and Maconochie mocked that someone should bring forward a lawsuit against the DRC, confident that they had done nothing wrong.[111] The situation had blown up in Maconochie's face, and he was not willing to admit it.

Hart, bothered by the DRC's fainthearted apology and their shaming of Whitmore and Murchison, went even further, publishing the private letters

---

compulsory legislation and had outstanding sanitary oversight include the Aylesbury Dairy Company. See Steere-Williams, "Milking Science for its Worth."

109 "Editorial," *Times*, August 27, 1873, 7.
110 Murchison, "Typhoid Fever and the Public Health," 5.
111 Maconochie, "Dr. Murchison and the Dairy Reform Company," 3.

between Whitmore, Murchison, and the DRC in the *BMJ*. This brought DRC director William Hope back into the fray, and he threatened to sue Hart for libel. In his version of events, the DRC had not looked so bad. Hope, selling out his partners at the DRC, claimed that he had originally considered Whitmore's suspicions but had the "greatest difficulty in getting my colleagues to admit, or rather to discuss, for they would not admit, the possibility that our milk" was "poisonous." Whitmore had not even been sure of the milk theory, he added, and the DRC had afforded Radcliffe every assistance. They even hired Corfield and Morton to investigate in full. When they received Corfield's telegram on August 13, they accepted the evidence, Hope noted, and immediately stopped the sale of the Chilton Grove Farm milk. It was epidemiological inquiry that was needed, Hope noted, not the premonitions of "some doctors." In a curious way, Hope was privileging the professional expertise of Radcliffe at the Medical Department over the private investigation of Murchison and Jenner. Murchison and Jenner's letters had been, in other words, "not sufficiently authoritative," Hope boasted, and they had been "neither courteous, nor in the interest of the public."[112] Hart, who as editor of the *British Medical Journal* kept the last word for himself, called it a "gross attack" on Murchison. The whole conduct of the DRC was "blamably indolent," Hart concluded, and their letters "lamentable examples of perverted ingenuity and prejudiced statement."[113]

But it was Murchison in actual fact who gave the swan song to the Marylebone Milk Crisis. In late November 1873, as a presage to the private ceremony at his house on April 18, 1874, a group of "late customers of the Dairy Reform Company" presented Murchison with a testimonial that attested his "skill and perseverance" in tracing the outbreak to the DRC milk and lamented "the manner in which you have been publicly attacked by the manager and secretary of the Dairy Reform Company."[114]

112 W. Hope, September 3, see *British Medical Journal* (September 13, 1873): 337.
113 "The Dairy Reform Company and the Epidemic of Typhoid Fever in London," *British Medical Journal* 663 (20 September 1873): 360.
114 *Marylebone Mercury*, October 4, 1873; *Daily Telegraph*, December 13, 1873; *Observer*, April 19, 1874; *Medical Times and Gazette* (April 25, 1874). All clippings from RCP, Murchison Papers, MS 710.

Milk Purity Redefined

While it was Murchison who received public praise—no doubt because of the scandal in the press and his celebrity-like status—it was Radcliffe whose name was most closely remembered as the Marylebone Milk Crisis became a focal point in the history of Victorian public health. As the spat between Murchison, Whitmore, Hart, and the DRC faded, the epidemiological significance of the outbreak came into greater focus. *The Daily Telegraph* noted that "the light thrown by this report upon the powers of Science ought to arouse, and must arouse, the activity of those who are entrusted with the power to protect society."[115] Corfield, delivering a lecture titled "The Progress of Sanitary Science," before the Birmingham and Midland Institute in October of 1873, noted that with the discovery of the milk-borne route of transmission, typhoid was known with more etiological accuracy than any other infectious disease. The Marylebone Milk Crisis, he hoped, would elicit "one of the greatest sanitary improvements of the day."[116]

The Public Health Act of 1875 made the appointment of MOsH and public analysts compulsory throughout England and Wales, but that alone did not solve the milk problem. The series of compartmentalized laws, particularly the Contagious Diseases (Animals) Act of 1878, and the Dairies, Cow-Sheds, and Milk-Shops Order of 1885 went some way toward increased supervision of milk and dairy operations, but, in a moment of oversight, the legislation left the matter to police inspectors and veterinarians instead of MOsH. Compulsory legislation that covered the broad spectrum needed in order to prevent milk-borne outbreaks went unfulfilled until the early twentieth century, but the milk-borne studies at Islington and Marylebone were the first to raise widespread awareness and elevate public discourse on the milk issue. Murchison, playing down his part in the whole affair, agreed. The Marylebone investigation produced three highly beneficial outcomes: it gave publicity to the fact that milk-borne typhoid was not an etiological obscurity but a common occurrence, it encouraged preventive legislation to curb unsanitary milk practices, and it made milk consumers more aware of the potential dangers of adulterated milk.[117] There were powerful lessons to be learned, in other words, for sanitary science and for preventive public health.

---

115 *Daily Telegraph*, 1873. Clipping in RCP Murchison Papers, MS 710.

116 Corfield, "The Progress of Sanitary Science," 481.

117 *Medical Times and Gazette* (1874): 456, clipping in RCP, Murchison Papers, MS 710. Privately Murchison was obsessed with the entire incident. He kept

Knowledge and awareness of milk-borne typhoid became domesticated into the public health canon in the second half of the 1870s, as Ballard and Radcliffe were highlighted in manuals, handbooks, textbooks, and lecture courses. As lecturer on public health at St. Thomas's Hospital in the late 1890s and early 1900s, Edward Cox Seaton frequently lectured on the Marylebone outbreak as "one of the best" examples "to illustrate the methods of proper scientific epidemiological inquiry."[118] At the Medical Department, outbreak investigation shifted in subtle but important ways: it became standard practice while on outbreak investigation for typhoid, scarlet fever, and diphtheria to inspect the potentiality of a milk-borne route of transmission. Quite quickly the picture was becoming clear. W. H. Power, investigating an outbreak of typhoid traced to a contaminated milk supply at Eagley and Bolton in 1876, for example, briskly concluded, "The case is simply one more, and a serious one, added to those cases already on record which point to the urgent necessity for regulation and adequate supervision over the sanitary circumstances of dairy farms."[119]

By 1900 to qualify for the diploma in public health, the standard degree for MOsH, one had to answer sufficiently the following question: "What are the various circumstances that should arouse suspicion of an outbreak of infectious illness being due to the ingestion of specifically contaminated Milk or Water? Quote instances in support of your views."[120] There were many examples from which to choose, as by the 1880s knowledge about the transmission of epidemic disease through food (milk being the most important) was widely accepted. Francis Vacher, MOH for Birkenhead, noted in 1881 that food might spread disease in three ways: the food itself could be in a pathological state, the food could serve as a medium (or nidus) for the multiplication of disease germs, or the food could serve simply as a vehicle for germs.[121] This opened up the etiological door to considering an entire range of food- and water-related media, such as shellfish, ice cream, and raw vegetables. But epidemics of milk-borne typhoid continued, highlighting the

a scrapbook of newspaper cuttings and letters related to the Marylebone Milk Crisis, now held at the Royal College of Physicians, London.

118 Seaton, *Infectious Diseases*, 104.

119 Power, "Report to the Local Government Board on an Epidemic of Enteric Fever Occurring at Eagley," 7.

120 Examination Papers for Diploma in Public Health (1900), Wellcome Collection, MS.6807/17–23.

121 Vacher, "The Influence of Various Articles of Food," 489–90.

fractured state of English public health: urban versus rural sanitary authorities, the relative power of central versus local government, and a lack of combined veterinary, chemical, and epidemiological oversight.[122]

By the 1880s enough time had elapsed to start writing milk-borne outbreaks into the history of public health. It began with Ernest Hart, long a champion of the epidemiological gaze and the type of outbreak investigation common for a generation of epidemiologists at the Medical Department. In an address before the International Medical Congress in 1881, held in London, he read a paper titled "The Influence of Milk in Spreading Zymotic Disease," which was the first to collect, list, and tabulate a decade's worth of investigations of milk-borne typhoid. Hart listed fifty outbreaks of typhoid traced to milk and warned that stopping milk-borne outbreaks was "a question of urgent concern."[123] Sixteen years later, in 1897, at the end of his career in public health, Hart returned to the subject with a second study of "The Influence of Milk in Spreading Zymotic Disease," first published in the *British Medical Journal* and then separately as a pamphlet. By 1897 Hart listed forty-eight additional investigations of milk-borne typhoid, the majority of which were conducted out of the Medical Department, bringing the total to around one hundred in thirty years.[124]

The Islington and Marylebone outbreaks had illustrated some new problems of sanitary administration. Ballard's study was largely metropolitan; the dairy farmer assisted with the case, and Ballard had an intimate knowledge of both the local environment and the health of the population. In later studies MOsH had similar advantages, particularly in rural areas where population densities were low and networks of communication and the exchange of materials well known. Urban MOsH, particularly those whose constituents received milk from the countryside, widespread by the mid-1870s, had a much more difficult time conducting epidemiological studies. This was apparent to Marylebone's MOH John Whitmore in 1873, when his only recourse was to enlist the assistance of John Simon at the Medical Department. Appealing to the Medical Department—an advisory body— did not solve the jurisdictional problem, as rural sanitary authorities still maintained control over the production side of dairy farming. Parliamentary legislation, which was pushed by later public health advocates such as George

---

122 John Simon, Confidential Memo to the President of the Local Government Board, July 10, 1868, National Archvies, Kew, MH 113/2.

123 Hart, "The Influence of Milk," 494.

124 Hart, *A Report on the Influence of Milk.*

Newman, increasingly tried to nationalize the supervision of dairy production and milk transportation. It was only through epidemiological practices,
such as carefully tracking cases of typhoid fever in rural populations and
excavating drainpipes to search for leaks, that such legal and sanitary supervision was increasingly viewed as necessary. And it took high profile, sensationalized cases like the Marylebone Milk Crisis to bring about the change.

When we place the Marylebone outbreak alongside the Prince's near-death
typhoid bout in 1871 and the 1872 Thanksgiving, it is clear that typhoid
was one of the most important topics of concern in Britain. No doubt the
public discourse was being driven by class-based fears. Epidemiological studies at the Medical Department in the 1860s, like the ones highlighted in
chapter 1 that traced outbreaks of typhoid to sewer gases and sanitary defects
in middle- and upper-class homes had ignited a class-based association with
the disease. Outbreaks of milk-borne typhoid went even further to show, as a
review of Budd's 1873 *Typhoid Fever* in the *Edinburgh Medical Journal* noted,
that typhoid was "a fever which is pre-eminently fatal among the rich."[125]
Typhoid was becoming a model disease for sanitary reformers by the 1870s
in no small part because it was threatening burgeoning notions of middle-
class respectability. Newly installed water closets and pure milk were inexorably tied to middle- and upper-class identity by the 1870s, but these products
of so-called sanitary progress had also facilitated the spread of typhoid. The
epidemiological gaze, the developing methods of outbreak investigation, and
the performative ways that epidemiological knowledge was communicated
to professional and public audiences, had wrought a new kind of palpable
fear.

A comical leading article in the *Engineer* during the Marylebone Milk
Crisis suggested the bewildering sanitary responsibilities being placed on "the
careful man." "We live in troublous times," it began, "in fact we hardly know
whether we live at all . . . few things are more bewildering than the methods
of precaution prescribed." First it was the water, filled with contaminating
excreta. Water should be filtered and boiled, people are instructed, and cis-
terns emptied and cleansed each week. And then people learned that dangerous sewer gases lurked in drains. Look to the waterclosets, and "attend to
every foul smell" and "see that every stench-trap is in perfect order." Empty
the dustbins, strip away the arsenic-laced green paper. Be wary of alum in
your bread and chicory in your coffee. And now it was milk. "The careful

---

125 "Review of William Budd's *Typhoid Fever*," *Edinburgh Medical Journal* 19
    (1874): 820.

man . . . feels confident that whatever else may be wrong, he is at least supplied with lacteal draughts of the very finest quality . . . but the too confident householder turns almost as white as the contents of the milk jug, when he reads in the morning paper that this milk is strongly suspected of disseminating typhoid fever![126] Now milk, too, had to be protected. But it was not the last in the pantheon of the "careful man"—soon epidemiological expertise would show that shellfish and ice cream could spread typhoid fever as well. And, after the discovery of B. typhosus in the early 1880s, there was a new set of fears, particularly about the role and life cycle of microbes outside of the body. Typhoid prowled English soils, the subject of the following chapter.

---

126 "Sanitary Science and the Milk Panic," *Engineer* 36 (29 August 1873): 137.

Chapter Four

Soils, Stools, and Saprophytes

Epidemiology in the Age of Bacteriology

In the days surrounding Christmas 1874 Edward Klein was busy examining the stools of typhoid patients. Klein was working alongside John Burdon Sanderson—they were both subordinates of John Simon—in a special branch of the Medical Department colloquially known as "auxiliary scientific investigations."[1] On December 14 Klein received fresh stools of a patient who had been laboring for three weeks under the delirious fever spell of typhoid. On December 26, Boxing Day, he received more fresh stools from a second typhoid patient. They were "ochre-coloured, thin, composed of a clear fluid in which were suspended pale yellowish small and larger flakes and lumps," Klein observed, "the well-known" characteristics of typhoid excreta. Klein macerated the fresh stools, mixed them with water, and bottled the concoction. With the aid of a microscope, he found what he was after: colonies of isolated, spherical micrococci "of a very characteristic appearance" (figure 4.1, marked "M"). When incubated for 24 hours at 39 degrees Celsius, they grew in number. In ten days, they were still growing "to an enormous extent."[2]

Klein had been at this for over a year, ever since the Marylebone Milk Crisis in the fall of 1873. He was probably the most dogged typhoid researcher in all of Europe, experimenting in his London laboratory on typhoid nearly every year until his death in 1910. It had been known from the late 1830s that typhoid produced pathological lesions in the small intestine. But not enough attention had been paid, Klein believed, to the "minute

---

1   On the Brown Institute, see Wilkinson, *Animals and Disease*, 163–81.
2   Klein, "Report on the Intimate Anatomical Changes," 82–83.

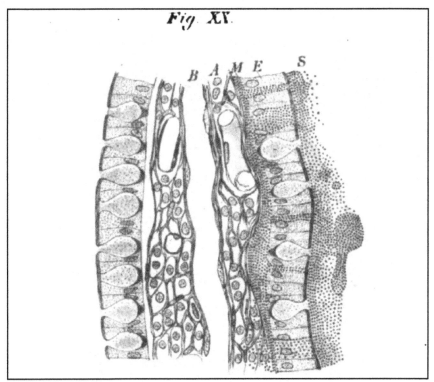

Figure 4.1 Supposed germs of typhoid fever. From Edward Klein, "Report on the Intimate Anatomical Changes in Enteric or Typhoid Fever," in Annual Report of the Medical Officer of the Local Government Board. Parliamentary Papers (London: Eyre and Spottiswoode, 1875), 105–6. House of Commons Parliamentary Papers, Crown Copyright.

anatomy" of the disease. To what was only slowly coming to be called "bacteriology." Armed with over a decade's worth of "clinical observation" and "etiological data," in other words, epidemiological evidence, Klein believed as did his department colleagues that "the contagion of enteric fever is a living organism."[3] It was an echo of Budd's widely cited claim from his 1873 study *Typhoid Fever* and a germ theory in line with other Darwin-inspired doctors like Burdon-Sanderson and James Russell. If the poison, or germ, was to be found anywhere, Klein presumed, it would be in excreta and in

---

3   Klein, "Report on the Intimate Anatomical Changes," 80.

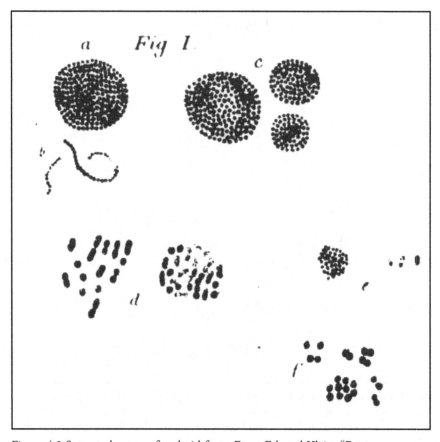

Figure 4.2 Supposed germs of typhoid fever. From Edward Klein, "Report on the Intimate Anatomical Changes in Enteric or Typhoid Fever," in Annual Report of the Medical Officer of the Local Government Board. Parliamentary Papers (London: Eyre and Spottiswoode, 1875), 105–6. House of Commons Parliamentary Papers, Crown Copyright.

and around the lesions in the small intestine. From September 1873 Klein had arranged with P. H. Mackellar to perform pathological dissections on recently diseased typhoid patients at the Stockwell Fever Hospital, the first built by the Metropolitan Asylums Board, in 1871. Collecting, preserving, and examining sections of hardened ileum with a Harnack's eyepiece from sixteen typhoid victims, Klein had found the same spherical micrococci in the epithelial cells that he was hunting after in typhoid stools a year later.[4] Klein had already reported his initial finding. But he did so first to the German medical community, in the September issue of *Centralblatt für die medicinischen Wissenschaften*.[5] It was a telling blow to the English scientific community, and Klein's research was only picked up domestically when he translated a preliminary notice to the *BMJ* in early December.[6] A full report came in 1875, in the annual report for the Medical Department, which had funded his research. Klein summarized that it was "highly probable that the presence of these organisms bears an important relation to the diseased parts, being perhaps the chief of the causes of the death—ulceration—of the lymphatic follicles."[7] It was hardly a triumphant statement for what might have amounted to one of the most important discoveries in medical science. Despite Klein's ambivalence, Simon lauded the work as a "discovery," as "the first time the contagium of enteric fever [was] something cognizable to the eye."[8] Hamlin has argued that Simon was quick to use the science of water analysis "to rationalize" his own "social reforms."[9] But as we have already seen, Simon and his inspectors at times dismissed evidence from the laboratory, demonstrating the rhetorical and performative ways that laboratory science was combined with epidemiological outbreak investigation.

---

4   There is some evidence that Klein was corresponding with Charles Darwin on the matter. Darwin's son Francis was studying under Klein at the Brown in 1873 and may have heard about Klein's typhoid research. Klein had visited Darwin's house in April 1874, and Francis wrote to his father on June 26, 1873, telling him to order a Harnack's eyepiece, one of Klein's favorite instruments in his typhoid research, from France. In a letter to Darwin on July 24, 1874, Klein described the smallest size of the *micrococci* he was studying. Darwin's letter to Klein has not survived, however. See, E. E. Klein to Charles Darwin, July 24, 1874, Darwin Correspondence Project. https://www.darwin-project.ac.uk

5   Klein, "Zur Kenntniss," 706.

6   Klein, "On the Minute Pathology of Enteric Fever," 699–700. He had also pronounced the discovery of the germ of sheep pox. See Klein, "Research on the Smallpox of Sheep"; Brunton, "Dr. Klein and the Pathology."

7   Klein, "Report on the Intimate Anatomical Changes," 80.

8   Simon, *Annual Report of the Medical Officer of the Local Government Board*, Parliamentary Papers (London: Eyre and Spottiswoode, 1875), 5. Simon especially praised that all of the microscopical illustrations were done by Klein himself.

9   Hamlin, *Science of Impurity*, 236–37.

Klein's supposed discovery of the "germ" of typhoid, including the explosive but ultimately short-lived debate it produced, is a useful window into the heated debate about germs, and the relative value between laboratory and field approaches to studying disease. It is telling that Klein's research, although ultimately a failure, originated and was supported by Simon at the Medical Department. When Klein spoke of the "etiological data" proving that typhoid was caused by a living organism, he was referring to the practical work of inspectors at the Medical Department, whose views by the mid-1870s were more aligned with Budd than Murchison. The episode represents the early failure of bacteriology in the 1870s to settle contentious debates over typhoid, which should come as no surprise considering the already cautious approach to water and milk analysis on the part of British epidemiologists. But from the 1870s, as the example of Klein's micrococci shows, epidemiologists studying typhoid had to contend with new evidence gleaned from the laboratory.

This chapter shows how they did so, by tracing the way in which epidemiological expertise interacted with and cautiously engaged the new science of bacteriology in the 1880s and the 1890s, particularly after the discovery of B. typhosus. Recall from chapter 2 that Thorne, in his investigation of Caterham in 1879, had disavowed laboratory evidence and relied solely on epidemiological expertise. Thorne's was probably the best example at the time of boasting for an epidemiological approach to outbreak investigation. And yet, in the last two decades of the century, it became increasingly difficult for British epidemiologists simply to ignore bacteriological practices. Even Thorne by the 1890s changed his tune toward laboratory expertise. As chief medical officer in the 1890s, Thorne was instrumental in orchestrating the integration of epidemiological and bacteriological practices into outbreak investigation. At the Medical Department the bacteriological work of Klein, along with a younger generation of bacteriologists such as Sidney Martin, A. C. Houston, Charles Creighton, and William Hamer, began to show what an integrated field and laboratory research agenda would look like. They relied on a new generation of epidemiologists who were also more willing to take laboratory findings in stride, such as H. Timbrell Bulstrode. The chapter begins by unraveling the English reception of European bacteriological research on typhoid in the 1880s, the product of which was the discovery of the Eberth/Gaffky bacillus, or B. typhosus. Even after the discovery of the bacillus, outbreak investigation in England remained wedded to traditional qualitative and quantitative epidemiological methods. This was in part because epidemiological expertise had more cultural capital than laboratory-based medical science and also a result of lasting confusion over the bacteriology of the disease. The chapter then moves on to consider two important case studies—by Frederick Barry in 1890–91 in the Tees Valley and by H. T. Bulstrode, in 1896 at Chichester—that demonstrate the cautious integration of the laboratory into outbreak investigation. I demonstrate how this collaborative spirit grew out of an interest in learning about the life history and viability of the bacillus outside of the human body, what was called at the time its "saprophytic existence." The crucial testing ground in the 1890s was soil-based research, which highlighted one of the most pressing public health problems that occurred in the second half of the century: sporadic but persistent outbreaks of waterborne typhoid, especially in rural areas. Soils had long been a concern for English epidemiologists, but in the 1890s, outbreak investigations of typhoid began to pair the practices of epidemiology and bacteriology to produce a decidedly ecological vision for public health.

The Tyndall-Typhoid Controversy

Edward Emanuel Klein was one of the most intriguing, enigmatic, and misunderstood figures in Victorian medical science. Slavonian born and Viennese trained in histology and pathology, Klein was lured to London by John Burdon Sanderson and John Simon in 1870. William Bulloch, his colleague and obituarist, called him "a bacteriologist malgré lui."[10] He had not trained in bacteriology but was thrust into the role of England's bacteriological leader both by his contemporaries and sometimes unfairly by subsequent historians. Most of his career was spent concurrently at St. Bartholomew's Hospital and the Brown Animal Sanatory Institution, but from his arrival in London he was also asked to conduct special investigations for the Medical Department. In the period from 1870 to his death in 1910, he produced nearly one hundred scientific works tied to medicine and public health for the department alone, nearly a quarter of them on typhoid fever. Steeped in European traditions of microbiology and always following Continental medical reports, Klein was on the cutting edge of scientific research as it applied to medicine. He probably trained more English bacteriologists than anyone else in the second half of the nineteenth century, and his 1884

---

10   William Bulloch, "Obituary for E. E. Klein." *Journal of Pathology and Bacteriology* 28 (1925): 684–97, 696.

Microorganisms and Diseases, which went through several editions, was a landmark bacteriological treatise in England. But Klein's career was marked by a series of prolific microbiological blunders. Before the Linnean Society in 1874 he mistakenly announced the discovery of the germ of sheep pox, which he sheepishly had to rescind in *Nature.* He was on the wrong side of history again in 1884 in disagreeing with Robert Koch over the discovery of the cholera vibrio in Egypt. His preliminary announcement in late 1874 and full report in 1875 on the discovery of the germ of typhoid fever suffered a similarly ignominious fate.

The initial reception of Klein's typhoid discovery in England was overwhelmingly positive. *The Practitioner* noted that although Klein had not fully proved that the micrococci were the cause of typhoid, all available evidence made it "exceedingly probable."[11] The scientist John Tyndall, who had jumped at the occasion of the prince's typhoid recovery in 1872 to defend medicine over prayer, examined in chapter 1, was quick to back Klein's work. What ensued, ironically but aptly leaving out Klein's name, became known as the "Tyndall-Typhoid Controversy." It began in the public pages of *the Times.* On November 9, Tyndall wrote an extensive article reviewing and supporting Budd's *Typhoid Fever* (1873), which he called "a masterly combination of observation and inference." Ending his review, and sparking the debate that ensued, was Tyndall's last sentence: "Dr. Klein has recently discovered the very organism which lies at the root of all the mischief, and to the destruction of which medical and sanitary skill will henceforth be directed."[12] It was an offhand remark and at the very least a repeat of what Simon said more emphatically in his 1875 annual report. Tyndall even acknowledged that it was his friend Simon who told him about Klein's typhoid research. Unknowingly, Tyndall had stirred up a vicious swarm of medical locusts, demonstrating just how entrenched the debate was in England at the time over the contagiousness of typhoid. Budd and Murchison had squabbled over the finer details for over a decade, but the so-called Tyndall-Typhoid Controversy brought the debate into yet another public spectacle over the filth disease.

Letters poured into the *Times,* including one authored by "A Promising and Potential Molecule," which attacked Tyndall, and by proxy Klein and Budd, for denying the spontaneous generation of typhoid. Popular sentiment

---

11   "Dr. Klein On the Pathology of Small-pox and Typhoid Fever," *Practitioner* 14 (1875): 10.

12   Tyndall, "Typhoid Fever," 7.

on the disease still needled toward Murchison's views, even if the vanguard of English epidemiologists were leaning toward Budd in practice. But English doctors on both sides of the Murchison/Budd debate saw this as an opportunity to attack Tyndall. Croydon physician and Murchison supporter Alfred Carpenter, for example, accepted in the *Times* that typhoid might be caused by a germ—although probably not Klein's micrococci—but that certainly the disease was not contagious and needed to undergo activation in the soil or a sewer.[13] The ire was palpable in the medical press, even among those who were favorable to Budd. Both T. Lauder Brunton, editor of the *Practitioner,* and Ernest Hart at the *BMJ* attacked Tyndall for suggesting that Budd's work was new. But at stake for both influential professional gatekeepers was that Tyndall did not have the expertise to weigh in on complex matters of etiology and sanitary science. Hart, who had been more sympathetic to Klein's "interesting observations" on November 11 in the *London Medical Record,* thought it was necessary to come to the aid of Klein, whom he clearly saw was caught in the middle of Tyndall's meddling. "Dr. Klein's researchers are still in embryo," Hart concluded, "and he himself would be the last, we believe, to make any such statement" as Tyndall had made.[14] At a meeting of the Pathological Society of London in May 1875, Murchison weighed in as well, echoing Hart's remarks in the *BMJ* that Tyndall's announcement of the discovery of the germ of typhoid was both "erroneous" and unjustified.[15]

Tyndall, in an attempt to popularize sanitary science and the germ theory, had come to the medical profession's defense during the prayer-gauge debate. But here, three years later, a branch of English doctors was attacking him. The Tyndall-Typhoid Controversy was hardly surprising considering the vociferous debates over germ theories in the early 1870s, as Worboys has shown. The episode dovetails with the public discourse on typhoid in the early 1870s explored in previous chapters. The public nature of the prince's sickness, the Marylebone Milk Crisis, and a class-based discourse on the disease all provided a critical context for a vocal science popularizer like Tyndall to jump at the opportunity to praise Budd's work and subtly twist Klein's

13 Carpenter, "Typhoid Fever," 3.

14 Brunton, "Another Aspect"; Hart, "Typhoid Fever," 621; Hart, "Dr. Klein's Researches," 720. Worboys argues that the negative reaction to Tyndall in the medical press was largely a continuation of a backlash against an address he made at the Belfast meeting of the British Association for the Advancement of Science earlier that year. See Worboys, *Spreading Germs,* 135.

15 Murchison, "The Germ-Theory of Disease," 621.

research into a critical discovery. As an early advocate of a singular germ theory and Darwinian ideas of evolution by natural selection, Tyndall desperately wanted Klein's micrococci to be a model example, another success for English science. But the Tyndall-Typhoid debate was as much about the messenger as about the message; Simon was not castigated for more vocally advocating for Klein, but he had done so in the less publicized reports of the department. Within months the whole debate fizzled, however. Klein's micrococci were, Charles Creighton observed in the course of his own research on cancer for the Medical Department, just "some albuminous matter."[16] Simon quickly changed his tone in his next annual report, calling Klein's organisms "curiously fallacious microscopical forms" and instructed him to get back to work on identifying the real germ of typhoid.[17]

The Uneven Road to Bacteriological Clarity

By mid-1875 Klein knew he had failed to link the spherical micrococci found in the stools of typhoid patients to the infective process of the disease. But he was anything but deterred and turned his focus to comparative pathology, spending the next two years conducting a series of experiments on typhoid fever in pigs. The move was not surprising, considering that Klein was originally trained in comparative pathology and had been brought to England largely to work on animal diseases at the Brown. Long interested in using comparative pathology to unravel the etiology of typhoid, Budd had been researching pig typhoid from the 1860s. In August 1865 Budd received a letter from John Gamgee in Edinburgh, reporting an outbreak of pig typhoid and inquiring whether Budd was interested in receiving specimens. Although Gamgee packed the dead pig in ice and shipped it to Bristol, upon opening the carcass Budd noted that it "stank so badly as to put my pathological zeal to a test of no common severity." Budd's findings were that the typhoid fever in pigs was remarkably similar to that of humans, "the exact counterpart," he observed.[18] Up until 1875 that view continued to be

---

16 Creighton, "Note on Certain Unusual Coagulation," 140–41.

17 Simon, *Annual Report of the Medical Officer*, 1876, 3.

18 William Budd, "Typhoid (Intestinal) Fever in the Pig," London School of Hygiene and Tropical Medicine Archives, London, William Budd papers, GB 809 Budd. In 1865 Budd also studied typhoid in Ox. See Budd, *The Siberian Cattle-Plague*.

accepted among leading English veterinarians like James Beart Simonds and J. Wortley Axe.[19] But Klein in 1875, collaborating with veterinary surgeon W. Duguid at the Brown, was not seeing in the intestinal lesions of dead pigs the same disease he had researched in humans. Klein agreed that pig typhoid was highly contagious; he produced typhoid in a number of healthy pigs by inoculating them with matter taken from the ulcerated intestines of those sick with typhoid.[20] But on all other matters the earlier researchers had been wrong. What he had demonstrated, of no small value to medical and veterinary science, was that swine typhoid was pathologically distinct from typhoid in humans. In the next year he continued animal research, and in 1877 Klein successfully discovered the germ of pig typhoid.[21] Following the methods of Koch's discovery of anthrax in 1876, Klein had successfully culti- vated a "specific schizomycete, spire-yielding rods and filaments" to an eighth generation incubated in the aqueous solution of a rabbit's eye.[22] Injecting the germ into healthy pigs, he was able to induce typhoid and extract the specific microorganism, fulfilling what would later be known as "Koch's Postulates." He had arrived at both a new methodology and a full-blown germ theory of disease: "Each distinct zymotic disease is in its essence an invasion of the ani- mal body by a distinct, extremely minute, living and self-multiplying thing." [23] By 1880 it was the standard view, as Francis Vacher, MOH for Birkenhead noted at the Public Health Section of the British Medical Association meeting at Cambridge, during a discussion titled "What Diseases are Communicable to Man from Diseased Animals Used as Food?"[24]

Klein's success with "Pneumo-Enteritis," as Klein renamed the disease in his final report, was a boon to English veterinary science and animal hus- bandry. But it was still unclear how such research might translate to human diseases. Klein got his chance in 1880, when departmental colleague Edward

---

19 Wortley Axe had been the president of the Royal College of Veterinary Surgeons, a professor at the Royal Veterinary College, and an inspector to the Surrey County Council.

20 Klein, "Report on the So-Called Enteric or Typhoid Fever of the Pig," 91–101.

21 Waddington has also shown that Klein was instrumental in comparative research on bovine tuberculosis and tuberculosis in humans. See Waddington, *The Bovine Scourge*, 43.

22 Klein, "Report on the Sso-Ccalled Enteric or Typhoid Fever of the Pig," 91–101.

23 E. Klein, "Report on Infectious Pneumo-Enteritis of the Pig."

24 "British Medical Association" *Veterinary Journal* 11 (1880): 349.

Ballard was sent to examine an extensive outbreak of food poisoning at the Duke of Portland's estate at Welbeck, Nottinghamshire. Around two thousand people from the surrounding area had attended a timber and machinery sale on the estate, and over seventy came down with what Ballard called "diarrheal illness," with vomiting, nausea, and stomach pain. Ballard interviewed many of those sick and examined the statistics of the outbreak, which helped him narrow in on the cause. It was overwhelmingly men who had been attacked, and during the estate sale predominately men partook of the food. Those who were sick had consumed and complained of the ham. Familiar with his work on the microorganisms of disease, Ballard turned to Klein for assistance, sending him samples of the suspected ham to London. Klein found a specific species of bacillus that when inoculated into healthy animals produced disease. Hardy has argued in her recent *Salmonella Infections* that "although Klein's conclusions were unspecific, Ballard was convinced"[25] and set out in the subsequent years to trace, with Klein's assistance, a series of precedent-setting outbreaks of food-borne illness. But here, as before with water and milk analysis, Klein's laboratory research of the hams was secondary and merely confirmatory to Ballard's epidemiological field-based approach.

Laboratory evidence continued its backseat status throughout the 1880s, in spite of a number of important discoveries. In 1880 Karl Eberth, studying the spleen and mesenteric glands of a dead typhoid patient, succeeded where Klein had failed in 1874. He described the rod-shaped organisms that quickly took his name—Eberth's bacillus—but contemporaries also used the bacteriologically reinvigorated moniker *bacillus typhosus*, shortened as *B. typhosus*. Hart favorably reviewed Eberth's findings in the *BMJ* but concluded that it was a subject "still occupying competent investigation," and such findings, he cautiously noted, "should be carefully scrutinised."[26] Four years later, in 1884, the same year Robert Koch identified the bacillus responsible for cholera, German bacteriologist Georg Gaffky isolated *B. typhosus* in a pure culture.[27] Gaffky's discovery, too, was covered in the English medical press but only translated by the New Sydenham Society two years later in 1886. The bacteriological moment had finally arrived for the filth disease—or

---

25   Hardy, Salmonella infections, 88.

26   Hart, "On the Bacillus of Typhoid Fever," 877.

27   Koch's well-known lecture before the Imperial German Board of Health, in Berlin, was published in full in the *British Medical Journal*. See Koch, "An Address on Cholera," 403–7.

so it seemed. The discoveries of Eberth and Gaffky, Hardy argues, "did not resolve the etiological problems surrounding typhoid. Although the existence of the bacillus initially suggested a relatively simple model of causation, the picture rapidly clouded."[28] This was particularly true after Gartner's 1888 discovery of bacillus enteritidis (*Salmonella enteritidis*), obtained from a man who ate the meat of a sick cow, confused matters even more. Some observers in England had successfully replicated Eberth and Gaffky's work, but *B. typhosus* was a tricky laboratory subject, and many in England remained wedded to Hart's scrutiny of new laboratory findings. For example, Klein's *Microorganisms and Disease*, already in its third edition by 1886, was skeptical of the recent typhoid discoveries. Klein argued that it was "doubtful whether these bacilli can be considered as necessarily and intimately connected with typhoid fever."[29] But by 1888 even Klein had acquiesced to the Eberth/Gaffky bacillus, replicating their findings of the bacillus in the mesenteric glands and spleens of typhoid patients, but not in their blood. He only grudgingly accepted the causal role of *B. typhosus* in the late 1880s, while testing the microbe-destroying properties of perchloride of mercury and heat, but it was still a tepid approval.[30]

Although the laboratory had supposedly provided clarity about the nature of typhoid, confusion reigned. What had been known as typhoid from the 1830s might not, indeed, be a singular thing, but rather, as Hardy has shown, a wider "typhoid group" whose members shared "morphological and cultural characteristics"[31] The confusion and the difficulty of the bacillus as a laboratory object help explain the cautious approach among English epidemiologists toward laboratory evidence and the continued reliance on epidemiological methods of outbreak investigation. The suspicion thrown upon new laboratory findings in Britain was so acute that many, like Lyon Playfair in an address on public health before the Social Science Association in Glasgow in 1889, took refuge in the old dictum "wash and be clean." "What is quite certain," Playfair concluded in what was a common sentiment in the still-contentious debates over germs, "is that if filth be entirely prevented" infectious diseases could find no hold.[32]

---

28 Hardy, *Salmonella Infections*, 24.

29 Klein, *Microorganisms and Disease*, 122.

30 Klein, "Further Observations on the Influence of Perchloride of Mercury," 448; Klein, "Report on the Influence of Heat," 450.

31 Hardy, *Salmonella Infections*, 89.

32 Playfair, *Subjects of Social Welfare*, 12–13.

	Unpolluted samples.			Polluted samples.		
	Dupré.	Frankland.	Wanklyn.	Dupré.	Frankland.	Wanklyn.
The stool obtained from William Cox on the morning of the 6th March.	Unpolluted Lambeth Water drawn on the 4th of March. Sent on the morning of the 8th for analysis.			Lambeth water, two litres of which had been polluted with the soluble portion of ·1 grm. of Typhoid stool known to contain ·0061 grm. of solid matter. This is in the proportion of 0·21 grm. soluble solid matter added to each gallon. Sent on morning of the 8th for analysis.		
Appearance	Clear	Clear	—	Very slightly turbid.	Clear	—
Colour	Pale brownish green.	—	—	Pale brownish yellow.	—	—
Deposit	None	—	—	None	—	—
Nitrous acid	None	—	—	None	—	—
Phosphoric acid	Strong trace	—	—	Strong trace	—	—
Colour of residue	Pale brownish.	—	—	Pale brownish.	—	—
Behaviour of residue on heating.	Blackens perceptibly.	—		Blackens perceptibly.	—	
Grains per gallon.						
Oxygen absorbed from permanganate.	0·2415	—	—	0·2312	—	—
Total dry residue	22·68	22·568	Not stated	23·24	22·96	Not stated
Consisting of { volatile matters.	0·70	—	—	1·96	—	—
{ fixed salts.	21·96	—	—	21·28	—	—
Chlorine	1·015	1·12	1·3	1·015	1·05	1·3
Nitric acid, N_2O_5	0·924	0·7722	—	0·770	0·8202	—
Ammonia	0·0011	0·	0·0014	0·0016	0·	0·007
Albuminoid ammonia	0·0090	—	0·0056	0·0100	—	0·007
Organic carbon	—	·2114	—	—	·2205	—
Organic nitrogen	—	·0371	—	—	·0399	—
Total hardness	—	15·26	18·	—	15·82	18·
Temporary	—	8·96	—	—	10·22	—
Permanent	—	6·3	—	—	5·6	—

Figure 4.3 Results of experiments of sewage contaminated water. From Robert Cory, "On the Results of the Examination of Certain Samples of Water Purposely Polluted with Excrements from Fever Patients, and with Other Matters," Eleventh Annual Report of the Medical Officer of the Local Government Board 1881, 142. House of Commons Parliamentary Papers, Crown Copyright.

So how did bacteriological evidence shape epidemiology? Klein's failure in 1874 to discover the typhoid bacillus had set things back and made many English researchers hesitant to accept laboratory discoveries, although Koch's anthrax discovery went some way toward reducing skepticism. Some authorities still believed that water analysis might hold the key to bolstering outbreak investigation and ultimately reducing the incidence of typhoid, which although the annual death rates had declined from 1870 onward, would not take a steep plunge until after 1900. In 1880 and 1881 Robert Cory began an interesting set of investigations into typhoid and potable water for the Medical Department. Cory, from the Cumbrian town of Carlisle, studied medicine at Cambridge and St. Thomas's Hospital. He remained closely tied to St. Thomas's for his entire professional career and is mostly remembered for his research on smallpox vaccination. His obituarist noted that Cory preferred "experiment to ordinary observation," no doubt leading to his death in 1900 resulting from a self-inflicted vaccination experiment.[33] In March 1880 Cory obtained the stools of a sixteen-year-old typhoid patient named William Cox at St. Thomas's Hospital. Cory mixed the stools with freshly drawn Lambeth water and bottled the concoction in three clean Winchester quart bottles. He took three additional clean quart bottles and only added Lambeth water. Carefully labeling each, he sent the samples (one of each type) to the leading chemists of water analysis in London, Alfred Wanklyn, August Dupre, and Edward Frankland, who reported back on their analytical findings (figure 4.3).[34]

And although Cory pored over the results, there was little of "practical interest" for sanitary science, Chief Medical Officer George Buchanan noted.[35] Cory did not mention Eberth's recent discovery or even test for the presence of microorganisms. He, like other English observers, recognized that stools of typhoid patients were critical test subjects for laboratory research, as they had long been assumed to contain the dangerous part of the disease. Typhoid, it seems, was also a model disease for analytical chemists, even if a not altogether useful one. But ultimately Cory failed where administrators like Buchanan wanted such tests to succeed. There was no way of knowing, via water analysis, that a given sample had been contaminated by the stools of a typhoid fever patient or the stools of a healthy individual. "The lesson is taught afresh," Buchanan concluded, "we must . . . go beyond the laboratory for evidence of any drinking water being free from dangerous organic pollution." It was best to stick to the epidemiological methods of outbreak investigation, in other words. He added that "the chemist can, in brief, tell us

---

33 "Obituary for Robert Cory," *St. Thomas's Hospital Reports* 29 (London: J.&A Churchill, 1902): 320.

34 Cory, "On the Results."

35 George Buchanan, *Annual Report of Medical Officer for 1881,* xix. Cory argued that Frankland's combustion process, of determining carbon and nitrogen in the organic substances in water as indicative of contamination, was the best test of water purity.

of impurity and hazard, but not of purity and safety."[36] Chemistry still could not produce what epidemiology could, and to adduce the point Buchanan cited as proof Thorne's 1879 Caterham study, where epidemiology had succeeded without chemical expertise. Reviewing Cory's investigation in the *Sanitary Record,* Charles Cassal and B. A. Whitelegge went even further in lamenting that in the laboratory the "absolute safety" of drinking water "is unknown and unknowable."[37]

Outbreak Investigation in the Early Age of Bacteriology

Throughout the 1880s, both chemical and bacteriological studies of typhoid failed to make a significant impact on outbreak investigation. So limited was their influence that Buchanan was still lamenting in 1888 the "increments of knowledge" in chemistry and bacteriology that could be applied to sanitary science. "As a rule," he concluded, "chemists have taken little heed of the operations of the bacteria of drinking waters, while, as a rule, bacteriological examination has extended little further than to the counting the number of colonies."[38] The Medical Department stood Janus faced. From the late 1860s Simon had initiated the program of auxiliary scientific research, consistently championing the study of microorganisms and disease by Burdon Sanderson and Klein and vouching for the inconclusive chemical findings of J. W. Thudichum and the inconsistent analyses of August Dupre.[39] The subsequent chief medical officers, Seaton and Buchanan, from the late 1870s through the 1880s took a similar approach, but few strides were made. Looking back, Sir Arthur Salusbury McNaulty noted in his history of English public health that the "great value" of the laboratory research at this time "lay not so much in the results achieved . . . as in the principles won."[40] Buchanan at least recognized the sea change that was to come with bacteriology and gave Klein, Charles Creighton, and a host of younger bacteriologists—Wooldridge, Cash, Lingard, Hamer—the time and space needed to

36   George Buchanan, *Annual Report of Medical Officer for 1881,* xxi.
37   Cassal and Whitelegge, "Remarks on the Examination of Water," 482.
38   Buchanan, *Annual Report of the Medical for 1887,* xvii.
39   In the 1870s Dupre was constantly having to fight for getting paid for all of his analyses conducted with outbreak investigations. See MH 32/106, National Archives, Kew, Medical Inspectors Correspondence.
40   MacNalty, *The History of State Medicine,* 40.

pursue cutting-edge research on microorganisms. Simon, too, even after he left the department, remained a vocal public supporter. In 1881, for example, in a landmark address at the International Medical Congress in London, Simon was confident that "all practical medicine . . . has been undergoing a process of transfiguration under the influence of laboratory experiments."[41] At the department, except for Sanderson and Klein, the bulk of bacteriological research in the 1880s comprised laboratory studies of disinfection, replicating the results of French or German bacteriologists, particularly on anthrax, typhoid, and cholera.

What is striking is that while department-backed bacteriological research grew in the 1880s, Buchanan and the inspectors still pushed back against the integration of the laboratory into outbreak investigation.[42] The laboratory, it seems, was still "auxiliary" to the field. Buchanan, writing a private memo to the Treasury in 1886, called such laboratory research "directly ancillary" to outbreak investigation.[43] When cholera threatened England once again in 1884, Buchanan mentioned Koch's discovery of the cholera bacillus, but, like most English sanitary leaders, he was skeptical. "With all the aid that the micropathologist can afford," he noted, "a better understanding on these points will remain to be gained through the application to the study of cholera of those methods of careful inductive research which sanitary inquirers, particularly in England, have learnt to apply to the study of their own domestic diseases."[44] It was yet another touting of epidemiological methods and in particular the extensive knowledge gained on the etiology of typhoid since the last visitation of cholera in 1866. Buchanan even reissued Radcliffe's 1865 investigation of cholera at Theydon Bois, Essex, as an exemplary model should cholera once again strike Britain.

There was little difference in department-sponsored outbreak investigations of typhoid fever in the 1880s from what had been established in the 1870s. Under Buchanan's leadership the department subtly shifted focus

---

41   Simon, "An Address Delivered at the Opening of the Section of Public Medicine."

42   This pushes back against Olga Amsterdamska's argument that British epidemiologists in the late nineteenth century were "uninterested with the new field of bacteriology." See Amsterdamska, "Demarcating Epidemiology."

43   George Buchanan, "Memorandum as to the Duties of the Board's Medical Department as at Present Constituted," 1886, National Archives, Kew, MH 78/1.

44   George Buchanan, "Cholera in Europe," xxx.

away from highlighting typhoid, and the annual reports tended to promote investigations of anthrax, tuberculosis, diphtheria, scarlet fever, smallpox, and the threat of cholera. It was in some ways understandable. Typhoid had dominated the department's work in the 1870s, and much of the etiology of the disease was thought to have been unraveled. And the results were being seen. With the implementation of more efficient sanitary infrastructure in urban areas, typhoid rates were decreasing, albeit slowly. Epidemiological methods of outbreak investigation of typhoid had also become standardized by this period, so much so that John Spear, tracing an explosive outbreak at Mountain Ash, Wales, said he merely had to look at three factors to find the cause of the mischief: sewage-contaminated air, an infected milk supply, and polluted water.[45] Frank Henry Blaxall, a retired naval surgeon and member of the inspectorate, traced an outbreak at Melton Mowbray in 1881 to excreta-laced sewer air in the main sewer drain. Page went to Grimsby in 1881 to unravel a widespread outbreak and could only point to the distribution of cases having in common their proximity to unventilated sewers. Shirley Murphy, one of the rising stars of English epidemiology, uncovered a milk-borne outbreak of typhoid at St. Albans in 1884; however, like the earlier work of Ballard and Radcliffe, she had to rely on supposition in the end to show how the milk had originally become infected. Most frequently in the 1880s, like before, epidemiological investigations pointed to infected water supplies. Hubert Airy, during an outbreak at Blackburn in 1881, traced the cause to the oozings of an excreta-infected privy pit into the public reservoir. Spear, in 1887, traced an explosive outbreak of over five hundred cases of typhoid in the Mountain Ash Urban District of Glamorganshire, Wales, to houses in three villages on the bank of River Cynon. He went some way to prove that the water service was infected with typhoid excreta. Buchanan, reviewing Spear's investigation, had yet another jab at bacteriology, noting that "while the infective material of enteric fever is not capable of recognition . . . it was rightly considered that the relation of the water-service to the disease would be adequately demonstrated, if opportunity were found to exist for the entry of any excremental matter into the water-pipe at the designated place." Spear had used basic case-tracing and experimentation—one of few such cases in the 1880s.[46] He dug up the area around the public water main

---

45   Spear was particularly keen to argue in this period on the dangers of an intermittent water supply. See Spear, "The Dangers of Water-Contamination."

46   Page, investigating an outbreak at Houghton-le-Spring in 1889, used another basic experiment to unravel the case. In that instance he proved that a local

that supplied the infected houses and found it was both leaking and located "immediately above, alongside, and even through old rubble drains." It was receiving "liquid filth from soil and sewer."[47]

But just as the methods of Radcliffe, Thorne, Ballard, and Buchanan were coming to fruition, the department brought on a younger generation of aspiring epidemiologists who often struggled with outbreak investigation. In some ways the epidemiological studies of typhoid in the 1880s were less impressive than the innovations of the 1870s. Fewer diagrams and maps were used, and complicated differential statistical studies would not come until the 1890s. This was probably the result of epidemiological methods becoming routinized. And the slowdown was also generational, as there was a unique kind of stubbornness in the cultural moment of the 1870s on the part of Radcliffe, Ballard, Buchanan, and Thorne to discover the index case of outbreaks, minutely trace and map an outbreak, and vocalize their findings to broader lay and professional audiences. Edward Cox Seaton, MOH for Surrey County Council and lecturer on public health at St. Thomas's Hospital, looked back on the epidemiological studies of the 1870s and called the group "practical epidemiologists," who possessed "the spirit of practicality and precise statement"[48] The same impulse was there in the 1880s, but it was less dogmatic. The frustrations of the newer inspectors were apparent in several cases. Page, on outbreak investigation in 1888 at the village of Mytholmroyd, West Yorkshire, could not find a specific cause. There were too many problems to enumerate, and he spent the report lamenting that four different sanitary authorities managed the village. Often, as was the case with D. A. Gresswell at Cradley in 1889, an inspector was sent to a location long investigated by the department, which brought its own kind of complications. Ballard had investigated an outbreak at Cradley in 1873, and Franklin Parsons had done another in 1880. Gresswell himself was there in 1886, and not much had changed. In the end, his 1889 report pointed to air and water being infected, but it was mostly a condemnation of "the great variety of unwholesome conditions," so that "the persistence of [the] filth disease is almost a matter of course."[49] The decade concluded, in

---

water supply had been contaminated by a sewer drain through a fissure in the ground through pouring salt in the drain and testing chloride levels in the water.

47   Spear, "Report on an Epidemic of Typhoid Fever," viii.

48   Seaton, "Evolution of Sanitary Administration," 1638.

49   Gresswell, "Report on the Sanitary Condition of Cradley," 55.

other words, with epidemiological studies of typhoid tending to confirm, as Buchanan did, the continued "simple neglect" and "blundering on the part of sanitary authorities"[50] It was a long-standing sentiment among members of the department. Corfield in 1871 had made the same claim in 1871 while investigating the sanitary state of Biggleswade and Potton in Bedfordshire, noting that the causes of typhoid and scarlet fever "are not far to seek, and most of them at any rate might easily be remedied were it not that the local authorities are afraid of incurring expense."[51] A host of other problems persisted as well, such as the lasting diagnostic confusion between typhoid and typhus. For example, from 1885 to 1887 Spear, who had made a name for himself earlier in the decade for his epidemiological prowess tracing anthrax, or woolsorter's disease, was instructed to inquire into the large uptick in typhus throughout England and Wales, particularly in the northern regions. He found extensive evidence throughout the country that typhus was still being confused with typhoid, not just by poor villagers but also by MOsH. It was a result of "diagnostic failure" and "mis-information."[52]

And yet for all of the mediocrity of the 1880s, the epidemiological study of typhoid once again surged into the national spotlight in the early 1890s. Frederick Barry's investigation of a violent outbreak of typhoid in the northeast of England, in the Tees Valley, was a landmark example of late Victorian epidemiology, helping to push typhoid back onto the national scene. Barry's study demonstrates the dominance of traditional, field-based methods of outbreak investigation established in the 1860s and 1870s but also the important ways that epidemiological expertise had grown and adapted since that earlier period. Barry's epidemiological gaze was not limited to a single city, town, or village, or even to a sudden or fulminating outbreak but instead focused on a broader geographical scale, its water supply, and the interconnectedness between urban and rural areas over an extended timeframe. This approach became common at the Medical Department from the early

---

50   Buchanan, *Annual Report of the Medical Officer for 1888*, v.

51   W. Corfield, *Report on the Sanitary State of Biggleswade and Potton (Bedfordshire), Especially with Regard to the Prevalence of Scarlatina, Measles, and Typhoid Fever*, National Archives, Kew, MH 113/4, Buchanan Office Papers.

52   Spear, "Report on Appearances of Typhus Fever," 269. Radcliffe had argued the same in an 1871 investigation of typhoid in Bradford. See, National Archives, Kew, MH 113/10.

1890s.[53] Epidemiological studies of the 1860s, like Radcliffe's cholera investigation at Theydon Bois, Essex, and Thorne's at Terling, explored in chapter 2, narrowed their gaze to the minutiae of sanitary facts—about the environment, the movement of people, and infrastructure—to prove the spread of typhoid. The more narrowly focused their studies were, they believed, the greater the chance of establishing important etiological facts. By the 1890s a younger generation of epidemiologists, such as Barry and H. T. Bulstrode, as we will see, widened their epidemiological gaze to regions and even to the entire nation, shifting an economy of scale in British epidemiology. They did this while maintaining many of the traditional field-based methods of interviewing, statistical inference, and simple experimentation. Much of the methodology remained the same. Theodore Thomson, for example, when sent to investigate an outbreak of typhoid in Penrith in 1891, compiled a simple chart to unravel the epidemic. He used columns listing onset of disease, name, residence, milk supply, water supply, and sanitary condition of the individual's house.[54] The minute tracing of cases would have looked familiar to department inspectors in the 1860s.

The Marylebone Milk Crisis of 1873 provided a critical precedent: that the health of those in urban areas—two thirds of the English population— was often dependent on the sanitary behavior of those living in rural ones. The Public Health Act of 1872 had divided the country into Urban and Rural Sanitary Districts; what was needed was an interconnected system of sanitary supervision, something still lacking in the 1890s. Barry's Tees Valley investigation, focusing, as we will see, on the water supply of the area, helped to highlight the disjointed sanitary system in England. In the age of a burgeoning bacteriology, it was traditional field-based investigations like Barry's that provided a nascent ecological understanding of typhoid and a growing national picture of the persistence of the disease.

---

53 Two important examples of a regional approach, including regional mapping that followed Barry's Tees Valley study were R. Bruce Low's "Report on the Circumstances of the River Trent in Lincolnshire and Part of Nottinghamshire," 1893, and T. W. Thompson in "Memorandum on the Recent Prevalence of Enteric Fever in Certain Areas within the County of Durham in 1895," National Archives, Kew. Low's report is contained in MH113/30. Thompson's report is contained in MH 113/31.

54 Theodore Thomson, "Table of Cases of Typhoid Fever," from April 18 to August 26, 1891, National Archives, Kew, MH 113/28.

Typhoid in the Tees Valley

Frederick Barry had spent the bulk of 1890 on duty for the Medical Department in the north of England. He investigated the isolation hospital in Keighley Union and the general sanitary arrangements of Rawdon, both northwest of Leeds. In September he traveled to Middlesbrough for a routine inspection of the area. He found that cases of typhoid had suddenly sprung up throughout town. The MOH even said that typhoid was simultaneously in the neighboring areas, particularly the registration districts of Stockton and Darlington. Barry wrote to the area's MOsH asking for information about recent cases of typhoid, and what he found was staggering. In ten different registration districts comprising thirty-two sanitary districts in the counties of Durham and Yorkshire—practically the whole valley of the River Tees—there were 570 cases of typhoid from early September to early October. Barry was occupied for months in the investigation and became embroiled with local officials over the cause of the outbreak. His Tees Valley study was a model epidemiological investigation to later observers, long remembered in the tradition of Victorian epidemiology.

Frederick William Barry was born at Scarborough in 1850 and educated at Edinburgh University, taking an MD in 1876. A year later he obtained the new mark of epidemiological credentialing, a diploma in public health from Cambridge. His first post, as the MOH for the Craven District in Yorkshire, lasted two years, and in 1880 he was appointed sanitary commissioner and quarantine superintendent for the British government in Cyprus. That post also lasted two years, and in 1882 George Buchanan hired him at the Medical Department. Barry discovered he had a knack for epidemiological investigation and stayed with the department until his death in 1897, being appointed senior inspector in 1892.[55] Like a surprising number of the inspectorate in the second half of the nineteenth century, he died of work-related causes.[56] In 1897 he was on outbreak investigation in Yorkshire and hit his head on a stone doorway, severely damaging his skull, which laid him up in bed for sixteen weeks. He did not work for seven months, and when he came back, while on duty in Birmingham, he suddenly died in a room at

55 Memo from Richard Thorne Thorne to F. W. Barry, December 14, 1892. National Archives, Kew, MH 113/29. Barry also took a law degree from Middle Temple in 1894 and was an examiner in medical jurisprudence and public health at Aberdeen and Edinburgh Universities.
56 Harries, Page, and Spear all died as a result of work-related injuries or illnesses.

the Grand Hotel. In his nearly two decades at the department he filled the vacancy left by Radcliffe in examining foreign epidemics and the supervising ports. His sudden death was mourned by the public health community: "At present juncture," the *Sanitary Record* observed, "so valuable an officer can ill be spared."[57] Barry's obituarist said he had "a wonderful faculty for collecting statistics and drawing valuable conclusions from them." The Tees Valley study was ample proof.[58]

Barry's Tees Valley investigation had really begun with clever statistical work. Compiling the number of typhoid cases in the year 1890 from local MOsH, he had instantly recognized the localized uptick across the area in the six-week period from September 7 to October 18, which saw a total of 570 cases. Most of this data was supplied through the new Infectious Diseases Notification Act of 1889, but Barry found that the act was not in operation in all areas of the Tees Valley, so he supplemented his data by reaching out to local practitioners, particularly in rural areas. Barry believed attack rate alone was an imperfect index, so he went through the extra trouble of calculating house attack rate. To do so he separated cases by household into what he called the "Area of Inquiry," in other words, into thirty-two sanitary districts of the Tees Valley. These included urban areas (which he divided into wards) and rural areas (which he divided by townships and villages). The 570 cases had occurred in 550 houses spread throughout the valley, "from the house of the poorest labourer to the mansion of the county Member."[59] From the statistical data Barry turned to social conditions and the traditional methods of outbreak investigation. The elevation of houses did not correlate, the milk supply was not common to cases, and the sewage systems were unique and confined to particular areas. Through induction Barry narrowed in on the water supply. About half of the entire valley was supplied by two main water companies, the Stockton and Middlesbrough Water Board and the Darlington Waterworks, and the other half got water from elsewhere, mainly private wells. The two companies supplied urban and rural areas, and while they had separate sand and gravel filtering facilities and lines, Barry learned that they both drew from the River Tees at the same location, at Broken Scaur, two miles upriver from Darlington. It was a critical finding in his investigation. Barry obtained a list of houses from the two waterworks

57 "Notes," *Sanitary Record* 20 (October 15, 1897): 407. Richard Thorne Thorne arranged for a memorial in Barry's hometown of Downe.

58 "Obituary of Dr. F. W. Barry," *Lancet* 3868 (October 16, 1897): 1016–17.

59 Barry, "Interim Report on an Epidemic Prevalence of Enteric Fever," 70.

companies and narrowed the search even further using his self-fashioned index of house attack rate. It was 12 per 1,000 from houses whose inhabitants drank Tees water and less than 1 per 1,000 for houses whose inhabitants did not. Tees water, then, was the "carrier of the disease," he argued. But even after the bacteriological birth of *B. typhosus*, Barry still called it the "enteric fever poison," indicating his reluctance to conform to laboratory lingo.[60] Through statistical sleuthing Barry had pointed to the water supplied by the two water companies that drew from the same source at the same spot. But how had the water become infected?

Barry turned upstream to find the answer, relying on the traditional methods of outbreak investigation. He visited village after village on both sides of the River Tees, going as far as Eggleston and Middleton-on-Teesdale, about twenty miles away. Local newspapers, like the *Teesdale Mercury*, reported that Barry's visits were an "all-absorbing topic."[61] He found plenty of sanitary faults. Most of the villages either emptied their sewer lines directly into the Tees or into nearby agricultural ditches, where sewage accumulated until heavy rainfall pushed it into the Tees. There were particularly offensive nuisances at Barnard Castle, a market town of around six thousand inhabitants, where sewer and privy outfalls dumped directly along the banks of the Tees, half a mile below the town. All along the Tees at Barnard Castle there was a thick, sewage-caked foreshore. There had previously been a weir, or dam, at the lower part of town, which brought the water level up and meant that sewage flowed directly into the river. But a flood had recently broken the dam, and what remained was "a mass of stinking abominations," which Barry sensorially observed had "to be seen and smelt to be appreciated."[62] The timing of the flood, qualifying for the time it might take for excremental matters to flow down to the intake in Darlington, neatly matched the incubation period for typhoid and the dates of the first cases. It was not an index case, but Barry treated it as such.

One local paper called Barry "the learned expert" who had adopted "the microbe or germ theory" in condemning the Tees water, which is interesting because Barry did not directly adduce germ theory language or rely on bacteriological specificity.[63] The evidence was not lacking that the Tees water, where it was taken up by the two water companies in Darlington, was

60 Barry, "Interim Report on an Epidemic Prevalence of Enteric Fever," 71.
61 "Stray Arrows," *Teesdale Mercury*, October 29, 1890, 4.
62 Barry, "Interim Report on an Epidemic Prevalence of Enteric Fever," 71.
63 "Barnard Castle," *Teesdale Mercury*, November 5, 1890, 4.

excessively contaminated with sewage, and the conditions at Barnard Castle were especially appalling. But, as Buchanan noted, it was circumstantial evidence. How had the water caused the limited outbreak? Why hadn't this happened before? Barry thoroughly examined the two waterworks stations but could find no plausible reason to suspect foul play with a lapse in the filtration process. He also considered, turning briefly to bacteriological evidence, that sand and gravel filtration might be insufficient to protect against typhoid. But here, too, concrete laboratory evidence was lacking. Barry turned to meteorological data to suggest an answer. Examining the local rainfall data from the area, he found that there had been heavy rainfall in the second half of August, directly preceding the outbreak. From there, in his preliminary report to the Medical Department, he pieced together what he believed had occurred. In the summer of 1890 typhoid-laced excreta had accumulated on the banks of the Tees, lurking in the soil, where it remained until excessive rain and subsequent flooding had flushed the sewage into the river and down toward the intake, where it spread to the customers of the two companies. It was a powerful and broad vision, a protoecological explanation for the environmental factors involved in the spread of typhoid. And yet it was a logical extension from earlier explanations by epidemiologists like Thorne and Radcliffe, who had narrowed the cause of typhoid epidemics to the excremental pollution of shallow wells in the 1860s and 1870s. Eminent water analysts like Edward Frankland had even forewarned that such a thing might happen from the 1870s. Frankland in 1877, for example, noted that in towns and villages across England the custom was to drink water from rivers and shallow wells that received the soakage of sewers and cesspools. "Immense numbers of the population are thus daily exposed to the risk of infection from typhoidal discharges," Frankland cautioned.[64] The situation was an ecological maelstrom in 1890 in the Tees Valley and continued throughout the 1890s to be, as Frank R. Blaxall opined, "a matter of considerable moment."[65]

In Barry's Tees Valley case, the statistics, particularly the house attack rate, made the theory plausible, but how had the outbreak originated? Here Barry had little to say beyond presumption. He could not find a concentrated number of cases of typhoid in the villages or towns upstream in July or August, and hence no index case. But, he argued, it was a "matter of common knowledge" that typhoid cases could be slight and undetected. Besides,

---

64   Frankland, *Experimental Researches,* 558–59.
65   Blaxall, "The Relations of Bacteriology to Epidemiology," 171.

he suggested, places like Barnard Castle, which had a seasonal market and a summer military training camp, had a "floating population," and it was too late to recognize those transient cases. And he also entertained a third hypothesis to locate the index case, a class-based explanation that "a steady stream of tramps is continually passing through the district."[66] Local opinion in Barnard Castle was inclined to blame tramps, but for Barry the class-based explanation was insufficient. A leading editorial in the *Teesdale Mercury* in October of 1890 praised Barry's "gaze," which might, they hoped, exercise "a wholesome reflex influence on the dirt-loving and yet palsied residuum of society."[67] But quickly local opinion turned on Barry and the intrusion from the government. Barry concluded his preliminary report saying that he had "personally no hesitation" in attributing the outbreak to the Tees water distributed by the two companies and warned people in the area to boil water before drinking. A full report would also come shortly, he noted, with "the detailed consideration of a number of complex facts."[68]

After his return to London with the interim report in press, cases of typhoid once again exploded in the Tees Valley, and Barry headed back to northeast England. He once again contacted the local MOsH and found a strikingly similar pattern to that of his first investigation: that cases were confined to the houses supplied with water by the two companies, and had especially stricken—to the sum of 91 percent—the districts of Darlington, Stockton, and Middlesbrough (figure 4.4). Examining the meteorological data once again, he found that a second flood had occurred in early December. It was more confirmation.

Barry's full report elaborated on the early statistical analysis he had developed in the interim report but expanded to include a wider scope and provided calculations for attack rate, house attack rate, and death rate in the sixteen-month period from January 1890 to March 1891. What is especially significant about the full report is the extent to which Barry used visual evidence to marshal his epidemiological claims. He relied on quantitative visuals, such as statistical charts and graphs like figure 4, which depicts attack

66 Barry, "Interim Report on an Epidemic Prevalence of Enteric Fever," 77. The public health aspects of vagrancy were the special subjects of both a meeting of the Society of Public Health and the British Medical Association in 1893. See "Proceedings of the Incorporated Society of Medical Officers of Health," *Public Health* 6 (1894): 130–36.

67 "Stray Arrows," *Teesdale Mercury*, October 29, 1890, 4

68 Barry, "Interim Report on an Epidemic Prevalence of Enteric Fever," 63.

SOILS, STOOLS, AND SAPROPHYTES &◆ 197

TABLE III.

The Ten Registration Districts selected for Inquiry.		16 Months (Jan. 1890 to Mar. 1891).	Two Periods, each of Six Weeks, Collectively.	First Six Weeks' Period (7th Sept.—18th Oct. 1890).	Second Six Weeks' Period (28th Dec. 1890—7th Feb. 1891).
		ATTACKS per 10,000 Population in each instance.			
THREE REGISTRATION DISTRICTS.	DARLINGTON	59·0 ⎱	41·2 ⎱	28·3 ⎱	12·9 ⎱
	STOCKTON	92·1 ⎬ 98	50·8 ⎬ 53	26·0 ⎬ 29	24·6 ⎬ 24
	MIDDLESBROUGH	117·4 ⎰	59·4 ⎰	31·4 ⎰	27·9 ⎰
OTHER SEVEN REGISTRATION DISTRICTS.	Teesdale	2·9 ⎱	2·4 ⎱	1·4 ⎱	0·9 ⎱
	Auckland	11·2	3·4	4·7	0·7
	Hartlepool	18·3	5·4	3·6	1·8
	Northallerton	2·7 ⎬ 12	0·9 ⎬ 5	0·9 ⎬ 3·5	0·0 ⎬ 1·5
	Stokesley	7·2	4·5	1·8	2·7
	Guisbrough	14·5	8·0	4·3	3·8
	Richmond	8·7 ⎰	1·6 ⎰	1·6 ⎰	0·0 ⎰

Figure 4.4 Statistical comparison of typhoid cases in the Tees Valley. From Frederick Barry, Report on Enteric Fever in the Tees Valley During 1890–91. Supplement to the Report of the Medical Officer of the LGB for 1891 (London: Eyre and Spottiswoode, 1893), 6. House of Commons Parliamentary Papers, Crown Copyright.

rates from those using Tees water compared to those not using Tees water (figure 4.5). But he also employed a variety of geographical forms of evidence, including diagrams of the waterworks and a series of spot maps of the region that marked houses invaded by typhoid as well as circling houses that were supplied with Tees water (figure 4.6).

Particularly striking was Barry's use of qualitative forms of evidence, central to communicating knowledge about outbreak investigation in the late Victorian era. Barry hired the printer Judd & Co. in London to produce a number of lithographs, which he included in the full report. The images were visual representations of the sanitary defects in towns and villages upstream of the waterworks intake in Darlington. Particularly in the limelight were the conditions in Barnard Castle, which was a central part of Barry's argument as to the origins of the outbreak. One example, figure 4.7, depicted a scene in Barnard Castle, with houses abutting the River Tees and a bevy of house drains, privy drains, yard drains, slop drains, and middens all accumulating on the banks of the river. Barry even labeled the lithographs in the style of contemporary anatomical atlases. The unsanitary city anatomized, and visualized, Barry believed, could help strengthen his claims. Seeing the stinking mess might make up for the lack of a true index case. The visuals, reprinted in summary reports in the *British Medical Journal*, were not surprisingly bemoaned by local Tees Valley rate payers as "highly problematical," and

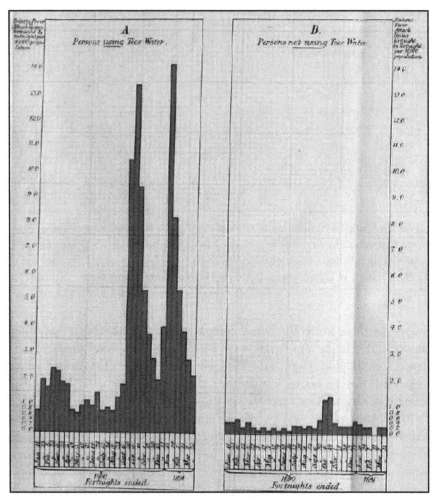

Figure 4.5 Chart showing the incidence of typhoid amongst Tees Valley water drinkers. From Frederick Barry, Report on Enteric Fever in the Tees Valley During 1890–91. Supplement to the Report of the Medical Officer of the LGB for 1891 (London: Eyre and Spottiswoode, 1893), 46. House of Commons Parliamentary Papers, Crown Copyright.

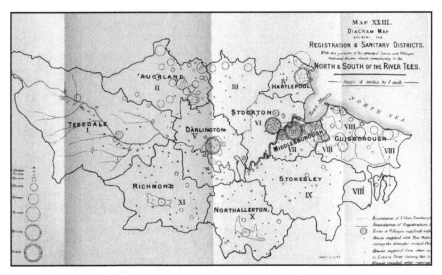

Figure 4.6 Map of the incidence of typhoid fever in the Tees Valley. From Frederick Barry, Report on Enteric Fever in the Tees Valley During 1890–91. Supplement to the Report of the Medical Officer of the LGB for 1891 (London: Eyre and Spottiswoode, 1893), 46. House of Commons Parliamentary Papers, Crown Copyright.

locals complained that the scenes at Barnard Castle "sent broadcast to the world" the private matters of their town.[69]

Combined, Barry's two reports on the outbreak of typhoid in the Tees Valley made for a powerful marshalling of both qualitative and quantitative evidence. But in the end Barry still had to rely on inference and weak causality. The Tees River had been heavily polluted, he had shown, and the incidence of the outbreak had been overwhelmingly confined to those who drank Tees water supplied by the two water companies. But the scope of his study, for all of its innovation, lacked what an earlier generation of British epidemiologists often demanded to know: the earliest cases of the disease, particularly the index case.

Barry's study also lacked laboratory confirmation. It was, to borrow a phrase from Hardy, "on the cusp" of a bacteriologically proven set of

69   "The Report on Enteric Fever in the Tees Valley," British Medical Journal 1725 (January 20, 1894): 13238; "Barnard Castle," Teesdale Mercury, January 31, 1894, 4.

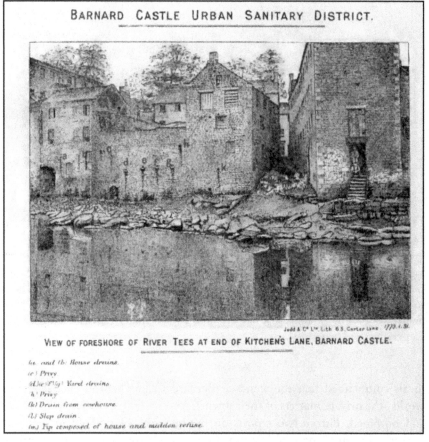

BARNARD CASTLE URBAN SANITARY DISTRICT.

VIEW OF FORESHORE OF RIVER TEES AT END OF KITCHEN'S LANE, BARNARD CASTLE.

(a. and (b. House drains.
(c) Privy
(d)e(f)(g) Yard drains
h. Privy
(k) Drain from cowhouse.
(l) Slop drain.
(m) Tip composed of house and midden refuse

Figure 4.7 Photograph of sewage faults at Barnard Castle. From Frederick Barry, Report on Enteric Fever in the Tees Valley During 1890–91.Supplement to the Report of the Medical Officer Of the LGB for 1891 (London: Eyre and Spottiswoode, 1893), 55. House of Commons Parliamentary Papers, Crown Copyright.

epidemiological claims.[70] Unlike Thorne at Caterham, Barry did not ignore chemistry and bacteriology, including in his final report an appendix with copious studies of Tees water by six different well-known analysts. But the results were not altogether helpful in proving the case against Tees water. In fact, the laboratory results in part seemed at odds with Barry's findings.

---

70   Hardy, "On the Cusp."

W. F. K. Stock, for example, public analyst for Durham, on two different occasions—late November 1890 and early February 1891—tested samples of unfiltered Tees water alongside water from the Darlington Waterworks Company. On each occasion he found the unfiltered water contaminated with excremental matters but the filtered water to be "good and wholesome drinking water." Edward Frankland had done the same at the request of D. D. Wilson, general manager of the Stockton and Middlesbrough Water Board, testing filtered and unfiltered Tees water in August and December of 1890. He found the filtered water "of excellent quality for dietetic and all domestic purposes." Alfred Allen, former president of the Society of Public Analysts weighed in as well for the Corporation of Middlesbrough and found the filtered water free of complaint. So, too, did A. C. Wilson, borough analyst for Stockton, who tested the water bacteriologically and found it "remarkably free from animal pollution."[71] But the bacteriological tests at least cast some doubt. The filtration systems at Darlington were filtering 85 percent of river water microbes, compared to Percy Frankland's published London rates of 98.5 to 99 percent. It was not proof, and Barry took little notice of the results other than that they might be suggestive. The lack of chemical or bacteriological evidence of specific contamination of the Tees water with B. typhosus was not surprising, considering the conclusions of E. Ray Lankester and G. S. Woodhead in evidence before the Royal Commission on Metropolitan Water Supply in 1893, the bacteriological analysis of water was "in its infancy."[72] Reviewing Barry's report, the Practitioner echoed the same sentiment, noting that "the bacteriology of typhoid is an obscure subject."[73] Hamlin has said as much of this period as well: the "bacteriological revolution" had not changed Edward Frankland's dictum from the 1860s and that it was too risky to use polluted water for public consumption "however completely it had been purified."[74]

71 Barry, Report on Enteric Fever in the Tees Valley, 120–30.

72 Royal Commission on Metropolitan Water Supply, 452, 503.

73 "Remarks on the Epidemic of Enteric Fever in the Tees Valley During 1890–91," Practitioner 52 (1894): 61.

74 Frankland in 1877 called the epidemiological evidence that the poison of typhoid was contained in the excreta from persons suffering from the disease and spread via infected water "abundant and strong as to be practically irresistible." See Frankland, Experimental Researches, 554–55. Hamlin, Science of Impurity, 125. Henry Letheby had long argued that water filtration and purification might be insufficient to prevent the germs of disease from spreading via water. See Henry Letheby, "Notes Accompanying the Monthly Reports on

It took a remarkably—in some ways embarrassingly—long time for Barry to complete the final report, much longer than was normal at the Medical Department. *Enteric Fever in the Tees Valley* did not appear until 1893, but when it did it had ballooned from a brief interim report into a 150-page, separately published supplement. The delay was partly because Barry was waiting to include demographic data from the new census, which did not appear until the fall of 1891. Barry was also busy conducting a sanitary survey of English ports in anticipation of epidemic cholera, so the Tees Valley study took longer than even he expected to complete. But much like other epidemiological investigations in the Victorian period—Radcliffe at Marylebone, Thorne at Caterham—Barry's Tees Valley investigation took on greater significance due to a debate that ensued after it was published. In his testimony before the Royal Commission on Metropolitan Water Supply in June 1892, Shirley Murphy, MOH for London County Council, mentioned Barry's interim report on the Tees outbreak report as one of the most important instances where typhoid was spread by filtered river water. Murphy believed it was an urgent matter that should be investigated in London, and perhaps the commission should speak with Barry after the full report was published.[75] To get a more thorough understanding of the particulars, the commission first examined David Doull Wilson, manager of the Stockton and Middlesbrough Waterworks, who had been carefully and methodically gathering evidence against Barry's indictment of the Tees water. He had been waiting for an opportunity to attack Barry publicly and got his chance in in June 1893 before the commission.

Wilson's testimony was merciless and at times pedantic. Barry had too closely followed the sentiment of local, incompetent MOsH, he argued, who had too eagerly narrowed their focus to the Tees water. Barry was more interested in blaming the water companies, Wilson argued, than figuring out the origin of the outbreak. If he had been careful, Barry would have examined the full history of typhoid in the Tees Valley and the local sanitary and climatic conditions. The linchpin of Barry's claim, the sewage-tainted foreshore at Barnard Castle, was a ruse, according to Wilson. He even produced a number of photographs—qualitative retribution—going back to 1884 that depicted the same foreshore as in Barry's 1893 visuals. Furthermore,

the Composition and Quality of the Metropolitan Waters, in the Year 1870," Wellcome Collection, SA/SMO/K.33.

75 *Royal Commission on Metropolitan Water Supply*, evidence of Shirley Murphy, June 28, 1892, 182–85.

Barry's insistence on the "trifling floods" was "insufficient" and "extremely convenient."[76] For all of the pettiness of his attack, Wilson had gathered a mass of statistical data, producing his own maps, charts, and graphs, which he carefully laid before the Royal Commission. The evidence contradicted Barry's claim that the outbreak was mostly isolated to those who drank Tees water. The small Birmingham village of California, for instance, received Tees water, but the 150 or so houses escaped the outbreak. Wilson tried to debunk many of Barry's attack rate calculations, highlighting small errors in Barry's figures, which he said were due to too much reliance on compulsory notification returns. In other words, Barry's statistical evidence was under-reported and thus skewed toward a waterborne theory. There were plenty of opportunities for "local" infection, Wilson maintained, and for the "spreading" of the disease from person to person through the traditionally convenient scapegoats of dung heaps and sewer gases.

A week later the commission called Barry to testify, and it was clear that Wilson's full-blown indictment had caught him by surprise. He began with an outright defense of both his argument and methodology. His report had "established the strongest possible presumption short of absolute proof." Wilson had merely attacked the fringe of his central argument—the outlying cases, not the core of the evidence. Asked how he came to regard water, *prima facie*, as the cause of the outbreak, Barry responded that he did so "by a method of exclusion" common to Victorian epidemiology. "As a rule I should first of all examine into all the sanitary circumstances," he explained, "and if I did not find that those gave me sufficient grounds, I should exclude first one and then another."[77] His defense, then, was that he had considered a variety of etiological factors and only settled on the Tees water after seeing the comparative incidence between those who drank Tees water and those who did not. He was repeating nearly verbatim what Thorne had done in 1879 in championing an epidemiological gaze. But Barry was also able to speak to the holes in his logic. There was enough evidence, he argued, to indict the Tees water without sleuthing for an index case, which was probably not even possible given the scale of the study, but the admission opened up more doubt than even Wilson had provided. The commissioners pushed Barry on the lack of confirmatory chemical and bacteriological evidence. Why, they wondered, had Frankland's chemical analysis found the Tees water

---

76   *Royal Commission on Metropolitan Water Supply*, evidence of D. D. Wilson, 503.

77   *Royal Commission on Metropolitan Water Supply*, evidence of F. Barry, 537–38.

pumped by the water companies "unimpeachable": "If one were to judge by chemical results alone," Barry pushed back, the water might be free of worry.[78] Epidemiological evidence had suggested otherwise, and so, too, had precedent, such as Thorne's 1879 Caterham study. In Barry's support, the *Practitioner* suggested looking at "the history of epidemics elsewhere," rather than "the behavior of the bacillus."[79] It was yet another case of privileging epidemiological expertise over laboratory expertise and of central governmental inspectors at odds with industry and local officials.

In the end Wilson's war against Barry had thrown enough suspicion, at least for the members of the Royal Commission, to caution against accepting Barry's ecologically driven waterborne theory as to the cause of the outbreak. Although the commission did not accept either theory, their final statement threw serious doubt on the Medical Department: Barry had not provided "conclusive evidence."[80] Wilson had other supporters. The local press in the Tees Valley, for example, reported that it was locally "a conviction, always well-founded" that the Tees water was not the source of the outbreak. *The Mercury* article noted that Barry's report "bore the impress of professional manipulation" and lacked evidence.[81] Another local report noted that it "was one-sided, misleading, and utterly unreliable." Central-local relations were muddled in mire, all because of the pesky, narrow-minded government inspector. The local press went so far as to call it a "Tees pollution craze."[82] Wilson had supporters in London as well. Following the Royal Commission's report, protrade journal *the Gas Journal* celebrated the findings, rejoicing that "the London Water Companies have received no harm from Dr. Barry."[83]

But the medical community came to Barry's support in droves. Ernest Hart, in a report for the Parliamentary Bills Committee of the British Medical Association, wrote an extensive review of Barry's findings, also including one of Barry's Barnard Castle photographs. Hart castigated the Royal Commission for not backing Barry, which, he argued would "do

---

78   *Royal Commission on Metropolitan Water Supply,* evidence of F. Barry, 549.

79   "Remarks on the Epidemic of Enteric Fever in the Tees Valley During 1890–91," *Practitioner* 52 (1894): 62

80   *Final Report, Royal Commission on Metropolitan Water Supply* (London, 1893), 66.

81   "Barnard Castle," *Teesdale Mercury,* June 28, 1893, 4.

82   "Stray Arrows," *Teesdale Mercury,* October 4, 1893, 5.

83   "Water and Sanitary Affairs," *Gas Journal* 62 (4 July 1893): 11.

harm to sanitary progress."[84] The *Practitioner*, in a direct reply to the Royal Commission, stated that Barry's evidence was "definite and unmistakable."[85] *The Dublin Journal of Medical Science* echoed as much: Barry's case was "clearly proven."[86] *Public Health*, the literary arm of MOsH, went even further than the *British Medical Journal* or the *Practitioner*, praising Barry's investigation and shifting the controversy into one of "national importance." While the connection between a contaminated water supply and the outbreak of typhoid was not new, *Public Health* commented that it had "not in this country been previously so nearly demonstrated." Arthur Newsholme, the editor and later chief medical officer, took an opportunity to slam Wilson, saying that "if the statistical evidence on which Dr. Barry's important and far-reaching conclusions are based is to be considered inconclusive, it is doubtful if statistical evidence can in any such case be considered to be convincing." Newsholme described the feud as between "a layman interested in the reputation of the company he serves against that of a distinguished hygienist, an expert in statistical inquiries, who has no other interests to serve but those of scientific truth."[87] The case mirrored what Radcliffe, Murchison, and Jenner faced with the Dairy Reform Company in 1873. In the years that followed, Barry's Tees Valley investigation was highlighted in textbooks, handbooks, and histories as one of the most important investigations to link typhoid to filtered river water. With the laboratory analysis of fecally contaminated water still inconclusive, Barry's study was a rallying cry for professional epidemiology. More recently, Hardy has called Barry's Tees Valley study a "classic" of Victorian epidemiology, which "reaffirmed and established the importance of unpolluted water supplies . . . and generated a renewed interest in typhoid incidence at the Medical Department . . . right up until World War I."[88]

Barry's Tees Valley study and the debate that ensued brought to the fore the excessive pollution of English rivers used as drinking water sources. Perhaps it was the reason for the continuance of endemic typhoid, despite declines in urban areas. This was not a debate new to the 1890s, but the

---

84   Hart, "Waterborne Typhoid," 1446–1147.

85   "Remarks on the Epidemic of Enteric Fever in the Tees Valley During 1890–91," *Practitioner* 52 (1894): 58.

86   "Enteric Fever in the Tees Valley," *Dublin Journal of Medical Science* 97 (1894): 49–53.

87   Newsholme, "Enteric Fever in the Tees Valley."

88   Hardy, "Methods of Outbreak Investigation," 200–201.

slow converging of epidemiology and bacteriology in that period meant that the topic received renewed interest. The investigation also threw into doubt, Hamlin has argued, confidence in sand filtration and the reassurance that bacteriological tests that showed low microbe counts in a sample of water meant typhoid-free water.[89] It demonstrated to a broad audience in Britain the lagging and uneven implementation of compulsory notification. But Barry's findings were anything but isolated. The whole Tees Valley episode was repeated in 1893 when Bruce Low, Barry's colleague at the department, traced an outbreak of typhoid in Lincolnshire to the polluted tributaries of the Trent River. There, too, local authorities along the Trent denied that contaminated water had caused the outbreak. More evidence poured in from the inspectorate that same year from Theodore Thomson, who showed that a fulminating outbreak at Worthing—over a thousand cases and nearly two hundred deaths—was caused by sewers leaking into the area's wells. In the Worthing case Klein had even discovered colonies of both *B. coli* and *B. typhosus* in a local contaminated well that Thomson's epidemiological sleuthing had pointed toward. Perhaps the laboratory and field could be merged.

From the mid-1870s Klein had been stubbornly working on the bacteriology of typhoid, but progress had been slow and unsteady. Thorne noted in his annual report of 1897 that the field epidemiologists of the department were eager to learn from laboratory evidence about the nature and behavior of *B. typhosus* outside of the body, particularly the microbes changing virulence. But for the most part, he noted, epidemiology had "obtained little encouragement from the labours of the bacteriologist."[90] The Worthing case had presented an opportunity to solve a problem with which European and North American bacteriologists were struggling—the supposed coidentity of *B. typhosus* and *B. coli*. French observers Rodet and Roux, in 1889, had argued that the two were varieties of the same bacterium. They might even be interchangeable. It was yet another example of the lack of laboratory clarity that remained after the discovery of *B. typhosus*. What was even more unclear was how to incorporate such knowledge into outbreak investigation. It had not worked for Barry in 1890, but by 1893 Klein, as the Worthing outbreak showed, was getting close. Klein was especially interested in the practical application of bacteriological knowledge. What was needed, Klein knew, was laboratory evidence of the action of the microbe outside of the body, just as Barry's epidemiological sleuthing had suggested. From the mid-1890s, the

89   Hamlin, *A Science of Impurity,* 284–85.
90   Thorne, *Annual Report of Medical Officer for 1896–1897,* xxi.

epidemiological problem was coming into sharper focus, particularly the role of infected soils leaching into waterways and drinking water. Klein had been experimenting on rodents with injected *B. typhosus* in 1892 and 1893 but was unsuccessful in reproducing the disease in the laboratory. The following year he turned to experimental studies with monkeys, feeding two of them the typhoid bacillus in a milk broth and inoculating the bacillus into eight other monkeys' groins. Three of the inoculated monkeys showed postmortem signs of an enlarged spleen, and in those cases Klein was able to recover *B. typhosus*. In another set of experiments in 1893 Klein injected four calves with the bacillus, and was able to recover it in abundance, postmortem from the inguinal glands.

In an ingenious set of experiments to sort out the supposed coidentity of *B. typhosus* and *B. coli*, Klein devised two tests. He first cultured and isolated both *B. typhosus* and *B. coli* from human sources. He then let them grow in both tap water and distilled water to see the vitality of each outside of the body in a natural growth medium. He extracted and isolated each colony and found that they remained distinct. In a second test Klein extracted both bacilli from polluted public water supplies. He then transferred each from peritoneum to peritoneum of several guinea pigs to observe their development in an animal subject. Here, too, as in the first test, *B. typhosus* remained *B. typhosus,* and *B. coli* remained *B. coli*. The two, in other words, were not the same bacillus but were different morphologically and biochemically outside of the body. Both organisms, Klein found, grew abundantly in water for extended periods—up to a month.[91] It was an important practical finding that became routinized in the everyday practice of public health in England. By 1900, for example, one of the examination questions for candidates wishing to obtain the diploma in public health was to describe the characteristics that differentiate *B. typhosus* from *B. coli*.[92].

European observers had widely speculated on the viability of *B. typhosus* outside of the human body, with some claiming five days and others over a hundred. In 1894 and 1895 Klein was determined to bring the issue more clarity through experimentation.[93] So, too, was Percy Frankland, Edward Frankland's son and England's leading expert on the bacteriology of water in the last two decades of the century. On behalf of the Water Research

---

91 Klein, "Further Report on the Etiology of Typhoid Fever," 457–68.

92 Examination Papers for Diploma in Public Health (1900), Wellcome Collection, MS.6807/17–23.

93 Klein, "On the Abilities of Certain Pathogenic Microbes," 411–28.

Committee of the Royal Society, Frankland had conducted a similar experiment with the typhoid bacillus in 1894, injecting a series of cultures with drops of Thames water, Loch Katrine water, and water from a deep well. Frankland found the typhoid bacillus viable in river water for up to thirty-three days and slightly longer in well water.[94] Though their methods were similar, Klein argued that Frankland had experimented on too small a scale, obscuring the practical question of when typhoid colonies completely disappear—not just diminish—in water.[95] Testing the matter himself in 1894 and 1895, Klein found the bacillus still viable in distilled water after six months and in Thames water after eight weeks. Separating B. typhosus from B. coli was an important laboratory finding for outbreak investigation. In other words, there were still numerous problems in the bacteriology of typhoid. But by the late 1890s bacteriologists in Britain and America were using the presence of B. coli as an indicator of excrementally polluted water, a helpful practical laboratory guide to outbreak investigation.[96]

Although they were converging, epidemiology and bacteriology had yet to come together successfully to solve a problem in outbreak investigation. That changed one year later, during an outbreak of typhoid in 1896 at Chichester. Investigated by H. Timbrell Bulstrode, the Chichester study demonstrated a new model of outbreak investigation; although guided by traditional field-based methods, Bulstrode relied extensively on bacteriology. He worked closely with Klein, who examined the bacteriological counts in the Chichester water supply, and Sidney Martin, who analyzed the presence of typhoid bacteria in samples of Chichester soils. Considering Klein's steady progress on the practical aspects of typhoid bacteriology in the early 1890s, the time was ripe. Contemporaries praised the epidemiological investigation at Chichester as another startling revelation of the continuing endemic threat of typhoid as the century came to a close. Bulstrode's epidemiological practices were braced by bacteriological tests of soil and water.

---

94   Frankland, "The Behaviour of the Typhoid Bacillus."

95   Klein cited the Thomson's Worthing outbreak, where he had discovered b. Typhosus, but only when he sampled twelve hundred cubic centimeters of well water. Had he only analyzed the typical ten to fifty cubic centimeters, he maintained, he probably would not have found the particulate matter of typhoid bacilli.

96   See, for example, Reynolds and Branson, "Report on a Bacteriological Examination of a Sample of the Horsforth Public Water Supply," October 9, 1896, National Archives, Kew, MH 113/34. Victor Vaughan in America was doing this as well. See Adler, Victor Vaughan, 42.

The Chichester investigation was important for two reasons. It showed that the shoe-leather practices of epidemiology at the Medical Department that began in the 1860s and 1870s, emblematic in Radcliffe's Marylebone and Thorne's Caterham investigations, remained largely unchanged by the end of the century. The field-based, statistically informed, and population-centered epidemiology of midcentury was essentially that of the 1890s, suggesting a powerful continuity of epidemiological practice that was at the center of the professional identity of working epidemiologists in England. The second is that despite a relative continuity of practice, the performance of epidemiology was changing by the 1890s. Bulstrode sought to establish his credibility and authority at the Medical Department, and by extension the credibility of epidemiology, in a disciplinary and historically reflexive way, one that was especially politicized. Bacteriology might not just be a handmaid to epidemiology, to borrow a phrase from Alfredo Morabia.[97]

H. Timbrell Bulstrode and the Chichester Typhoid Study of 1896

By the late 1890s Chichester held a poor sanitary reputation among the staff at the Medical Department. The city possessed, as A. C. Houston later noted in 1904, "the unenviable reputation of being one of a number of places in England and Wales in which enteric fever prevails in endemic and epidemic form to a notable extent."[98] Edward Seaton, one of the department's earliest inspectors, was the first to investigate the sanitary state of Chichester, in 1865. Seaton, no doubt seeking to shock his readers, noted in his report that the "death-rate which, for a small city well situated, not overcrowded, but comprehending within its bounds even fields and open country, in which no large manufactures are carried on, gives strong evidence of something radically amiss in the sanitary conditions of the place."[99] As of 1865 Chichester had no system of drainage and no extraneous water supply; Seaton found nuisances of every sort, in no small part due to Chichester's large cattle market, held every other Wednesday. Several years later, in 1879, when Seaton

---

97   Morabia, "Epidemiology and Bacteriology in 1900," 617–18.

98   Houston, "Report on the Chemical and Bacteriological Examination of Tunbridge Wells Deep Well Water," 581.

99   Seaton, "Report on Circumstances Endangering the Public Health of Chichester," 220.

replaced Simon as chief medical officer, Hubert Airy visited Chichester to investigate an explosive outbreak of typhoid fever. Airy's investigation localized the 1879 outbreak to an infected milk supply; he ended his report by noting that "there yet remain grave defects in the sanitary condition of the city."[100]

Between 1870 and 1890 vital statistics from the registrar-general's office showed that the death rate from typhoid fever in Chichester was one of the worst in England and Wales. During both decennial periods—1871 to 1880, and 1881 to 1890—Chichester had the highest death rate of all the registration districts in Sussex. Moreover, compared with all of England and Wales, only 31 of 630 districts had a higher death rate from 1871 to 1880. Chichester was worse off in the decade 1881 to 1890, when the city ranked in the top twenty districts with the highest incidence of typhoid fever. Therefore, when the mayor of Chichester wrote to Thorne, then chief medical officer, in July 1896 to ask for assistance with an explosive outbreak of typhoid fever, Thorne quickly responded by sending H. Timbrell Bulstrode, a member of his epidemiological staff.

Herbert Timbrell Bulstrode served as an inspector at the Medical Department for nearly twenty years, from 1892 until his sudden death from heart failure in 1911. Thirty years old and fresh from a medical degree at Cambridge, Bulstrode was the first inspector Thorne brought on when he became chief medical officer. "He had a notable characteristic of independently investigating" his obituarist noted, and he was part of a cadre of epidemiologists who—following in the footsteps of Ballard, Radcliffe, Buchanan, and Thorne—considered themselves professional epidemiologists. Though perhaps less well-known today, Bulstrode is best remembered for providing epidemiological confirmation of the role of shellfish in transmitting typhoid fever, and, as Morabia and Hardy have shown, for using novel methods of epidemiological inquiry such as questionnaires.[101]

In 1896 the population of Chichester stood at just over ten thousand. While typhoid was a common occurrence, between July and August over one hundred new cases of the disease were reported, most of which occurred "were the same as those which had been attacked when Seaton reported on the city 30 years ago."[102] Bulstrode's Chichester investigation began much

---

100 Airy, "Report to the Local Government Board on an Outbreak of Enteric Fever in Chichester," 9.

101 Morabia and Hardy, "The Pioneering Use of a Questionnaire."

102 Thorne, "Enteric Fever at Chichester," xii.

like the hundreds of others the inspectorate of the department conducted. He convened with Mr. E. Prior (the mayor), Mr. Davy (the board's general inspector), members of the local sanitary committee, and with the chairman of the water company, all of whom combined to provide Bulstrode with an up-to-date list of fever cases, their addresses, and the sanitary condition and source of water supply of each house. Such assistance from local officials—though not always forthcoming—was a central feature of late nineteenth- and especially early twentieth-century epidemiological investigations. Bulstrode visited and interviewed individuals on the list and also inspected the public waterworks.

Bulstrode's initial focus was on the water supply and drainage of Chichester. The city was supplied, he found, with water from both private shallow wells and the Chichester Waterworks Company. The shallow wells, "imperfectly protected against filth soaking through the soil," were of particular concern, as many were located near privies or cesspools and fitted with loose, wooden lids.[103] Chichester possessed a recently constructed sewer system, but privies were still in wide use, Bulstrode found, and even in places where household privies had been abandoned, "the privy vaults had, together with their contents, perhaps the accumulation of some years, been simply filled in, and not, as they should have been, carefully emptied, their bricks removed, and their sites carefully cleansed."[104] "Chichester must, I fear," Bulstrode lamented in his report, "still be regarded as not differing substantially from an undrained city."[105]

Bulstrode found nothing illuminating as to the distribution of the disease via sex, though he noticed that 63 of the 111 victims were between the ages of 5 and 20.[106] The public water supply was largely free from suspicion, a conclusion Bulstrode reached using epidemiological, chemical, and bacteriological evidence. Of the 682 houses within the walls of Chichester, 494 were supplied by the public water company. Of that number, Bulstrode found, only three were invaded by typhoid. Altogether, of the 76 houses invaded, 39 were supplied by private wells (2.9% case incidence) and 37 (2.6% case incidence) with water from the public company. Though the epidemiological evidence was too inconclusive to indict the public water supply, Bulstrode

---

103 Bulstrode, "Report Upon Prevalence of Enteric Fever," 93.

104 Ibid.

105 Bulstrode, "Report Upon Prevalence of Enteric Fever," 92.

106 Though a higher incidence in children and young adults suggested dissemination via milk, Bulstrode found no evidence that milk played a role.

sent samples of Chichester water to Klein. On July 29, 1896, with the incidence of typhoid fever in Chichester on the rise, Klein, at his laboratory at
St. Bartholomew's Hospital, performed three routine bacteriological tests on
the Chichester water. He first made a gelatin plate with one-fourth c.c. water
to determine the number of aerobic microbes. After a forty-eight-hour incubation period the plate yielded only 23 colonies, or 92 aerobic microbes per
1 c.c., a small number of harmless bacteria.[107] Klein then took 1,200 c.c. of
Chichester water and forced it through a Berkefeld filter, using gelatin culture media—phenolated broth, phenolated gelatin, and iodised potato gelatin—to test for the typhoid bacillus. He found no typhoid microbes. Lastly,
Klein took the 120 cc particulate matter and tested it for the presence of
anaerobic microbes, none of which he found. Klein ended his report, which
was compiled at the end of Bulstrode's, by soundly declaring that "the sample
of water delivered here was of excellent quality as far as bacteriological tests
go."[108] Klein's bacteriology, in other words, was sufficient in guiding epidemiological practice—it took Bulstrode's attention away from the waterworks
company. But insofar as it applied to epidemiology, bacteriology was only
used here to confirm epidemiological methods.

Bulstrode's rhetorical strategies at Chichester relied on a historical epidemiological claim, emphasizing that typhoid prevailed in 1896 in the same
places it had in former years. Neither the construction of a new sewerage system nor the public provision of water to parts of the city effected the preventive change necessary to curb outbreaks of the disease. Seemingly progressive
sanitary improvement, Bulstrode suggested, had failed to prevent the disease.
"There would, indeed," Bulstrode concluded, "appear from consideration of
the past history of Chichester in respect to enteric fever, no need to seek out
in explanation new agencies of dissemination, such, for instance, as the public water supply, or the recently constructed sewerage."[109] It was clear that
typhoid fever was endemic in Chichester; but its cause, Bulstrode feared, "is
not easy to determine." With filthy cesspools and privies still in abundance,
Bulstrode declared that "not until the cesspits and cesspools of the place have
been abolished, and their sites and the soil in the neighbourhood thoroughly
cleansed, can it be hoped that enteric fever will be banished from the city."[110]

---

107 Klein, "Report of Bacteriological Analysis," 105–6; Bulstrode, "Report Upon
Prevalence of Enteric Fever," 105.
108 Klein, "Report of Bacteriological Analysis," 106.
109 Bulstrode, "Report Upon Prevalence of Enteric Fever," 104.
110 Ibid.

Compared to Thorne's 1879 Caterham investigation or Barry's Tees Valley study, Bulstrode's Chichester study failed to elicit a dramatic response from local authorities. This was partly, it seems, due to the rhetorical and performative strategies Bulstrode used to communicate his study. Like Thorne, Bulstrode provided a list of recommendations to the Chichester town council, issued July 21, 1896. He included generic sanitary suggestions, such as the removal of all "accumulations of filth," and specific remedial measures increasingly used to combat infectious diseases, such as the removal of early cases to the local isolation hospital. Bulstrode's chief concern was the state and preponderance of privies in Chichester. He noted in his report that the Chichester Sanitary Committee adopted a formal resolution to "carry out these recommendations in their entirety," but further epidemiological study in 1900 by Theodore Thomson indicated that such measures largely went unfulfilled.[111]

In the course of Bulstrode's investigation bacteriology was relied upon but only in an ancillary way. Klein's analysis of the Chichester public water supply failed to detect the specific germs of typhoid fever and hence all but ruled out suspicion of the company. But Bulstrode's statistical analysis led him to the same conclusion. In this way, the new methods of bacteriology had yet again failed to push the boundaries of disease investigation. It was rather the opposite; the defining feature of Bulstrode's 1896 Chichester investigation was that epidemiological methods had localized the outbreak to Chichester soils. It was not too different from the protoecological conclusion of Barry just a few years earlier condemning the Barnard Castle foreshore. Thorne, for example, in his summary highlighted that Bulstrode's study "goes to show that enteric fever, though mainly distributed in epidemic form by means of water or of milk, is by no means always a 'water-borne' disease; and it raises anew the question as to how far recurring prevalences of enteric fever in one town or spot can be due to the persistence in more or less active form in certain soils of the organism of that disease."[112] Contemporaries such as William Henry Corfield saw Bulstrode's 1896 study as a powerful example of the endemicity of typhoid fever and one that provided etiological clarity on the role of soil in transmitting the disease.[113] It was epidemiological investigation—the methods and practices exhibited by both Barry in 1890 and Bulstrode in 1896—that pushed etiological boundaries and pointed to the

---

111 Thomson and Marsh, "Enteric Fever in the City of Chichester."

112 Thorne, "Enteric Fever at Chichester," xiii.

113 Corfield, *The Aetiology of Typhoid Fever*, 125.

role of soil in maintaining outbreaks of typhoid fever. J. Lane Notter had argued before the Epidemiological Society of London in 1895 that "certain factors situated in the soil itself, must furnish not only material for its origin, but also for the continuance of typhoid sickness."[114] In the late 1890s soil-based research was becoming clearer, yet this was a matter left up to bacteriology and microbiology to further investigate in the twentieth century.

It is worth reflecting on the performative aspects of Bulstrode's 1896 Chichester investigation, especially as it compares to Thorne in 1879 at Caterham and Barry in 1890–91 at Teesdale. The shoe-leather practices of Victorian epidemiology—what Ballard called the "*via exclusionis*" method— was still at the center of disease investigation as the nineteenth century came to a close. And while we usually claim that the "new" public health of the early twentieth century was obsessed with individuals—and the resultant public health practices of isolation and disinfection—Bulstrode's epidemiology was firmly population-centered. Unlike Thorne in 1879, but more like Barry in 1891, Bulstrode was keen to use epidemiological findings to engage in politicized arguments. Perhaps it was because earlier epidemiologists like Thorne at Caterham and Radcliffe at Marylebone were successful in cajoling local authorities into action using only epidemiological evidence. Bulstrode, however, used the rhetoric of historical epidemiology to substantiate the conclusions to be drawn from his 1896 Chichester study. This positioning had important methodological and performative ramifications and indicates that while the methods of epidemiological inquiry had not substantially changed from the 1860s to the 1890s, the way in which epidemiologists at the Medical Department substantiated epidemiological ways of knowing were changing. Of particular interest are three maps Bulstrode prepared for his 1896 report (figures 4.8, 4.9. 4.10).[115]

The maps depict the registration counties of England and Wales: Map 1 shows the annual death rate of typhoid fever per 100,000 persons during the decade 1871–80, with the rates on different counties indicated by five sets of colors, ranging from 70 deaths or more per 100,000 to under 30 deaths per 100,000. Map 2 provides the same data for the period 1881–90; what is

114 Notter, "The Influence of Soil," 103.

115 Medical geographers have recently made cogent claims about the epistemic role of epidemiological maps in making arguments about the causation and spread of disease. See Koch, *Disease Maps*. Some historians of medicine have recently done so as well. See Arnold-Forster, "Mapmaking and Mapthinking"; Mooney and Tanner, "Infant Mortality, a Spatial Problem."

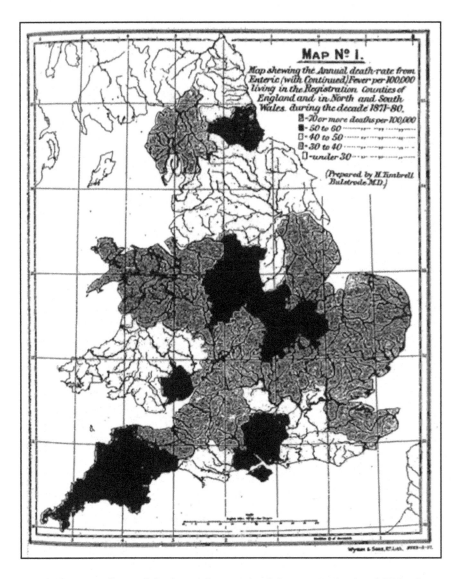

Figure 4.8 Map of annual death rate from typhoid fever in England and Wales from 1871-1880. From H. Timbrell Bulstrode, "Report Upon Prevalence of Enteric Fever in the City of Chichester," in Twenty-Sixth Annual Report of the Local Government Board, Supplement Containing the Report of the Medical Officer for 1896–97, 107. House of Commons Parliamentary Papers, Crown Copyright.

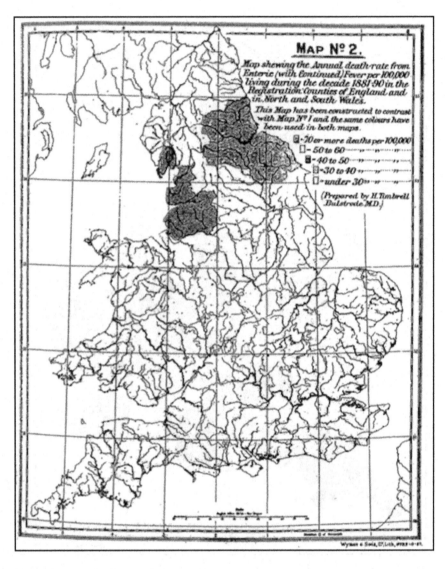

Figure 4.9 Map of annual death rate from typhoid fever in England and Wales from 1881-1890. From, H. Timbrell Bulstrode, "Report Upon Prevalence of Enteric Fever in the City of Chichester," in Twenty-Sixth Annual Report of the Local Government Board, Supplement Containing the Report of the Medical Officer for 1896–97, 108. House of Commons Parliamentary Papers, Crown Copyright.

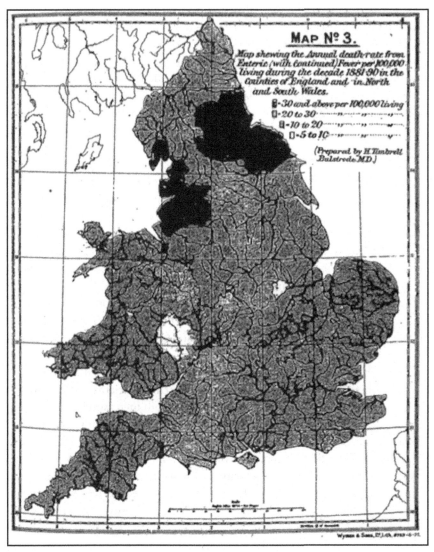

Figure 4.10 Map of annual death rate from typhoid fever in England and Wales from 1881-1890. From, H. Timbrell Bulstrode, "Report Upon Prevalence of Enteric Fever in the City of Chichester," in Twenty-Sixth Annual Report of the Local Government Board, Supplement Containing the Report of the Medical Officer for 1896–97, 107. House of Commons Parliamentary Papers, Crown Copyright.

striking was that only two of the five colors in the first map remained, as three of the highest incidences of death had altogether disappeared. Bulstrode, and by extension Thorne, used the tools of epidemiology—including cartography—to depict what was seemingly a successful narrative of Victorian public health: namely, the dramatic decrease in the incidence of typhoid fever from 1860 to 1900. The rhetorical claim behind the use of such representations was that epidemiology, as the central science of state medicine, was in part responsible for the decrease in the disease. Yet, Bulstrode used to construct a rather different public health argument; it showed those registration districts in the period 1881–90 that had the highest incidences of typhoid fever and were thus lagging behind the general trend.[116] This, too, was no doubt part of Bulstrode's attempt to situate and self-present his epidemiological practices at Chichester, and by extension, what he saw as the continual forging of the relationship between epidemiology and bacteriology. In his *Annual Report*, Thorne noticed that they served "to indicate that whilst enteric fever has been undergoing enormous diminution in this country, the areas of both its maximum and its minimum incidences have remained practically the same during the 20 years 1871–90."[117] The rhetoric of condemnation here is particularly interesting, especially in light of Keir Waddington's analysis of practices and conceptualizations of rural public health in late Victorian Wales.[118]

Thorne played a significant role in guiding the surge of soil-based studies of microorganisms in late nineteenth- and early twentieth-century Britain from his perch at the Medical Department. Though increasingly bacteriological, these studies remained committed to furthering epidemiological claims, although, as Thorne noted in his *Twenty-Sixth Annual Report* in 1897, "there has been rather discouragement" of bacteriological evidence confirming epidemiological suspicion.[119] During the Chichester study, Bulstrode—at Thorne's orders—sent samples of soils thought to be infected with typhoid microbes to Sidney Martin, the Jamaican-born University College London and Vienna-trained bacteriologist working on a part-time basis for the

---

116   Graham Mooney has argued that "mortality comparisons between countryside and town became a particularly useful tool for demonstrating the shocking conditions of urban life." See Mooney, "Professionalisation in Public Health," 53.

117   Thorne, "Enteric Fever at Chichester," xiii.

118   Waddington, "It Might Not Be a Nuisance."

119   Thorne, "Enteric Fever at Chichester," xxi.

SOILS, STOOLS, AND SAPROPHYTES 6♠ 219

department. The role of soil in spreading infectious diseases such as typhoid fever was not new to the 1890s but resurged as a result of epidemiological studies such as Barry and Bulstrode's.

From the late 1860s, as we saw in chapter 2, epidemiologists at the Medical Department—Ballard, Radcliffe, and Buchanan—argued that outbreaks of waterborne or milk-borne typhoid fever were the result of dangerous germs gaining access to water supplies through the medium of the soil. The connection between soil and sewage was far from new. Polemical chemist Alfred Smee of Croydon, for example, maintained from the 1870s that cows fed with sewage-contaminated grasses could spread typhoid through their milk.[120] Smee's etiological theory combined Murchison's and Pettenkofer's belief that disease-causing germs had to undergo a period of fermentation, or incubation, in the soil to become infective.[121] Early theories such as Murchison's and Petterkofer's, which were environmentally driven, have been chalked up to the lasting strength of localist doctrine in the late nineteenth century. As Worboys has shown, there was a multiplicity of germ theories. It was still etiologically viable, after all, to suggest that the germs of typhoid and similar diseases multiplied in favorable soil conditions rather than in the bodies of patients, a view that had crucial public health implications for stopping the spread of infectious diseases through disinfection and isolation practices.[122] Yet it would be misleading to think of soil-based etiological theories that persisted into the 1890s (aligned with the Murchison/Pettenkofer camp), as etiological holdouts that maintained a belief in spontaneous generation long after it was scientifically fashionable. Instead, the vanguard of British bacteriologists—Sidney Martin, A. C. Houston, and

---

120 Smee, *Milk, Typhoid Fever, and Sewage;* Smee, *Sewage, Sewage Produce, and Disease;* Carpenter, *Some Points in the Physiological and Medical Aspects of Sewage.* Smee's interest in the matter can be dated to the late 1850s, when he sent a series of letters to John Simon, then MOH for the City of London; See Letters from Alfred Smee to John Simon, December 19, 1859 and December 20, 1859, Royal College of Surgeons of England, John Simon Collection, 67.h.5 Letters & Papers, re: College Affairs.

121 Pettenkofer, "Boden and Grundwasser." Bacteriological research in the 1880s and 1890s on the relationship between soil and anthrax may have also contributed to Houston's interest. On anthrax, see Stark, *The Making of Modern Anthrax;* Jones, *Death in a Small Package,* especially chapter 1.

122 Etiological debates on typhoid were at the center of the Section of Medicine at the Annual Meeting of the British Medical Association in 1879 held in Cork. See Carpenter, "A Consideration of Some of the Fallacies," 79–81.

Edward Klein—undertook soil-based research and sought to prove more exclusivist etiological theories and to explore fundamental biological questions about the life cycle of germs.[123] It was only in the 1890s that the role of soil was again considered, but it was in light of epidemiological specificity.

With the soil samples he received from Bulstrode at Chichester, Martin began to test what soil conditions—temperature, soil bacteria, water levels—were productive or inimical to the development of *B. typhosus* outside the human organism.[124] Martin's research demonstrates cooperation between epidemiologists and bacteriologists at the Medical Department. Martin received eight samples of soil, half were from houses where typhoid had been extensively present during the 1896 Chichester study and the other from houses free of the disease.

Martin found that the typhoid bacillus could remain alive and virulent for long periods in sterilized cultivated soils (normal garden soil, for example, that might be found near households), but that "in virgin, uncultivated soil it rapidly dies."[125] Bacteriological testing of *B. typhosus* in soils was a confirmation of John Burdon Sanderson's long-held doctrine that certain diseases "possess the wonderful property of passing into a state of persistent inactivity or latent vitality, in which they perform no function, but can at any moment be wakened up into active function, whenever they are brought under favourable circumstances."[126] Reflecting on the importance of Martin's soil-based studies of typhoid in his *Annual Report* for 1897, Thorne noted that "whilst much of the diminution in enteric fever has gone hand-in-hand with the abandonment of water services which, being subject to receive specific pollution, served for wide diffusions and sudden outbursts of enteric fever—much of the persistent prevalence of that disease is associated with those systems for the disposal of excreta and refuse which still find favour in certain parts of this country, and which inevitably involve organic pollution of the soil."[127]

---

123 Houston, "Enteric Fever in its Public Health Aspects," 468–69.

124 Martin, "Preliminary Report on the Growth of the Typhoid Bacillus in Soil."

125 Martin, "The Growth of the Typhoid Bacillus in Soil"; Martin, "Further Report on the Growth of the Typhoid Bacillus in Soil," 525–48.

126 Thorne, "Remarks on the Origin of Infection," 240. It was also the belief of Glasgow MOH and Darwinist James Russell. See Russell, *Lectures on the Theory and General Prevention*, 2–3, 39.

127 Thorne, *Annual Report of the Medical Officer for 1896–1897*, xiv.

Soil-based research highlighted one of the most pressing public health problems that occurred in late nineteenth-century Britain, namely, sporadic but persistent outbreaks of endemic diseases such as typhoid fever. This was, as Hardy has claimed, originally a "specific epidemiological problem" and one that "bacteriology had failed to provide the answer."[128] Yet, in the last decade of the nineteenth century bacteriological studies at the Medical Department on disease-causing organisms in soil and in water succeeded in elucidating further etiological clarity and reinforcing remedial measures in public works. This confirms Worboys's claim that a "seed and soil" botanical metaphor dominated the understanding of germs in the second half of the nineteenth century.[129] Yet "seed and soil" was more than simply a metaphor; it guided epidemiological as well as bacteriological practice. Whereas Hardy has seen the failure of bacteriology to confirm the etiological role of soil in spreading typhoid as a plausible rationale for the growing "uneasiness" between the two groups of practitioners, it is more likely that this episode confirms that epidemiological rather than bacteriological practices dominated the Medical Department.

In his annual report for 1897, Thorne summarized Bulstrode's epidemiological research alongside Martin's fledgling bacteriological research, noting that

> these facts go to indicate the need for systematic study of a question which has gradually come to acquire considerable importance, and which may be put thus—What are the local conditions by reason of which certain areas, whether registration counties, town, or villages, have, for at least a generation, become identified with such persistence or periodic recrudescence of enteric fever, as has continued to secure for them death-rates from that disease in excess of other districts with some at least of which they may not unfairly be compared?[130]

Epidemiological practices played a key role in answering Thorne's call to activism, but so, too, did the new practices of bacteriology, particularly water- and soil-related studies that sought to understand the survival of germs outside the human body. That Bulstrode actively yoked his epidemiological fieldwork to the practices of bacteriology signaled a shift in the performance of

---

128 Hardy, "On the Cusp," 343.
129 Worboys, *Spreading Germs*, 6–7.
130 Thorne, *Annual Report of the Medical Officer for 1896–1897*, xiv.

public health at the Medical Department. By the 1890s epidemiologists like Bulstrode could not claim, for example, that they had "little acquaintance" with the laboratory as Thorne had done at Caterham. Increasingly, bacteriology and epidemiology together sought to answer the tough questions in public health, such as the persistence of typhoid fever. "We have the aid of laboratory," Shirley Murphy triumphantly declared in his inaugural presidential address before the Epidemiological Society of London.[131] Hardy has shown that in the twentieth century laboratory methods were incorporated into outbreak investigation studying the wider *Salmonella* group, particularly in foodborne outbreaks. Ultimately, however, from the perspective of professional identity, Bulstrode's inclusion of bacteriology only muddied the etiological waters of his epistemological claims. Though he sought to "receive support at the hands of the bacteriologist," he ultimately found little value in bacteriological justification.[132] Epidemiology had suggested the endemicity of typhoid in the Chichester soils, and bacteriology was too immature to provide more than preliminary causal evidence. Unlike Hardy's claim, this was not by itself reason for fissure between epidemiology and bacteriology. Hence Bulstrode's recourse to historical epidemiology and to the aesthetics of nationwide mapmaking. Relying on the traditional posturing of epidemiologists, intelligible to Thorne and Bulstrode, the Chichester study could be used to make a politicized argument that denounced laggard local authorities such as those in Chichester, and perhaps throughout England, as Barry had done in the Tees Valley. So as much as epidemiology was changing, its disciplinary identity clung to established ways. Describing the history of epidemics and epidemiology in late nineteenth-century England in 1911, Edward C. Seaton, in *Infectious Diseases and Their Preventive Treatment*, argued that even after the Notification of Infectious Diseases Act of 1889, what had been needed to curb the endemic threat of typhoid was the "collective investigation" of typhoid between the field and the laboratory.[133] From his perch in 1911, Seaton could see that although typhoid was on the decline, more work was needed, as there were still between eight thousand and ten thousand cases each year. Nevertheless, the precedent was set.

Klein, for his part, remained a tenacious typhoid laboratory scientist. Following his limited success in the mid-1890s in researching typhoid

---

131 Murphy, "On the Study of Epidemiology," 24.
132 Bulstrode, "Report Upon Prevalence of Enteric Fever in the City of Chichester," 101.
133 Seaton, *Infectious Diseases*, 92

outside the body, he began to turn his attention to the afterlife of typhoid *in* bodies. In June 1898, for example, he was busy injecting *B. typhosus* into the abdomen of guinea pigs. After the guinea pigs died, about a day later, he carefully placed them in wooden coffins and buried them in an experimental burial box filled with normal garden soil he took from Wandsworth Common. There the typhoid corpses sat for thirty-one days, until Klein exhumed the bodies, took up a scalpel, and opened the abdominal cavities, looking for colonies of *B. typhosus*. Klein had a new obsession, the fate of microbes in animals—and by extension human corpses. Klein's experimental interests were driven by what he called a "general and popular belief that the microbes of infectious disease retain their vitality and power of mischief within dead and buried bodies for indefinite period."[134] Klein's corpse research was widely published in British and European journals, and he was not alone in this period in turning to experimental studies of the behavior of germs within bodies. In fact, the turn toward typhoid in bodies—particularly the idea that bodies (like water, milk, or soils) could serve as media in the spread of the disease—dominated research on the disease in the early twentieth century. Before the debate on typhoid shifted to so-called healthy carriers, or Typhoid Marys, the discourse on typhoid in England in the last years of the nineteenth century and the first years of the twentieth was already centered on the body, particularly the body of the male soldier. As typhoid declined at home, one final Victorian public calamity brought about by the filth disease erupted overseas, turning what had been an English problem into a British imperial problem. Typhoid was on the rise among troops in India. And most importantly, during the South African War, over seventy-five thousand Britons were struck with the disease and over ten thousand died in three years. It was the single largest incidence of the filth disease in the Victorian period. The typhoid outbreak during the South African War, as explored in the final chapter, produced a palpable anxiety over the relationship between imperialism and disease. It threw into doubt the ability of the nation to protect the health of its citizens, which might be done at home but not abroad. And it proved yet another arena for an already-seasoned debate over the relative merits of epidemiology and bacteriology, particularly around Almroth Wright's antityphoid vaccine developed in 1896.

---

134 Klein, "Report on the Fate of Pathogenic and other Infective Microbes," 345–49.

Chapter Five

Typhoid in the Tropics

Imperial Bodies, Warfare, and the Reframing of Typhoid as a Global Disease

In the thick of the most expensive war during Queen Victoria's reign, on June 29, 1900, the American-born Conservative MP for Westminster, William Burdett-Coutts, stood before the House of Commons and retold a shockingly solemn scene from his recent wartime travel to Bloemfontein, South Africa:

> After the railway was opened, there was one of the hospitals containing typhoid patients which had no disinfectants of any kind, and another in which the corpse of one of the patients who had died during the night had been stuffed into the only lavatory there was in the hospital. It was found by the patients who went to use the lavatory in the morning.[1]

Klein's research less than a year prior, on the infectivity of the animal typhoid corpse, had a corporeal corollary of striking proportions on the South African veldt. In January of 1900 Burdett-Coutts sailed for South Africa as a special war correspondent for the *Times*, writing to his Westminster constituents days before departing that "too much information cannot be given to the public" about the condition of sick and wounded British troops.[2] In February he arrived in Cape Town, from there moving inland to join the combined British forces in Bloemfontein, the center of the most heated

---

1 Burdett-Coutts, *The Sick and Wounded in South Africa*, 57.
2 Burdett-Coutts, *The Sick and Wounded in South Africa*, 3.

battle with the Afrikaner Boers and with the typhoid bacillus. In March he published the first in a series of seven sensational articles in the *Times* entitled "Our Wars and Our Wounded." His story of a typhoid corpse stuffed into a lavatory highlights the emergence of yet another intense moment in the Victorian history of the filth disease. So concerned were members of Parliament that on July 19, 1900, in response to Burdett-Coutts's typhoid claims, they established a royal commission—that preeminently Victorian response to real or imagined crisis—to investigate the care and treatment of the sick and wounded in South Africa.

Although Burdett-Coutts's story of typhoid corpses was sensational, by mid-1900 stories like his were not uncommon. It was clear to anyone reading the press in Britain that far more British soldiers, officers, and medics were dead or dying from typhoid than from battle. "Typhoid," noted an anonymous medical officer in the *British Medical Journal* in July 1900, is "the most deadly of our enemies" in South Africa.[3] In many ways the typhoid epidemic *was* the defining experience of the military conflict, whether lived on the veldt by British soldiers, lived through in reports read in Burdett-Coutts's *Times* journalism. On top of stories were new visual forms of mediated communication, "grim photographic evidence of stretcher bearers carrying away hundreds of British corpses," in the periodical pages of *Black and White, the Sphere,* and *the Illustrated London News.*[4] In his widely read reports Burdett-Coutts highlighted "growing scenes of neglect and inhumanity."[5] While mortality figures resonated with a Victorian public enamored, as Ted Porter has argued, with statistics, Burdett-Coutts's journalism struck the heart of the British public through thick descriptive moralization.[6] It was a late Victorian public well aware and receptive to moralizing about the filth disease, as we saw in chapter 1 with the sickness of the Prince of Wales and in chapter 3 during the Marylebone Milk Crisis. The raw data of a soldier down with typhoid in Burdett-Coutts's reporting was transformed into a corpse stuffed into a lavatory. More than just the figure of the corpse, corpselike sufferers came to the fore as alarming incidents were reported where men were struck "in the worst stages of typhoid, with only a blanket and a thin waterproof sheet . . . between their aching bodies and the hard ground, with no milk and hardly any medicines, without beds, stretchers, or mattresses, without

---

3   "Medical Aspects of the War," *British Medical Journal* 2062 (7 July 1900): 51.

4   Morgan, "The Boer War and the Media," 9

5   Burdett-Coutts, "Our Wars and Our Wounded," 4

6   Porter, *The Rise of Statistical Thinking.*

pillows, without linen of any kind, without a single nurse amongst them."
Some lay lifeless, Burdett-Coutts pressed on, with "flies in black clusters
too weak to raise a hand to brush them off," while others wandered around
camp half-naked in a typhoid-induced delirium.[7] At a time heightened by
both jingoist proimperial bravado and growing antiwar agitation in England,
the stark reality of war in South Africa painted by Burdett-Coutts shocked
late Victorian sensibilities. Burdett-Coutts's stories of emasculated typhoid
bodies and desecrated typhoid corpses struck a chord in Parliament, particularly in antiwar Labor MPs, but more importantly, perhaps, it tugged at the
heartstrings of the Victorian social body. There had been no quick defeat of
the Afrikaner forces, as many in England foretold, and from late 1899 and
early 1900 the British forces had lost key battles at Ladysmith, Mafeking,
and Kimberley. Though the *Times* called it "more than any other in modern times . . . a popular war," the South African War was quickly becoming
embarrassing and costly.[8] It was also dangerous to the health of British soldiers and ergo to the imperial might of the nation. Added to the unsettling
mix were the recruiting statistics at home, particularly the dramatic figures
from Manchester, where eight thousand out of eleven thousand men were
rejected for service as unfit.[9] It was a crisis, one yet again with typhoid at its
center.

This time, as the century came to a close and Queen Victoria's life and
reign was coming to an end, the public anxiety over typhoid was decidedly
both nationalistic and imperial. The near-death experience of the prince in
1871 had brought the English nation together to grieve under the auspices
of the filth disease. The view had also extended to the British Empire, with
celebratory sermons in India, Australia, Canada, and Ireland. But in the
decades that followed typhoid was largely framed as a local, endemic disease
that was the responsibility of local sanitary administration in England and
Wales. It was as if the disease percolated in the 1870s, 1880s, and 1890s as a
problem of English sanitary administration and municipal sanitation, bubbling away in the form of small-scale outbreaks and bursting from time to

---

7   Burdett-Coutts, "Our Wars and Our Wounded," 4.
8   "The Addresses to their Constituents Sent Out," *Times*, September 21, 1900,
     7. On the antiwar movement in British popular culture, see Smith, *Drummer
     Hodge*, 19
9   Vanessa Heggie has argued that the Manchester statistics only became a "cliché
     chant for reformers" after early military defeats in South Africa. See Heggie,
     "Lies, Damn Lies, and Manchester's Recruiting Statistics."

time in epidemic form.[10] At least this was the perspective of many English public health authorities, including those at the Medical Department, who believed by the late 1890s that typhoid was slowly coming under the control of progressive sanitary policy.

The outbreak of war in South Africa in October 1899 with two independent Boer republics—the South African Republic (or Transvaal), and the Orange Free State—set the stage for yet another palpable anxiety over the filth disease. In the course of three short years around 75,000 Britons were struck with typhoid in South Africa and over 10,000 died from the disease, whereas less than 8,000 were dead from direct combat.[11] It was the single largest outbreak of typhoid in the Victorian period, closing the nineteenth and opening the twentieth century with another stark reality as to the ravages of typhoid fever. The staggering rates of typhoid sickness and death among British troops in South Africa, then, represented a challenge to British imperial might but also in deeply embedded ways challenged an emerging discourse about the strength of English public health. The epidemic led to two independent commissions focused on the typhoid outbreak in South Africa. The first, spurred by Burdett-Coutts's journalism, was the Royal Commission on the Care and Treatment of the Sick and Wounded. The internal fears over typhoid within the War Office led to the creation of a second commission, appointed by the secretary of state for war: the Royal Commission on the Nature, Pathology, Causation, and Prevention of Dysentery and its Relationship to Enteric Fever.

In this chapter I argue that the typhoid epidemic during the South African War was a critical public calamity that brought the filth disease to a new level of public consciousness, elevating typhoid from local and national to imperial concern. The outbreak highlighted the role of infectious disease in thwarting the implementation of British colonial policy and called into question the mission of colonial public health. It also brought to the fore a particularly racialized understanding of the global spread of the disease. The second half of the chapter closely follows the two commissions and the

---

10 Welshman, *Municipal Medicine.*

11 Such statistics are probably a poor reflection of actual deaths, considering they only counted white British military and civilian volunteers, not Afrikaner or indigenous African deaths. Conan-Doyle put the figure of those who suffered from the disease at more like two hundred thousand. See Conan-Doyle, "The War in South Africa," 49; Hardy, *Health and Medicine in Britain Since 1860,* 48–49.

framing of the outbreak as an epidemiological problem for the empire. But there was a longer legacy in British military medicine of thinking about and researching typhoid fever in colonial locations. In the first half of the chapter I trace the uneven and complex history of typhoid in colonial India from the 1870s. Epidemiological and bacteriological research on so-called tropical typhoid collided and converged in the lead-up to the South African War, particularly around the testing and bumpy implementation of Almroth Wright's antityphoid inoculation. The epidemic in South Africa during the war represents in large part the failures both of new bacteriological practices and in implementing long-standing epidemiological principles that had emerged at the Medical Department, as we have seen. The case studies of research on typhoid in colonial India and South Africa demonstrate both the uneven adoption of English epidemiology and bacteriology into military medicine and the complex webs of knowledge circulation on typhoid fever in the late Victorian era, which was often funneled through organizations like the Epidemiological Society of London and through military training at the Royal Victoria Military Hospital, Netley.

Typhoid as "Tropical": The Filth Disease in British India

Patrick Manson, in his vastly popular and nearly thousand-page 1898 tome *Tropical Diseases: A Manual of Diseases of Warm Climates*, declared that

> Typhoid now ranks not only as a common disease in the tropics but, to the European there, as one of the most commonly fatal. Little is known about typhoid as a disease of natives, beyond the fact that it does attack them; as a disease of Europeans it is only too familiar to the army surgeon in India and to the civil practitioner in most, if not all, parts of the tropical world.[12]

Both the chronological part (i.e., that typhoid *now* ranks as a common disease) and the geographical part (i.e., that typhoid is ubiquitous in all parts of the tropical world) had long been controversial in British military medicine. Manson, in framing typhoid as common within tropical medicine was obscuring a long-standing debate about the existence of the disease in British

---

12 Manson, *Tropical Diseases*, 193.

tropical hygiene circles.[13] Until the 1870s it was either blatantly denied that typhoid existed in British colonial environments such as India or Africa, or British military medics in the 1880s commonly believed that a typhoid-like disease existed in tropical climates, albeit one substantially distinct from the disease at home. As Pratik Chakrabarti has recently observed, the historiography on tropical medicine across the British Empire has been dominated by parasitology, especially the work of Manson and Ross.[14] Debates around what I call "tropical typhoid" reveal a more complex picture of the networks of epidemiology within public health in the tropics.

"Even now," army medical staff surgeon-captain H. R. Whitehead wrote in 1893, "considerable doubts exist in the minds of some whether the so-called typhoid fever in India is really the disease known under the name in Europe"[15] There was a prolonged history of typhoid denialism in British India, and, as David Arnold has shown, a localist, environmentally driven paradigm dominated the approaches of British medics in India throughout the nineteenth century. In the first edition of his *Clinical Researches on Disease in India* (1856), Charles Morehead, influential professor of medicine and principal of Grant Medical College in Bombay, for example, emphatically stated that typhoid fever as described by William Jenner was "unknown in India."[16] Four years later, however, in the second edition, he backed off his position, saying that reports in the *Indian Annals of Medical Science* by Joseph Ewart (of the Bengal Medical Service), and J. B. Scriven (surgeon-major in Lahore) had convinced him that typhoid at least occasionally occurred in India.[17] But Morehead doubted it was the same typhoid as in England. Even when typhoid was considered in India, most medics believed the disease was due to the unique local climate of tropical and subtropical India. In the 1860s the Army Medical Department recorded few cases of typhoid, and it was only from 1870 that typhoid, also referred to as "enteric fever" as it was in England, systematically appeared in British Army records

---

13   On the distinction between tropical medicine and tropical hygiene see Harrison, "Tropical Medicine in Nineteenth Century India."

14   Chakrabarti, *Bacteriology in British India*, 8.

15   Whitehead, "Tropical Typhoid Fever," 251.

16   Morehead, *Clinical Researches on Disease in India*, 307.

17   Ewart's early typhoid research in the 1850s, at the Ajmeer jail, Rajputana, and attached to the Megwar Bheel Corps, Kherwarrah, Rajputana, detailed typhoid amongst Indians, not just Europeans. Ewart, *The Sanitary Condition and Discipline of Indian Jails*.

in India, first in Hyderabad. The *Indian Medical Gazette* noted, for example, that until 1870 typhoid fever either "did not exist" or "remained concealed" in British India.[18]

The statistical naissance of typhoid in British India was due in large part to a wide-ranging statistical analysis of the Bengal presidency by Surgeon-Major James Lumsdaine Bryden, statistical officer with the sanitary commissioner of the Government of India. Bryden, examining the ten-year period 1860–69, argued that what had for years been labeled "remittent," "intermittent," and "continued" fever in India was true typhoid fever. But, Bryden argued, in India the disease appeared sporadically, due in large part to the impact of heat on the unacclimated. It was another affirmation to the environmentalist paradigm. But even then Bryden's claim came with a racialized twist. Typhoid only extended to white Europeans: "I know of no single record of the existence of typhoid among the native population," he noted.[19] Managing typhoid, at least to those like Bryden in the early 1870s, only extended to white European bodies. The Indian body, not believed to be at risk of contracting typhoid, was not to be colonized, to borrow Arnold's metaphor, on account of the filth disease. A similar debate played out with regard to the use of pharmaceuticals in British India, particularly the use of cinchona, Rohan Deb Roy has recently shown.[20] Racialized exceptionalism would precipitously change in the 1890s as Indian bodies became the chief focus of the British epidemiological gaze. But more than an etiological claim, Bryden's statistical analysis in the 1870s was one of the first to raise a new red flag to British officials in India. Typhoid was not just misdiagnosed. It was the most common cause of sickness and death among young soldiers recently arrived in India. More than a statistically manufactured crisis, Bryden's finding not only became a mantra among medics in India but a rallying cry for preventing typhoid in cantonments and ushering patients to convalescent hill stations.[21] From 1870 typhoid appeared in the statistical returns throughout British India, with two serious revelations. The first was confirmatory: that Bryden's observation about age and length of service seemed to ring true throughout the country. The second was that typhoid

---

18   "Surgeon-General Gordon on Enteric Fever in the European Army of Madras," *Indian Medical Gazette* 1 (October 1878): 276.

19   Bryden, *On Age and Length of Service*, 53.

20   Deb Roy, *Malarial Subjects*.

21   Kennedy, *The Magic Mountains*.

was the number-one cause of mortality of British troops in India. There was a sharp increase in the mid-1880s, and again in the late 1890s.

The British military medical elite in India quickly picked up Bryden's finding. The fourth and fifth editions of E. A. Parkes's *Manual of Practical Hygiene*, the *de facto* handbook for British military medics serving in India, for example, listed Bryden as the authority on the subject.[22] In Parkes's *Manual* Bryden's findings were stitched together with the English epidemiological work of the Medical Department, Budd, and Murchison; typhoid could be spread via air or water and was at least a specific disease. But in India the etiological questions remained obscure for the last three decades of the century, more so than in Britain. One group of British medical officers in India followed Murchison's pythogenic theory that typhoid was not directly contagious, and long after the *de novo* or spontaneous origin of typhoid was settled in England it remained a viable etiological position in colonial spaces. Murchison, after all, had been attached to the East India Company in Bengal and Burma, and, as Margaret Pelling argues, drew his theory of typhoid from colonial experience.[23] But more common in British India was a centrist approach: that typhoid in India was similar to that of England but spread due to nonspecific, climate-induced causes. A variant of the latter camp believed that it was a disease concomitant with malaria, the so-called typho-malarial fever. The etiological maelstrom in British India in the 1870s dovetails with what Arnold argues was the unique self-fashioning and professional angst of British medics in India at the time.

C. A. Gordon, surgeon-general of the Army Medical Department, was representative of Indian exceptionalism built on typhoid denialism. In 1875 the Indian Government called upon him to investigate Bryden's claims as to the existence of typhoid fever among troops in the Madras presidency. It apparently caused him "all the troubles of mind and body," and he concluded, contra Bryden, that "the cases alluded to were of climatic endemic fever, and not the specific disease due to a specific cause." But even for his clinging to climatological origins, Gordon at least acknowledged that what he had found there was an etiological mess. In 1878 Gordon published his full account, a *Report on Typhoid or Enteric Fever in Relation to British Troops in the Madras Command*, in which he went against Bryden and the authority

---

22   For more on Parkes's *Manual* and how it was used by colonial physicians, see Harrison, "Tropical Medicine in Nineteenth Century India."

23   Pelling, *Cholera, Fever, and English Medicine*, 288.

of Parkes to deny the existence of typhoid in India.[24] Gordon had examined the records of 175 cases of typhoid returned from medical officers throughout the Madras and also had personal case notes on around 150 supposed typhoid patients. He concluded that his colleagues were wrong. The disease looked like typhoid clinically, some observers had even found pathological lesions in the ileum of the small intestine. But it was not typhoid because he could find no specific cause related to filth. Instead, Gordon noted, they were "fevers of the country" of India, "endemic and climatorial."[25] His position was in line with other top-ranking officials, such as Surgeon-General J. M. Cunningham, who Arnold has shown was a waterborne cholera denialist at the time. In an attempt to settle the matter, and presumably to gain support for his position, in 1879 Gordon gave the Madras government five hundred rupees, not an insignificant sum at the time, to be given as a prize for the best essay "on the several points in relation to the disease called 'enteric' fever on which want of unanimity existed."[26] Three years and numerous submissions later, the prize committee was still not satisfied that the question had been answered, and they sent Gordon back his money, without interest, and without the backing he desired. But in going against Bryden, Gordon had stoked an etiological fire, one that had ramifications across international networks of epidemiological practice on typhoid. This was anything but an esoteric debate among British military officials in India.

The existence of typhoid in India was the central topic at a series of meetings of the Epidemiological Society of London (ESL) in 1879 and 1880. The ESL had long been a hub for the self-fashioning of an epidemiological identity in England. It was probably the single most important node in a complex web of epidemiological knowledge circulation. Recall that Simon was an early member and advocate, and the first generation of English epidemiologists—Radcliffe, Buchanan, Seaton, Thorne, Ballard—had all been prominent members, secretaries, and presidents of the organization. Many of the reports of the inspectorate, moreover, were discussed and debated at ESL meetings. But from its inception the ESL had endorsed a global brand of epidemiological practice, publishing reports from the far reaches of the

---

24   Gordon, *Report on Typhoid or Enteric Fever.*

25   Gordon, "Enteric or Typhoid Fever in India," 97–98.

26   Gordon, "Enteric Fever in India," 540; Gordon, "Prize For Essay on Fevers," 673.

British Empire.[27] No doubt the international flair of the ESL was pushed by leading members such as the irascible Scot and transimperial epidemiologist Gavin Milroy, president from 1864 to 1866. In the 1880s and 1890s the ESL elected a number of high-ranking colonial epidemiologists who had practiced in India as president, starting with Sir Joseph Fayrer in 1879, Norman Chevers in 1884, Sir Thomas Crawford in 1889, Joseph Ewart in 1891, and J. Lane Notter in 1897.

Fayrer opened the 1879 meeting of the ESL with a full-blown call for imperial epidemiology. "The *raison d'etre* of this Society," he argued, "is the investigation and development of our knowledge of disease in motion . . . whether among the people of a house, a ship, a village, a city, a province, or a continent."[28] Disease had to be studied "not only by the bedside of the metropolitan hospitals, but in all climates, in every quarter of the globe, in the army, navy, colonies, and in our Indian empire."[29] Fayrer was in a unique position to make such an appeal for extending the epidemiological gaze. He had been appointed to the Indian Medical Service of Bengal in 1850 and served in a number of posts, including at Lucknow and at the Medical College of Calcutta. In the early 1870s he returned to England, where he served on the Medical Board of the India Office from 1874 until 1895. Fayrer spent the bulk of his address discussing the entrenched debate in India over typhoid. He was decidedly in line with Bryden that typhoid "is an important cause of mortality among our young European soldiers in India."[30] But Fayrer waffled, occupying a centrist position that became common in 1870s British India. "Very frequently it is exactly identical" to typhoid in England, but, he admitted, "as frequently, or more so, it is not." Fayrer's typhoid hybridism was "a form of fever exactly like European typhoid, except in its etiology . . . it is due to climatic causes, not to filth or specific causes such as give rise to it in England."[31] He had more than one platform to make his localist claims. In 1882, before the Royal College of Physicians of London, Fayrer delivered the Croonian Lectures, a series of three talks dedicated to the "Climate and Fevers of India," where he fully

---

27 The international circulation of epidemiological knowledge in the early to mid-nineteenth century is an unexplored topic addressed in the forthcoming Downs, *Empire's Laboratory.*

28 Joseph Fayrer, "Inaugural Address," 268.

29 Fayrer, "Inaugural Address," 265.

30 Joseph Fayrer, "Inaugural Address," 268.

31 Joseph Fayrer, "Inaugural Address," 269.

expressed his ideas on the unique spread of typhoid in the tropics. Neither Budd's nor Murchison's theories sufficed to explain typhoid in India, which was due, he again argued, to climate and individual predisposition.[32] It was not typhoid denialism like Gordon's, but it amounted to a rejection of English epidemiology.

For all of Fayrer's celebrity status, he had detractors. Also weighing in on the tropical typhoid debate at the ESL meeting in February of 1880 was Deputy Surgeon-General Joseph Ewart, formerly of the Bengal Medical Service. Ewart had been in practice in India from the 1850s, and he believed from that time that typhoid was the same in India and England and presented in both Europeans and Indians. Ewart went even further than Fayrer or Bryden in dismissing climatological theories of the origins of typhoid and adhering to a position somewhere between Budd and Murchison. Typhoid was a specific disease, clinically and pathologically uniform "in all parts of the world, in the white as in the black races" and linked to a poison exuded in the excreta of persons suffering from the disease and spread via air, water, and food.[33] It was a filth disease, in other words, and researchers like Gordon—who he cited—who could not find the specific cause in unsanitary conditions were simply shoddy epidemiologists. Fayrer, the shrewd ESL president with the centrist views on typhoid, invited Gordon to give a paper replying to Ewart at the next meeting of the society, on April 29, 1880. Gordon's attack on Ewart was a summary of his earlier views. He maintained that what was being called typhoid in India was not the same as in England. It was instead a typhoid-like condition, similar clinically and pathologically, but due to climate and not a specific poison spread via the discharges of the sick. Gordon's was an interesting position. Clinical medicine and pathology were not to be trusted. But a particular kind of localist Indian epidemiology could be.[34] In the discussions that followed the papers of Fayrer, Ewart, and Gordon, Medical Department inspectors George Buchanan and John Netten Radcliffe were quick to jump in and provide their insight. Knowing their extensive experience investigating typhoid, it was no surprise that they sided with Ewart and against Fayrer and Gordon. Buchanan acknowledged that epidemiological methods of outbreak investigation were "difficult enough of accomplishment under the conditions of English society, but must needs be incomparably more difficult" in India. But the English way could prevail in

---

32 Fayrer, *On the Climate and Fevers of India.*
33 Joseph Ewart, "Enteric Fever in India," 290.
34 Gordon, "On Certain Views Regarding Fever in India."

the tropics: careful inquiry of cases, household inspection, discovering the index cases, inspecting air, water, and food. Radcliffe was more belligerent, clamoring that Gordon and Fayrer's notion of climatic causation could not logically be a "cause" of typhoid or any specific disease.

The networks of imperial epidemiology widened again a year later, in 1881, at the International Medical Congress, which assembled for the first time in England. The president of the section on medicine was none other than long-standing typhoid expert William Gull. During the course of the meeting an entire session was devoted to the etiology of typhoid in India. It began with a paper by William Campbell Maclean, influential professor of military medicine at Netley, "On the Prevalence of Enteric Fever among Young Soldiers in India." Maclean had a storied career in British military medicine. Educated at Edinburgh, he joined the Madras Army in 1838 and was a medical officer in the Indian Army until the 1850s, when he joined the Army Medical School. Maclean was certain, in line with Ewart, that typhoid was the same whether in India or England. Gordon's localism, he argued "had no weight with me."[35] Mclean followed Murchison's pythogenic theory of typhoid, which, while losing steam among elite epidemiologists in England by the early 1880s, was coming into prominence among some British military officials in explaining typhoid in India.[36] Mclean argued that medical officers in India had to look to the sanitary conditions of barracks, hospitals, and cantonments, particularly the water supply and the handling of excrement. Many stations had already abolished the latrine system and were employing what was called the "dry earth system," whereby excreta were buried in the soil outside of camp and used as fertilizer for growing vegetables. Once the sanitary conditions of European habitations were under control, he argued, officers should turn their gaze to "native bazaars and villages." "It cannot be carried into our barracks by sewer air, for we have no sewers there," Mclean argued, but it could be spread via water, milk, other beverages, food, or even clothing tainted by unsanitary natives.[37] And while

---

35 Maclean, "On the Prevalence of Enteric Fever among Young Soldiers in India," 528.
36 E. W. Goodall, Medical Superintendent of the Eastern Hospital of the MAB, argued that amongst general practitioners Murchison's theory held enormous influence until around 1900. See Goodall, "Introduction to a Discussion on the Infectivity of Enteric Fever," 169.
37 Maclean, "On the Prevalence of Enteric Fever among Young Soldiers in India," 531.

236   CHAPTER FIVE

Maclean maintained that his was a global argument—typhoid was spread in India in the same ways that epidemiologists in England had shown it operated at home—his recourse to a morality-fueled, racially based typhoid epidemiology in some ways reinforced another kind of Indian localism: a myth of Indian inferiority.

Maclean was not alone in this view and became representative of a group of British doctors in India who adopted a global theory of typhoid. In the discussion of Maclean's paper at the 1881 congress, his views on typhoid were vocally supported by Netley inspector-general J. D. Macdonald, J. B. Scriven (a medical officer in Lahore), and by Ewart. It was a telling turn in understanding typhoid in the tropics, but the climate-based, local understanding represented by Fayrer died a slow, cumbersome death. Surgeon-General A. C. C. DeRenzy, former sanitary commissioner of the Punjab, was outspoken in lamenting in the early 1880s that "there has been an apparent unwillingness on the part of many of the most distinguished medical authorities in India, to admit that the prevalences of such diseases as cholera and enteric fever are mainly due to the state of the water-supply." DeRenzy called for Indian officials to use "experience attained in England," in slowing the spread of typhoid, particularly maintaining a clean water supply, "for Nature," he argued, "does not work on one plan here and on another in India."[38] But there remained doubters to DeRenzy's vision. Sir Thomas Crawford, director-general of the Army Medical Service from 1882 to 1889, for example, in his inaugural presidential address to the Epidemiological Society of London in 1889, was still suspicious of both the causative role of *B. typhosus* and the global nature of typhoid at home and abroad. There were too many cases of isolated epidemics, he argued, and "neither the specific poison theory, now much favoured, nor the pythogenic theory alone, seems capable of accounting for these isolated cases." It all added up for Crawford, at least, to say that "there are facts encountered in practice, and especially in India, which it is difficult to reconcile with any of the theories favoured by European pathologists." The only recourse, Crawford believed, "is hardly explicable on any theory short of origin *de novo*."[39]

The lasting localism was increasingly meeting the ire of a new class of British medics in India like Maclean, DeRenzy, and J. B. Hamilton. Hamilton, statistical superintendent for the Government of India, and later health officer in Cape Town, South Africa, was instrumental in advocating

38 DeRenzy, "The Sanitary State of the British Troops in Northern India," 42.
39 Crawford, "Inaugural Address," 14.

for a global theory of typhoid in line with English observers in the 1890s. But to do so he still had to urge his colleagues in 1894 that with regard to "the disease itself as seen in tropical or sub-tropical climates . . . there is little or no marked variation between it and enteric fever as observed at home," which suggests that there were still plenty of Fayrer followers like Crawford left in British India.[40] They were often in the highest ranks of IMS officials. In 1889 the Sanitary Department of India set up a special commission to inquire into the increase of typhoid after explosive outbreaks occurred at Lucknow and Meerut, appointing Sir Benjamin Simpson (surgeon-general and sanitary commissioner with the Government of India), W. H. Thomson (surgeon-general and attached to the forces in Bengal), J. Richardson (deputy surgeon-general and sanitary commissioner for the Central Provinces), and D. D. Cunningham (professor of physiology at the Medical College in Calcutta).[41] Mark Harrison and David Arnold have shown the complex ways that Cunningham stubbornly influenced sanitary policy in nineteenth-century British India, particularly his resistance to the waterborne theory of cholera in favor of a localist, Fayrer-approved, theory of its origins.[42] The position had even led him head-on in opposition to Robert Koch's cholera discovery in the 1880s.

The 1889 Typhoid Commission unsurprisingly echoed earlier views of typhoid much in line with Cunningham's antiwaterborne understanding of cholera. They even went so far as to say that the increase in typhoid from 1870 was probably not even real but a statistical fallacy from overdiagnosis on the part of doctors at large cantonments.[43] If there was an increase, they surmised, it was because of the susceptibility of young, recently arrived troops to "cyclical variations in climatic conditions."[44] At both Lucknow and Meerut the commission could find no unsanitary causes in water supply, air, or food. It was yet another flag waving for the environmental view of tropical typhoid and a denial of the statistical epidemiology making inroads

---

40   Hamilton, "Enteric Fever in Tropical and Sub-Tropical Climates," 95.

41   *Report by the Committee appointed to Enquire into the Recent Epidemics of Enteric Fever in Lucknow and Meerut,* British Library, IOR/I/mil/7/303–6.

42   Harrison, "A Question of Locality"; Arnold, "Cholera and Colonialism in British India."

43   Cunningham's views were in line with those published by J. M. Cunningham. See Cunningham, "The Sanitary Lessons of Indian Epidemics."

44   *Report by the Committee Appointed to Enquire into the Recent Epidemics of Enteric Fever in Lucknow and Meerut,* British Library, IOR/I/mil/7/303–6.

into British India. But several observers, including Robert Pringle (a former medical officer in the Sanitary Department of the North West Provinces) attacked the commission's report. Before the Epidemiological Society of London in 1890, Pringle called into question the practical experience of the commission's members, saying they were too yoked to theory and not actual practice. Pringle, like Maclean and Hamilton, believed the increase to be real and due largely to unsanitary conditions at cantonments that led to the pollution of local water supplies. "Everything which would tend to originate or increase its impurity," he added, "has been allowed to exist, and continue; and hence an increase of enteric fever." The Sanitary Department of India was at fault.[45] It was a damning indictment, and one that several observers in the 1890s repeated.

Even among those like Pringle, Hamilton, and Maclean who sought to construct typhoid as a global entity, the remarkable epidemiological fact remained that "youth and recent arrival" were deterministic features of typhoid in India. Hamilton's statistical work in the 1890s, buttressed by similar investigations by Andrew Davidson for the Bengal Presidency, were confirmatory of long series of statistical revelations extending back to Bryden: typhoid predominantly attacked those twenty-five and younger who were in their first or second year of service. By the mid-1890s typhoid was again on the rise among British troops in India. In 1895, for example, the death rate of those under 25 was 8.51 per 1,000, while among those 30 to 34 the rate was 2.37 per 1,000. Among those in the first year of service the death rates were 11.31 per 1,000, while men who had served in India for six to ten years only had a 2.18 per 1,000 rate.[46] The decade 1891–1900, moreover, saw over fifteen thousand cases of typhoid alone return in the British Army, with over four thousand deaths.[47] The experience of India was a critical linchpin for a global view of the disease, but there were still unanswered riddles.

What was at stake in these debates was more than etiological grandstanding, despite the likes of Gordon and Cunningham's insistent typhoid denialism. Military expenditures were another very real concern. "Every soldier attacked by enteric fever is useless to the State for an average duration of

---

45 Pringle, "Enteric Fever in India," 116.

46 *Statement Exhibiting the Moral and Material Progress*, 19.

47 Major T. McCulloch, "Enteric Fever amongst the British Troops in India" (1902), Wellcome Library, RAMC Files, WC270. There was not a significant decrease in typhoid cases or deaths in British India until the first decade of the twentieth century.

six months," Hamilton noted in an 1890 article in the *BMJ*, estimating the governmental loss at thousands of pounds per annum and highlighting the need for a clearer etiological picture of the disease.[48] The debates were about resources and prioritization. Whether typhoid was local and climatic or spread via the discharges of the sick and unsanitary conditions manifestly mattered to the daily operations of barracks, hospitals, and cantonments. In theory, as ideas in British military medical networks coalesced around the global experience of typhoid at home and abroad, the epidemiological lessons from England were slowly implemented. Maintain a clean water supply. Disinfect excreta and ensure that they do not mix with sources of water. Vigilantly inspect food handling and transportation. It all added up to sound sanitary science. But that was theory. In practice, as Arnold and Harrison have previously suggested, there was a surge of race-based blame for the spread of typhoid in British India. Where before the existence of typhoid in natives of India had been flat-out denied, in the 1890s typhoid in the tropics became the exclusive domain of so-called filthy indigenous Indians, particularly those close to food and water supplies, and those laboring in conservancy.

By the 1890s the debate over typhoid in the tropics subtly but significantly shifted to the question of where typhoid originated: was it imported by British soldiers and settlers, endemic to native bodies, or a product of tropical environments? Some, like H. R. Whitehead, surgeon-captain of the Army Medical Staff of India, were coming to the uneasy conclusion that typhoid might be a European import. "Wherever Europeans have resided for any length of time," Whitehead noted in 1893, "we find the disease noted as present, and the cause of many fatal epidemics."[49] Admitting that typhoid was a product of colonization received less attention in this period, as we might expect, than the unsanitary habits of Indians. We saw in chapter 2 the complex ways in which John Simon and the Medical Department fueled a discourse on typhoid that relied on moralization and individual responsibility. An Indian corollary occurred in the 1890s. This was particularly the case after the discovery and acceptance of *B. typhosus*. But bacteriological tests that confirmed the existence of the bacillus did little to clarify the matter abroad as they did at home in England until the first decade of the twentieth century. The dream that "bacteriology promised a unique panacea in colonial

---

48   Hamilton, "Enteric Fever in India," 787–89.
49   Whitehead, "Tropical Typhoid Fever," 217–19.

medicine," as Chakrabarti contends, was often met with disillusionment.[50] Ernest Hanbury Hankin's laboratory at Agra was an exception; established in 1892, Hankin was bacteriologically examining samples of water, milk, and stools in search of *B. typhosus*.[51] He often failed to detect disease-causing microbes, as in the case of an outbreak of typhoid in 1893 but was at least working from a similar position as Klein at the Medical Department.[52] But in British India, combined with a military-skewed epidemiological gaze, bacteriological tests served to ignite a race-based discourse on typhoid. Fayrer's place blaming, it seems, gave way to Hamilton's race blaming. Here it was easy to dichotomize the sanitary cantonment with the filthy village bazaar, as Hamilton frequently did in the 1890s. The topic was at the center of the Section of Medicine and Therapeutics at the Annual Meeting of the British Medical Association in July 1890 at Birmingham. Hamilton there infamously quipped that "outside the cantonment limits India is exceedingly foul . . . I think the simplest description I can give of the sanitary position of our troops in India is—they reside in 'oases of cleanliness surrounded by deserts of filth.'" He went on the say at the same meeting that "it was clear that typhoid fever would spread terribly throughout Hindostan under the extremely filthy habits of the natives."[53] This epidemiologically specific but racialized view was echoed throughout British India. R. H. McPherson, surgeon-general in Delhi, thought British soldiers on the march were particularly vulnerable, being outside of the oases of the cantonment. Indians "are of very dirty habits," he warned, "are not particular as to how, or where, they relieve themselves . . . the following day the ground, thus soiled, may be occupied by the tents of a British officer or soldier, who may possibly remark that his tent has a bad smell in it, and at the same time lay the seeds of disease which may turn out Enteric Fever."[54] The new ethos of the likes of McPherson and Hamilton was that it was up to "the civilized nation,

---

50　Chakrabarti, *Bacteriology in British India*, 10.

51　*Report on the Sanitary Measures in India in 1894–95*, 45–46.

52　Letter from Administration Medical Officer of Jubbulpore to Principal Medical Officer, May 9, 1893, British Library, IOR/I/mil/7/303–6.

53　Hamilton, "Enteric Fever in India," 787. Hamilton was keen to implement the epidemiological methods of English practitioners. In 1889, for example, he traced an outbreak of typhoid to contaminated milk. See Hamilton, "Report on the Recent Outbreak of Enteric Fever at Bareilly," British Library, Colonial Office Records, IOR/I/mil/7/303/6.

54　R. H. McPherson to Dr. Taylor, April 17, 1889, British Library, Colonial Office Records, IOR/I/mil/7/303/6.

England, to teach the backward nations of the East the value of cleanliness and the theory of germs."[55]

The etiological debates over typhoid in India were significant in the history of the disease and held important ramifications for the study of British epidemiology. They also were a precedent for the practical administration of military medicine during the South African War. But in the three decades between 1870 and 1890 the debates over typhoid in the tropics were largely confined to military circles and the complex network of epidemiologists at home and abroad. Though the statistical returns from India showed an increase from the 1870s, there was little in the way of public concern until the late 1890s, when the tune began to change as epidemiological and bacteriological evidence made clear that typhoid was the most important infectious disease threatening the stability of British imperial interests in India. As the statistics came under greater scrutiny more British public health leaders spoke up. We saw how Pringle had done so before the Epidemiological Society in 1890. Ernest Hart, ever the typhoid spokesman, tried his hand at examining the typhoid problem in India in an address at the Section on Public Medicine of the Annual British Medical Association Meeting in London in 1895. Having just returned from a trip to India, Hart lambasted the long-standing "stolid resistance," and the "ignorant and monstrous opposition to the diffusion of our modern knowledge" of public health, particularly the waterborne nature of cholera and typhoid, among British officials in India.[56] Hart blamed mismanagement and despotism at the top ranks of the Indian Medical Service and the Army Medical Service and called for a complete reorganization of medical services in India. It was a damning report and in some ways unfair to a small group of Indian Medical Service and army medics who shared his vision for the control and prevention of typhoid. By the early 1890s many British medical officers in India had accepted the waterborne nature of typhoid and the role of *B. typhosus*, but Hart was correct in thinking they had been late in doing so. Parliamentary officials, too, began to speak up on the growingly visible typhoid problem in India. In the House of Commons, on February 27, 1896, George Hamilton, secretary of state for India, was asked to explain the increase of typhoid among troops in India. He was asked the same question a year later by General Russell on March 4, 1897, and again on May 5, 1898. There was growing worry, and Hamilton's replies showed the frustration on the part of the

---

55   J. B. Hamilton, "Enteric Fever in India, 788.
56   Hart, "Public Health Legislation and the Needs of India," 289.

Government of India about the typhoid problem. But at least they were no
longer denying typhoid's existence or its spread along well-known routes of
communication. Hamilton replied in 1897 that he had noticed "with regret"
the increase in typhoid and that attempts at improving sanitation and safeguarding the water supply of cantonments were coming under greater scrutiny.[57] Typhoid "is constantly engaging" official attention, he noted with
exasperation to both questions in 1896 and 1897. By 1898 he replied that
the focus was now on the improvement of the water supply, the provision
of pure milk and butter, and improved sanitation of camps, cantonments,
and barracks. One cantonment, Dagshai, where there had been serious outbreaks of typhoid, had been "completely evacuated for a year, pending the
installation of an improved water supply and the disinfection of the barracks
and their vicinity."[58] It was finally policy in line with sanitary legislation
in England, but even then the implementation in India was tinged with a
racialized epidemiological gaze. Just as the tropical typhoid controversy was
dying down and sanitary measures being implemented, there arose a poten-
tially easier way out than wholesale sanitary overhaul. It was hope from the
laboratory, a promise of a typhoid prophylactic produced by Almroth Wright
at Netley. Wright's antityphoid inoculation, it was believed, would finally
solve the problem of typhoid in the tropics; however, as we will see below, it
ushered in a new set of controversies around the filth disease.

The Fallacious Promise of Prevention: Almroth Wright's Anti-typhoid Inoculation

Just as English epidemiology was self-congratulating and writing its history on the back of success against typhoid at home, British bacteriology
was making a flurry of important inroads into the study and prevention
of typhoid fever. Two were intimately tied to the mercurial microbiologist

57   Hamilton was telling the truth. See, for example, the wealth of correspondence
     between the Government of India and local authorities regarding the installa-
     tion of piped and filtered water supply, British Library IOR/I/mil/7/303–6.
58   "Answer to General Russell's Question No. 16, 5th May 1898," British Library,
     IOR/I/mil/7/303–6. General Russell and George Hamilton, Enteric Fever
     (India), *Parliamentary Debates, March 4, 1897* (London: Merlow & Sons,
     1897), 1586. See also a draft memo of Hamilton's reply to Caldwell in 1896,
     British Library, IOR/I/pj/6/784.

Almroth Wright. From Yorkshire, Wright was educated at Trinity College, Dublin. He spent time in the bacteriological laboratories of Julius Cohnheim and Carl Ludwig in Leipzig, and Klein at the Brown Institution. After brief stints at the University of Cambridge and the University of Sydney, in 1892 Wright joined the Army Medical School, Netley—as a civil servant, not with military rank—teaching pathology to a legion of budding Army Medical Service and Indian Medical Service surgeons during the most heated debates over tropical typhoid. He remained at Netley until 1902, when he moved to London, attached for the remainder of his career to St. Mary's Hospital where he hovered over a generation of pathologists in the Inoculation Department for over forty years. Worboys has characterized Wright as representative of "the new breed of patho-physiologists or experimental pathologists."[59]

The first important laboratory discovery relating to typhoid in the 1890s was the Widal Agglutination Test, discovered in 1894 by two British students—Herbert Durham and Albert Grunbaum—in the laboratory of Max von Gruber in Vienna, and by the French bacteriologist Georges Fernand Widal, who developed it into a clinical diagnostic test and first published the results in 1896. The Widal Test was yet another seemingly powerful victory for laboratory bacteriology, echoing the promises of the discovery of the bacillus in the mid-1880s. It followed a similar line of agglutination work by Pfeiffer on the cholera bacillus. The obscure and uneven clinical manifestations of typhoid had long been debated, and the Widal Test offered diagnostic certainty in the clumping reaction of blood serum mixed with a solution of *B. typhosus*. Wright, alongside Surgeon-Captain F. Smith, were early trialists of the Widal Test in 1896 and 1897 among invalided soldiers sent back from military stations abroad to Netley. Wright instantly saw the power of the Widal Test in ending debates over tropical typhoid in British colonial locations and positively noted that it "will be everywhere welcomed."[60] He even made minor suggestions to improve the technique and extended the practice to Malta Fever. In 1895 Wright had made an important contribution to the study of typhoid, with real-world application to outbreak investigation, alongside his pupil David Semple, in confirming for the English medical community that *B. typhosus* could easily be found in the urine of patients suffering from the disease.[61] It was a logical extension of over a

59 Worboys, "Almroth Wright at Netley," 82.
60 Wright and Smith, "On the Application of the Serum Test," 656.
61 Wright and Semple, "On the Presence of Typhoid Bacilli in the Urine," 196–99; Smith, "On the Respective Parts Taken by the Urine," 1346.

half-century's worth of epidemiological evidence gleaned on typhoid and proved that Budd's fecal-oral route and three decades' worth of obsession with typhoid excreta were too exclusive in scope. Initially there was a flood of interest around the new diagnostic test. Wright and Smith had shown as much at Netley, but English epidemiologists also took notice.

David Davies, the energetic and outspoken MOH for Bristol, was probably the first epidemiologist in England to apply the Widal Test in the aid of outbreak investigation.[62] In 1897 an explosive outbreak of typhoid occurred in Clifton, and around the same time local practitioners noticed an uptick in influenza as well. Davies had heard about the new Widal Test from a colleague, Dr. George Parker, and saw a way to sort out which cases were indeed typhoid. He wrote to every physician in the area asking for blood samples of any doubtful cases and received forty-one samples in four days. In the course of his investigation Davies examined nearly two hundred blood samples, which was helpful in determining confirmed typhoid cases. Davies also brought in Klein from London to conduct postmortem analysis on five deceased individuals suspected of having typhoid. Klein found both the distinctive pathological lesions in the dead bodies, and colonies of B. typhosus in the spleens of each case. With front end, diagnostic, and back-end pathological evidence, Davies turned to routine epidemiology and masterfully traced the outbreak to a contaminated milk supply. It was a glowing example of a new kind of multidisciplinary outbreak investigation increasingly common in the twentieth century, and many MOsH throughout Britain enthusiastically took up the basic laboratory techniques of preparing and employing the Widal test. So much so that J. S. Tew, MOH for the West Kent Combined Sanitary District, noted in a meeting of the Home Counties Branch of the Society of Medical Officers of Health in 1898 that although the test was not "infallible," he had "obtained a positive reaction with monotonous regularity in decided cases."[63]

But there were plenty of problems. One was that patients sometimes presented all the clinical signs of typhoid but received a negative agglutination test. This was in part figured out in 1896 by two French observers, Achard and Bensuade, who isolated and named paratyphoid. But it was not until the early twentieth century that the paratyphoids A and B were distinguished, and the broader group of Salmonella was recognized. The other problems were the lack of standardization of the test and the stability and choice of

62 Davies, "On an Outbreak of Milk-Borne Enteric Fever in Clifton."
63 Tew, "The Agglutinative Reaction in Typhoid Fever," 185.

sera, problems that Hardy has shown lasted well into the twentieth century.[64] But Wright's interest in typhoid had really been prevention and not just diagnosis. Shortly after Wright's arrival at Netley, the Russian bacteriologist Waldemar Haffkine had visited to demonstrate his new, live-culture method of cholera inoculation, which he was soon to test in British India.[65] Haffkine had suggested to Wright that the same might be done to protect against typhoid fever. Little did Wright know at the time that research on typhoid inoculation would take up the next two decades of his career.

Wright and Semple broke from received Pasteurian wisdom and used a heat-killed bacilli vaccine instead of a living, attenuated vaccine as Haffkine had done with cholera. It was much safer, they argued, and equally effective. As Worboys contends, the move "established Wright's approach to immunity as that of a physiologist rather than a bacteriologist."[66] But ensuring the vaccine's success meant getting the dosage right, measured at the time by the number and virulence of bacilli present. In July and August of 1896 at Netley, Wright and Semple tested numerous strengths, on themselves and on staff, publishing their results in the *Lancet* in September, and more fully in January 1897 in the *BMJ*.[67] In the fall of 1897 Wright saw a chance to test the inoculation on a larger scale on the civilian population. The opportunity came with a sudden and serious outbreak of typhoid at Maidstone—the largest outbreak of the late Victorian period, with over fifteen hundred cases among a population of thirty-five thousand, and was traced to the contamination of the local water supply. Wright first sent Semple to the town to inoculate anyone who would volunteer. Hearing of cases at the Barming Asylum, Semple consulted the superintendent, Dr. A. M. Jackson, who agreed to let the medical and nursing staff volunteer (but not any of the patients). It was an interesting ethical choice, particularly considering later vaccine trials for the polio vaccine in America.[68] In total eighty-four members of the

---

64   Hardy, *Salmonella Infections*, 135.

65   Wright and Bruce, "On Haffkine's Method of Vaccination against Asiatic Cholera"; Chakrabarti, *Bacteriology in British India*, 185–86; Lowy, "From Guinea Pigs to Man."

66   Wright and Semple, "Remarks on Vaccination Against Typhoid Fever," 256. Wright later noted that the viability of a heat-killed vaccine was first suggested to him by Pfeiffer. See Wright, *A Short Treatise on Anti-Typhoid Inoculation*, 19. See also Worboys, "Almroth Wright at Netley," 88.

67   Simultaneously Pfeiffer and Kolle had produced a similar antityphoid inoculation and published their results in November of 1896.

68   Oshinsky, *Polio*.

medical and nursing staff at the asylum assented to Semple's inoculation, which occurred in early October. The results, as reported by local MOH J. S. Tew, were striking. None of those vaccinated at the asylum came down with typhoid, despite attending and nursing typhoid patients, and of the unvaccinated 120 nurses and attendants, sixteen contracted the disease.[69] The *Lancet* noted that "Dr. Tew's paper . . . should be read by every medical man. His results would certainly seem to show that 'anti-typhoid vaccination' has a most decided prophylactic or immunizing effect and the value of this fact in an epidemic like that of Maidstone or Lynn cannot be over estimated."[70] It was a telling result, albeit limited. As Hardy has shown, the vaccination did not reach or have an effect on the general population of Maidstone or on curbing the outbreak. But it was at least the kind of confirmatory evidence that Wright wanted. He even broached to the commander in chief the idea of vaccinating British troops.[71]

It was not long before Wright was presented with the opportunity to carry out another test of the vaccine, this time more extensive and within the military. Wright's expanding research program at Netley had landed him a spot on the government's India Plague Commission. In the fall of 1897, while Semple was trialing the vaccine in Maidstone, Wright was preparing to leave for India. Having heard of Wright's vaccine, on November 11, 1897, the Government of India wrote to the secretary of state asking for Wright's services for a four-month trial on a voluntary basis for those soldiers and officers at Netley about to leave for India. Historians have tended to overstate the "deeply ingrained resistance to the new measure in government circles and in the IMS," but all evidence points to one vocal and powerful objector: the secretary of state for war, Henry Petty-Fitzmaurice, Lord Lansdowne.[72] An internal memo of the War Office from January 1898, for example, noted that "Lansdowne does not feel that there is at present a sufficient agreement among the leading medical authorities as to the value of Prof. Wright's methods to justify him in giving his assent to the proposal of the Indian Gov't that either officers or soldiers even if willing to be experimented on should

69   Tew, "The Agglutinative Reaction in Typhoid Fever," 186.

70   "Agglutination in Typhoid Fever and "Anti-Typhoid' Vaccination," *Lancet* (March 19, 1898): 805.

71   Bruce, "Analysis of the Results of Professor Wright's Method," 244.

72   Harrison, *Public Health in British India*, 71.

be subjected to the requisite treatment at the public expense."[73] The official reply, and refusal, was sent to the Government of India and in turn to the principal medical officer. But they pushed back. In an April 7, 1898 letter the principal medical officer wrote to Secretary of State George Hamilton asking that the government reconsider the objection. "Typhoid," he argued, "most seriously affects the health and efficiency of the British Army in India." He noted the "extreme importance of the measure," and that it "does not cause any risk to health"[74] But the War Office would not budge. So instead the Government of India "misinterpreted" Lansdowne's objection, which was really about the safety of the vaccine, and believed the problem "applied rather to the formal authorization of inoculation at the public expense, than to voluntary operations at private cost."[75] It appears as though the Government of India turned a blind eye, and Wright, on duty with the Plague Commission, rolled out a widespread trial of the vaccine at various stations in India in 1898.

It was hardly at "private cost," as the vaccines had at least initially been prepared at Netley. It was onerous work, as Wright noted, "under great external difficulties." He often prepared new batches of the vaccine during railway journeys.[76] There was also the problem of convincing volunteers. As Worboys and Hardy have commented, Wright's first trial in India was through a number of "stump speeches," performatively cajoling officers and soldiers to volunteer for the vaccine. One local newspaper, the *Pioneer Mail,* recounted Wright's visit to Meerut, where he lectured about "his preventive serum," giving "very striking instances of the value of this treatment." He spoke of instances like the thirty-eight out of forty Indian soldiers who had been inoculated in one troop: none of the thirty-eight got the disease, while the two uninoculated soldiers did. Wright turned to the power of numbers, ironic because he would later detest statistical inference; about twenty-five hundred British troops had been inoculated, he reported, and none have since had

---

73 War Office Draft Minute, May 15, 1899, British Library, IOR/I/mil/7/304–7. See also the formal letter, from War Office to India Office, January 24, 1898, British Library, IOR/I/mil/7/304–7.

74 Principal Medical Officer, India to Sec of State, India, April 4, 1898.

75 W. S. A. Curzon, Edwin H. H. Lockhart, C. M. Collen, C. E. Rivaz, and T. Raleigh Dawkins to Lord George Francis Hamilton, Sec. State for India, May 25, 1899, British Library. IOR/I/mil/7/304–7

76 Tooth, "The Recent Epidemic of Typhoid Fever in South Africa," 647.

the disease.[77] The *Pioneer Mail* report noted that Wright inoculated troops at Meerut, but he was "not able to operate on anything like the number of those who volunteer," and he left the rest to Major Rennie of the RAMC.[78] No doubt Wright's early success in trumpeting the vaccine was braced by the earlier work of Haffkine, who had traveled throughout India to the same locations promoting his anticholera inoculation. But rather quickly the War Office got word of Wright's trials, even leading to a question on the floor of the House of Commons that embarrassed Hamilton, who did not know of Wright's "private" trial.[79] The result was that the Government of India was forced to issue official orders to Wright to "stop further inoculations." But the matter did not end there.

On May 25, 1899, the Government of India was again "pressing for permission" from the War Office to resume antityphoid inoculation on a volunteer basis, this time with governmental sanction. "We are very strongly of opinion that a more extended trial should be made of the treatment," they noted, "and we trust that Your Lordship will permit us to approve the inoculation, at the public expense, of all British officers and soldiers who may voluntarily submit themselves to the operation."[80] And for good rhetorical measure they turned to statistics and the pressing epidemiological problem of typhoid in India, which had increased from 1890 to 1898. Much as the existence of "tropical typhoid" had earlier centered on the white British male body, the corporeal framing dictated early debates around Wright's vaccine.[81] Haffkine, for example, noted before a meeting of the Royal Society in 1899 that Wright's vaccine "has a special interest for Europeans, as cholera has for the natives of India" particularly "soldiers of this country residing in India, and of white men in general in all tropical countries."[82] It was no doubt a racial double standard, British medics blaming the increase of

---

77   On Wright's disdain for statistics, and later feud with Major Greenwood, see Matthews, "Major Greenwood versus Almroth Wright."

78   Newspaper clipping, titled "Meerut," anon. *Pioneer Mail*, February 10, 1899, British Library, IOR/I/mil/7/304–7.

79   George Hamilton to Gov't of India, March 23, 1899, British Library, IOR/I/mil/7/304–7.

80   Curzon, Lockhart, Collen, Rivaz, and Dawkins to Hamilton, Sec. State for India.

81   On the broader antivaccination debates in nineteenth-century England see Durbach, *Bodily Matters*.

82   Haffkine, "Discussion on Preventive Inoculation," 15.

typhoid on Indians, but it was also focused on preventing the disease in Europeans. But the rhetorical pressure was enough that Lansdowne not only withdrew his objections but also changed his tune. In his eyes inoculation was "a considerable measure of protection from that dangerous disease [typhoid]."[83] And just like that the War Office had given in to the Government of India. James Jameson, director general of the Army Medical Services, wrote on May 31, 1899, that "all soldiers about to proceed to stations where the disease is prevalent (such as South Africa, India, Bermuda), should be given the opportunity of being inoculated on their volunteering to undergo the operation."[84] Jameson also noted that medical officers should lecture recruits about the benefits of the operation, particularly how "the immediate effects are not more inconvenient than those produced by vaccination." By June, officials in India were reporting to local medical officers that they could resume typhoid inoculation, and Wright himself recorded another 2,000 inoculations in India in 1899, bringing his total number of vaccines given to just under 5,000 in two years. Wright claimed to have personally performed 3,000 of them and that there was a less than 1 percent attack rate on those inoculated.[85] Another 6,000 were inoculated in India in 1900, and nearly 5,000 more in 1901.[86] Perhaps Wright's vaccine would finally solve the youth and recent-arrival problem of tropical typhoid that had plagued British India for decades. The evidence available from the vaccine trial in India was positive, but Wright sought even more confirmatory evidence. He and others had found minor problems with typhoid vaccine, including the proper dosage that would still be effective but minimize uncomfortable side effects. There was also the realization that a second dose of the vaccine was often required for maximum protection, and the issue of timing, or what was being called the "negative phase," whereby if troops were exposed to the bacillus soon after inoculation they would actually be more likely to get the disease instead of receiving the protective effects of

---

83 Draft of telegraph from War Office to Secretary of State, India, June 14, 1899, British Library, IOR/I/mil/7/304–7. See also E. Fleetwood Wilson, undersecretary of the War Office to Undersecretary of State, India, June 7, 1899, British Library, IOR/I/mil/7/304–7.

84 Memo from James Jameson, May 31, 1899, British Library, IOR/I/mil/7/304–7.

85 Tooth, "The Recent Epidemic of Typhoid Fever in South Africa," 647.

86 Secretary of State of India to Viceroy, July 4, 1899, British Library, IOR/I/mil/7/304–7.

the vaccine. But by mid-1899 Wright had at least overcome the political hurdle of government censure.

Café Enterique, Boulevard des Microbes: Wright's Vaccine in South Africa

Shortly after the government sanctioned another rollout of Wright's vaccine—a policy meant to appease the Government of India, Britain declared war on the independent Afrikaner republics of the Transvaal and the Orange Free State. It was another serendipitous stroke of luck for Wright, who returned to London having finished with the Plague Commission and quickly set to work mobilizing the typhoid vaccine for South Africa. It is impossible to know how many British soldiers, officers, and nurses were inoculated with Wright's typhoid vaccine, as neither he, the RAMC, nor the War Office kept accurate statistics on the distribution. There were scattered reports, particularly in the *Lancet* and the *BMJ* from the medical staff of field hospitals but little in the way of aggregate data. Wright claimed to have distributed four hundred thousand vaccines. Most officers and soldiers were inoculated *en route* to South Africa aboard passenger ships. Anthony Bowlby's experience in December 1899 is indicative of the lingering fears of the procedure. Bowlby, from St. Bartholomew's Hospital, had written *Surgical Pathology* in 1887, an early attempt to infuse bacteriology into post-Lister British surgery. At the outbreak of the South African War, Bowlby was named senior surgeon alongside Howard Tooth of the Portland Hospital, a private voluntary unit and the first civilian hospital sent to South Africa. In early December 1899 they set sail for Cape Town, and between musketry practice and playing cards, Tooth and Bowlby inoculated as many on board as would volunteer. There were forty-one total members of the Portland Hospital—it was supposed to care only for a maximum of one hundred sick soldiers, a totally inadequate number once they reached Bloemfontein in 1900. Four out of five of the medical staff were inoculated, twenty-four of the thirty-two noncommissioned officers, orderlies, and servants but none of the four nurses. Bowlby recorded in his diary for December 16, 1899, that at "6 P.M. we inoculated 8 of our men against typhoid and in the evening after dinner Tooth and Calverley were also victimized. Lots of the officers on board are anxious to be done."[87] The staff members of the Portland, inocu-

---

87   Diary of Anthony Bowlby, Wellcome Library, London, GC/181/C/2.

lated with fresh vaccine prepared by Wright and sent to the epicenter of the typhoid outbreak in South Africa, provide an interesting window into the efficacy of the vaccine.

Bloemfontein had been the capital of the Orange Free State, with a population of around seven thousand inhabitants. British troops arrived in February 1900 with nearly forty thousand troops, just before the arrival of the Portland Hospital. Within months the population surged to over seventy thousand, and the Boers in retaliation cut off the water supply to the town, so the British reverted to using formerly disused wells. What ensued was the single largest outbreak of typhoid during the war. Philip Curtin has argued that before April 1900 the health of British troops had rarely been questioned, with only about fifteen hundred dead from disease.[88] The rest of the year proved disastrous to British health, with Bloemfontein being the center of the outbreak; in the first half of 1900 the British reported a thousand troops dead from typhoid. The Royal Commission on Dysentery and Enteric, later found that the incidence of typhoid at Bloemfontein was 10.6 percent, with 4,280 cases in the course of seven weeks alone in 1900.[89] W. J. Simpson, one of three commissioners, called it an "extremely severe outbreak," while Arthur Conan Doyle, who spent several months in Bloemfontein as a medic attached to the volunteer Langman Hospital, echoed that it was the most lethal outbreak in modern warfare. "The whole hillside for the circuit of a mile around Bloemfontein was contaminated," exclaimed Portland Hospital's Bowlby.[90] Rudyard Kipling, who spent about a month in Bloemfontein as a correspondent for the *Friend*, a British propagandist newspaper, enshrined the epidemic in the 1903 poem "The Parting of the Columns" by calling it "Bloeming-typhoidtein," a chilling portmanteau that echoed throughout British popular culture.

Howard Tooth in 1901 recorded that ten members of the staff contracted typhoid, and one died. None of them had been inoculated. He had also kept records of those under treatment at the Portland in the previous year, 232 patients in total. Only a quarter of those had been previously inoculated, and four had died. Of the 178 not inoculated 25 had died. It was enough for Tooth and Bowlby to be "favourably disposed towards inoculation," but

88   Curtin, *Disease and Empire*, 212.

89   *Report of the Commission on the Nature, Pathology, Causation*, 62.

90   *Report of the Royal Commission Appointed to Consider and Report Upon the Care and Treatment of the Sick and Wounded*, 211

Tooth lamented that "inoculation has not yet had a fair trial."[91] Too many had refused the vaccine, he thought, and not enough careful statistics like his own were being kept. An official governmental investigation at Ladysmith had showed similar results: 2 percent death rate among those inoculated compared to a 14 percent rate among those not inoculated. But large-scale statistics were lacking. And the results were not as conclusive as Wright and Tooth made it seem. Many officers in South Africa reported cases of typhoid sickness and death among those inoculated, even with the double regime. It was not merely that too few Britons had volunteered for the vaccine, in other words. There were also scientific and practical problems. One was that Wright's vaccine was probably not effective against paratyphoid, as Hardy has argued, and that Wright had "not appreciated the full sensitivity of his vaccine to temperature changes while in storage" on ships to South Africa.[92] Freshly prepared vaccines seemed to be more effective than older ones. Colonel Henry Cayley, for example, medical officer of the Scottish National Red Cross Hospital, observed a natural experiment that had occurred under his watch. The Scottish Hospital's staff came to South Africa in two waves. The first ship, with sixty-one staff members left England on April 21, 1900. All but four of the members were inoculated while on board, twice given Wright's vaccine in the span of ten days. Cayley noted that he had personally received freshly prepared vaccine directly from Wright. A second staff group of eighty-two left England a month later in May. Nearly all of them were also inoculated, but the vaccine "was not so fresh," and most were only inoculated once.[93] Three months after arriving at Kroonstadt, where the Scottish Hospital was established, and where there had been an influx of typhoid cases, Cayley was approached by pathologist Dr. R. W. Dodgson, who was on a special assignment by the director-general of the Army Medical Department to investigate the effectiveness of Wright's vaccine in military hospitals throughout South Africa.

Dodgson's use of the Widal Test to examine a portion of the staff of the Scottish Hospital revealed that among those on the first ship, 21 of 23 gave clear positive sera reactions. But of the 22 tested on the second ship, inoculated only once with old vaccine, 11 gave a negative reaction, 9 produced a weak reaction, and only two gave a positive reaction. If the blood tests were not enough, Cayley had even clearer evidence: no members of the first

91   Tooth, "The Recent Epidemic of Typhoid Fever in South Africa," 645.
92   Hardy, "Straight Back to Barbarism," 273.
93   Cayley, "A Note on the Value of Inoculation Against Enteric Fever," 84.

ship had contracted typhoid, while five members of staff on the second ship had come down with the disease. It was anecdotal evidence, which defined both the earlier Indian trial and the massive rollout of the vaccine in South Africa. Dodgson, a St. Mary's Hospital graduate and later collaborator with Wright on an investigation of epidemic pneumonia among African laborers in the mines of Witwatersrand, spent eight months—from November 1900 to March 1901—traveling around South Africa in the midst of war trying to gauge the effectiveness of Wright's vaccine.[94] Dodgson's results were carefully studied by David Bruce, who had been given a postwar assignment in 1902 by a subcommittee of the Army Medical Services to study the effectiveness of wartime inoculation. There were suggestive results, like those of Tooth, Bowlby, and Cayley, but Bruce found the aggregate statistics lacking. Dodgson's sample sizes were also quite often small, Bruce argued, and of limited value. And some of the reports were not at all favorable, with case mortality rates similarly high between inoculated and uninoculated staff. It all added up, Bruce found, to the conclusion that "Dr. Dodgson's statistics . . . are of little or no value." It was a damning blow to the entire operation, and as Hardy has shown, it was concomitant with increased public outcry in England against the vaccine. "No trustworthy statistics can be hoped for from the troops employed in South Africa during the present war," Bruce concluded, "the future of anti-typhoid inoculation does not appear to be very bright."[95] While the army's inoculation problem continued in India and Egypt, after the publication of Bruce's report with the subcommittee to the advisory board, all antityphoid inoculations were put to a halt. The committee put Surgeon-General William Leishman, Wright's former assistant, in charge of reevaluating the entire inoculation protocol, and Hardy has detailed the continued turbulent history of the vaccine up until it was made compulsory before World War I. Wright, understandably, was furious, but he had already resigned from the Army Medical Service.

In 1902 Wright accepted an offer by the board of governors at St. Mary's Hospital to become chief pathologist. The move outraged army officials. The position in London would be "a minimum inroad on my time," Wright pleaded, and he had in fact tried to contact—three times—both Director-General William Taylor and Deputy-Director General Alfred Keogh to talk about the position at St. Mary's. He also was not aware that taking another

94 On British colonial efforts in the South African mines, see the classic account, Packard, *White Plague, Black Labor.*
95 David Bruce, "Analysis of the Results of Professor Wright's Method," 255.

position would violate his Netley contract. The chief reasons Wright gave, however, were practical. It was difficult to come by pathological material, he lamented, and he often had to rely on William Bulloch in London to supply him with specimens. It would be, furthermore, "to the advantage of the school" if he were connected to one of the metropolitan hospitals.[96] But his arguments were for naught. The advisory board would not assent, saying that holding the second position was "entirely incompatible with the due performance of his duties as Professor of Pathology" at Netley.[97] They gave Wright an ultimatum; Keogh wrote that they would be "glad of his decision by the 6th of Dec. as to which post he proposes to resign."[98] And so Wright did, leaving behind both his career at the RAMC and the prospects of the antityphoid vaccine, which he only picked up again close to World War I.[99]

Royal Commissions and Epidemiology on the Veldt

While the statistical evidence for the efficacy of Wright's typhoid vaccine was piecemeal and inconsistent during the South African War, what was not lacking were gross statistics and qualitative reporting on the mounting number of typhoid deaths. As the war dragged into late 1900 and early 1901, the increased media scrutiny at home, fueled by wartime journalism like that of Burdett-Coutts's reporting on typhoid corpses stuffed into lavatories, typhoid emerged as the central story of the war. How had such a massive epidemic occurred? Wright's vaccine, it was clear, had been of limited value, but the epidemiological question remained and demanded answers. It was a full-blown crisis during what amounted to Britain's most unpopular war in modern history. The response within the RAMC had been to appoint Dodgson to conduct a one-man investigation as to the efficacy of Wright's vaccine,

---

96 A. E. Wright to William Taylor, Director General of Army Medical Service, November 26, 1902, National Archives, Kew, WO 138/12.

97 Memo by Advisory Board to Alfred Keogh, November 28, 1902, National Archives, Kew, WO 138/12.

98 Memo by Alfred Keogh, November 28, 1902, National Archives, Kew, WO 138/12.

99 Leonard Colebrook, in his obituary for Wright says that Wright resigned because of lack of support from the War Office for his typhoid vaccine. The archival evidence suggests otherwise. See "Obituary for Almroth Edward Wright," *Biographical Memoirs of Fellows of the Royal Society* 17 (November 30, 1948): 298.

which had proved inadequate and ill-planned. The epidemic also elicited a parliamentary response, first in the form of a royal commission established in July 1900 to inquire into the *Care and Treatment of the Sick and Wounded*. It was, for all practical purposes, a typhoid commission and the result of wartime journalism from Burdett-Coutts. But it was not strictly a medical commission, comprising Robert Romer, a privy councilor and high court judge; David Richmond, a Glasgow businessman and lord provost; F. Harrison, an engineer and railway expert; and two physicians, William S. Church, president of the Royal College of Physicians, and D. J. Cunningham, professor of Anatomy at the University of Edinburgh.

The hospital commission, as it was sometimes called, was faced with the difficult prospect of untangling Burdett-Coutts's sweeping indictment. Was he a "superficial observer" and a "sensational publicist," as some politicians claimed, or were these the real scenes from South Africa?[100] The press coverage on the war was mounting. The illustrated weekly *Sphere*, for example, in the fall of 1900 published a series of stories and photographs entitled "The Hospital Scandals in South Africa."[101]

The commission spent nearly two weeks in London and at the Netley Hospital, interviewing military officials, wounded soldiers, and medics who had recently returned from South Africa. Twice Burdett-Coutts was called to testify before the commission. In August the group of five commissioners sailed for South Africa, where they traveled for three months observing firsthand the bell tents of field hospitals at Deelfontein, De Aar, Bloemfontein, and the battle sites at the Modder River. They interviewed lowly privates and commanding officers. Though they were charged with investigating the larger problem of hospital management and accommodation, the commissioners were particularly bent on assessing the reality of Burdett-Coutts's typhoid corpse. They made it a point to inquire "in all quarters to find out whether there is any foundation for" the allegation by Burdett-Coutts that a typhoid corpse was shoved into a lavatory.[102] It was a telling window onto the palpable anxiety around the filth disease during the war. And it was understandable. In gathering statistics from both military and private hospitals, the commission found that typhoid accounted for two to three times as many deaths as other forms of disease (figure 5.1). The soldier sick

---

100 Burdett-Coutts, *The Sick and Wounded in South Africa*, 8. For a critique of Burdett-Coutts see Asph, "The South African Hospitals Enquiry."

101 "The Hospital Scandals in South Africa," *Sphere* (September 8, 1900): 287.

102 Asph, "The South African Hospitals Enquiry," 44.

	Deaths due to General Causes.	Deaths due to Enteric Fever.
	Per cent.	Per cent.
Military Hospitals { Raadzaal, No. 5 Stationary	6·98	15·9
No. 9, General Hospital -	4·94	14·05
Private Hospitals - { Irish - - - -	7·83	13·16
Langman - - - -	7·15	18·78
Portland - - - -	7·33	14·07

Figure 5.1 Hospital figures collected during the South African War in 1900. From Report of the Royal Commission Appointed to Consider and Report Upon the Care and Treatment of the Sick and Wounded during the South African Campaign, 15. House of Commons Parliamentary Papers, Crown Copyright.

with typhoid and the typhoid corpse during the South African War came to stand as a potent symbol for military disorganization, ushering in significant changes in the British military leading up to World War I. On July 30, 1900, for example, one of the commissioners, Sir David Richmond, lord provost of Glasgow, directly asked Burdett-Coutts, "What is the suggestion when you say the corpse was stuffed into the lavatory; do you think it was put there to get the corpse out of the way?" Burdett-Coutts briskly replied, "Yes. Because probably they had no other place to put it."[103]

They interviewed Surgeon-Lieutenant John William Smith, practicing surgeon in Manchester, who was attached to the No. 9 General Hospital, first located in Cape Town and at the height of the typhoid epidemic in Bloemfontein. Asked if he had experience of typhoid corpses being thrown into a lavatory he replied "no, we had nothing of the sort. We had a mortuary the other side of the donga," a dry eroded land previously filled with water.[104] RAMC Principal Medical Officer R. Exham, who described his duties as

---

103 *Report of the Royal Commission Appointed to Consider and Report Upon the Care and Treatment of the Sick and Wounded during the South African Campaign*, 87.

104 *Report of the Royal Commission Appointed to Consider and Report Upon the Care and Treatment of the Sick and Wounded during the South African Campaign*, 256.

"the supervision of everything," might have been an authoritative source.[105] Interviewed on September 1, 1900, Exham, when prompted to answer about corpses put into lavatories, noted that "I have made careful enquiry into that point; and every medical officer in charge of every hospital here denies that any such thing occurred in their hospitals. I have sent round to special enquiries." Kendal Franks, vice president of the College of Surgeons, Ireland, equally denied Burdett-Coutts's claim that funerals were happening day and night at Bloemfontein, that "shapeless forms were being carried to unknown, nameless graves."[106] Franks argued that funerals were held from 3:00 p.m. to 5:00 p.m. daily. "There were great numbers of them," Franks admitted, but every grave was numbered and registered in the cathedral books.[107]

The hospital commission concluded that "Mr. Burdett-Coutts was misled by his informant."[108] They reported that even in Bloemfontein, where the typhoid deaths reached a staggering forty to fifty per day, each corpse was buried separately, away from camp, "with every respect and care, and each grave was numbered, and the number and name of the dead man registered."[109] Burdett-Coutts was quick to defend his assertion of what the commission called "a gruesome story." In the *Times* on February 13, 1901, he maintained he heard it from a "distinguished major-general, then a patient in a town hospital at Bloemfontein . . . anxious to give evidence before the Commission; but being away in the field it was impossible for him to attend."[110] And while the commission admitted that the chief difficulty with obtaining evidence as to "the true condition of affairs" in South Africa was that witnesses were either too partisan and in favor of the war, or,

---

105 *Report of the Royal Commission Appointed to Consider and Report Upon the Care and Treatment of the Sick and Wounded during the South African Campaign*, 259

106 *Report of the Royal Commission Appointed to Consider and Report Upon the Care and Treatment of the Sick and Wounded during the South African Campaign*, 261.

107 *Report of the Royal Commission Appointed to Consider and Report Upon the Care and Treatment of the Sick and Wounded during the South African Campaign*, 361.

108 *Report of the Royal Commission Appointed to Consider and Report Upon the Care and Treatment of the Sick and Wounded during the South African Campaign*, 361.

109 *Report of the Royal Commission Appointed to Consider and Report Upon the Care and Treatment of the Sick and Wounded during the South African Campaign*, 44.

110 Burdett-Coutts, "The South African Hospitals," 11. Coutts did forward to the head of the commission the name of his informant.

like many privates, were "very slow to make complaints," they nevertheless branded Burdett-Coutts's claims as exaggerated and misleading.[111] He was, to borrow Bernard Porter's phrase, just another "critic of empire."[112] The anxiety produced by the story of one typhoid corpse, perhaps *because* of its questionable authenticity, provides a rare glimpse into how fears over typhoid continued to influence popular discourse in Britain into the early twentieth century. It was because of the interrogation into the typhoid epidemic, for example, that the royal commission concluded that the RAMC was "wholly insufficient" in staffing, equipment, and planning.[113] Not enough nurses had been employed, first for fear of having female nurses at field hospitals, also because of the scant numbers of nurses employed at stationary hospitals, which had led to massive inadequacies. At the height of the war, about 220,000 troops, 1,000 medical officers, 7,000 hospital subordinates, and 900 nurses had been employed, and it was nowhere near enough to handle the staggering number of those sick and dead from typhoid. In other words, the filth disease had revealed the shortcomings of military medicine on an unprecedented scale. Combined with the onslaught of typhoid during the Spanish-American War, Vincent Cirillo has gone so far as to call both outbreaks "medical fiascoes."[114] And though the royal commission charged with investigating the care of the sick and wounded in South Africa had narrowed its gaze on the organization of the RAMC, it did not address the epidemiological problem of why typhoid was so rife in South Africa, or what might be done to curb the epidemic. Given the makeup of the commission they were not prepared to do so.

The War Office had instituted its own commission to inquire into the typhoid epidemic in South Africa. Appointed in August 1900—roughly the same time as the hospital commission—it was composed of three members: military epidemiologist James Lane Notter, tropical medicine specialist William John Simpson, and pathologist David Bruce. The group arrived in Cape Town in early September 1900 and agreed to split up the work along bacteriological and epidemiological lines. They first visited Bloemfontein and Kroonstad, two of the sites where typhoid had raged to an unprecedented

---

111 *Report of the Royal Commission Appointed to Consider and Report Upon the Care and Treatment of the Sick and Wounded*, 3.

112 Porter, *Critics of Empire.*

113 *Report of the Royal Commission Appointed to Consider and Report Upon the Care and Treatment of the Sick and Wounded*, 4.

114 Cirillo, *Bullets and Bacilli*, 138.

extent. From there they went to Pretoria, where Bruce set up a bacteriological laboratory in two rooms of the No. 2 Model School Hospital, intended to receive only cases of typhoid and dysentery. Simpson and Notter, meanwhile, traveled east to Komatiport, conducting epidemiological investigations of the sanitary conditions of nineteen military camps along the way. By early 1901 Bruce's laboratory had been operational for months, and the group was set to complete more sanitary investigations throughout South Africa. Then plague broke out in Cape Town. Simpson, considered an expert on plague, was ordered by the secretary of state for war to return to the Cape and assist MOH John Gregory. Earlier in 1900 Simpson had published *Memorandum on the Influence of Rats in the Dissemination of Plague*, a treatise based on his long-standing experience as health officer in Calcutta.[115]

Simpson, from Glasgow, had a medical degree from Aberdeen and a diploma of public health from Cambridge. He had served as Aberdeen's MOH in the 1880s, then as health officer for Calcutta from 1886, where he was in the vanguard of medical officers in India pushing for sanitary reform along the lines of what was occurring at home—but with a distinctly racialized bent. His reports, for example, show a detailed focus on reducing food and water contamination and on drainage schemes. However, they also blamed indigenous Indians for the spread of disease and issued orders for the wholesale disinfection and quarantine of Indians into segregation camps, as Aidan Forth has recently shown.[116] Simpson was a vocal reformer in calling for a reorganization of sanitary administration in India along civil rather than military lines, and he also established a bacteriological laboratory in Calcutta, where Haffkine's anticholera inoculations were tested on a wide scale. Simpson for several years edited the *Indian Medical Gazette*. However, owing to declining health, Simpson left Calcutta in 1897 and returned to London, where he was made professor of hygiene at King's College and helped to found of the London School of Hygiene and Tropical Medicine. Simpson led transimperial public health efforts in India and South Africa that were, as Projit Mukarji recently observed, "socially divisive, politically fraught, capital intensive, and usually underwritten by direct or implicit violence."[117]

---

115 Simpson, *Memorandum on the Influence of Rats in the Dissemination of Plague*, National Archives, Kew. CO 885/7/17.

116 Forth, *Barbed-Wire Imperialism*.

117 Mukharji, "Cat and Mouse."

With Simpson in Cape Town, Bruce and Notter carried on typhoid research, conducting more laboratory tests in Pretoria and in the spring of 1901 visiting military stations in Natal, the Orange Free State, and the Cape. As the threat of plague diminished in August 1901 and Simpson had set up strict quarantine rules and the forcible removal of indigenous Africans along the lines of what he had done in Calcutta, he was dispatched back to Pretoria to join Notter and Bruce.[118] But when he arrived Simpson was not satisfied with how Notter had conducted the epidemiological investigation and so insisted that he revisit several of the stations previously inspected. In early November 1901 the three returned to London and completed the report, a process that confirmed that the whole investigation had been a disaster.

The first part of the 1901 report focused on Bruce's laboratory research untangling the relationship between typhoid and dysentery. For at least two decades medical authorities had debated whether dysentery was a singular disease, like typhoid, or a symptom of a bowel-related disease like typhoid, cholera, or the ambiguous "summer diarrhea." In 1898 Japanese bacteriologist Kiyoshi Shiga, student of famed bacteriologist and Koch protégé Shibasaburo Kitasato, announced the discovery of *bacillus dysenterie*. Although Shiga was correct, many still questioned in 1900, when Bruce was investigating the matter in South Africa, whether dysentery might be caused by a virulent outburst of *B. coli communis*, which had only recently been unyoked from *B. typhosus*, particularly by Klein, as examined in the previous chapter. With a sharp rise in both dysentery and typhoid during the South African War, Bruce had hoped the influx of clinical material would lead to definitive answers. His work was doomed from the start, however, as he sourly noted in the final report that "on this rock the laboratory work . . . came somewhat to shipwreck."[119]

The No. 2 Model School Hospital, for starters, had been on orders from RAMC Colonel Stevenson to receive all of the typhoid and dysentery patients in Pretoria. It was a shortsighted plan, as there were far too many typhoid cases for the hospital to take in, and in the exigencies of war, cases of dysentery—clinically often mistaken for typhoid—were sent to the nearest hospital. "Very few suitable cases of dysentery found their way," Bruce lamented, and he was forced to travel from hospital to hospital, sometimes miles away, to obtain pathological material, which was often postmortem

118 White, "Global Risks, Divergent Pandemics."
119 *Report of the Commission on the Nature, Pathology, Causation, and Prevention of Dysentery, and its Relationship to Enteric Fever,* 8.

and studied in a field tent. Despite his efforts, Bruce could only offer weak conclusions. He was timidly skeptical of Shiga's bacillus, and in his South Africa research had identified multiple specific bacilli that might be responsible for the disease. It was definitely not typhoid, however, and Bruce used the Widal Test to confirm case after case of typhoid, beautifully illustrating the report with pathological and bacteriologically illustrations. But in the end, under the duress of war, Bruce's laboratory work with the commission yielded little in the way of clarity and much in the way of frustration.

It did not help matters that Bruce's colleagues, Notter and Simpson, were at odds with one another. It was in the second aim of the commission, the epidemiological investigation of typhoid, that matters came to blows. Simpson and Notter intended to jointly write part two of the report, but the two could not agree and so wrote separate reports. Notter was so furious with Simpson's interpretation of the epidemiological findings that he refused even to sign his name to the report, instead separately issuing a statement on his dissenting views. Part two was Simpson's blow-by-blow account of cities, towns, villages, and military stations throughout South Africa. It detailed case after case of excremental pollution of water and soil and unsanitary housing and hospital arrangements. Striking images of the conflict entered the public sphere, like figure 5.2, a sketch by RAMC officer Joseph Hinton, of soldiers suffering from typhoid in a makeshift field tent.

What is striking is the way Simpson infused race into epidemiological specificity in tracing the media of typhoid recognized by 1900. Native Africans, or "Kaffirs," the racialized slur common among British imperialists at the time, were responsible for polluting wells and otherwise pure springs with excremental matters. They were also dangerous distributors of typhoid-laced food and not to be trusted. If the search for the index case had been a particular obsession of English epidemiologists at home in tracking outbreaks of typhoid, in British colonial spaces the outbreak obsession was in Simpson's hands a racialized one, with an unscrupulous "careless and dirty" "Kaffir" at fault. "In the future sanitation of the country," the report noted, "it must be remembered that the Kaffir is a very important agent in the maintenance and spread of enteric fever."[120] Such a racialized construction of the filth disease mirrors the narrowing view of many medical officers in British India at this time, explored above. And as in India, military camps

---

120 *Report of the Commission on the Nature, Pathology, Causation, and Prevention of Dysentery, and its Relationship to Enteric Fever,* 65.

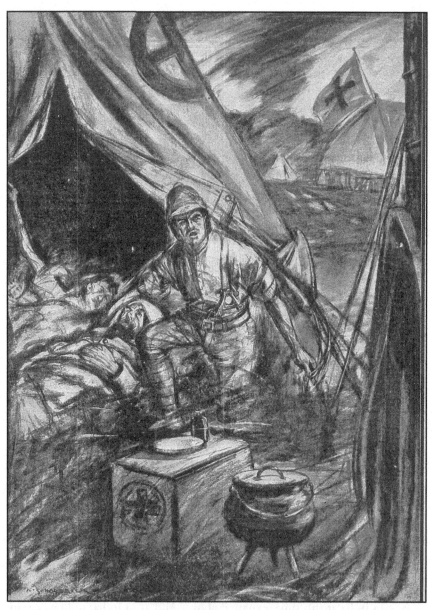

Figure 5.2 Boer War: an army medical officer, Joseph Hinton, pulling down the fly of a marquee in which lie soldiers with enteric fever. Process print after A. S. Hartrick, ca. 1900. Image courtesy of the Wellcome Library, London. Creative Commons Attribution only license CC BY 4.0.

were believed to provide sanitary protection, to be, as Hamilton noted above, "oases of cleanliness surrounded by deserts of filth."[121]

But typhoid had prevailed throughout the army in South Africa at unprecedented levels, and Simpson blamed both the enemy Boers—again in a racialized construction—who fouled the soil and water of British encampments and on RAMC officials for unsanitary camp arrangements that led to waterborne contamination. In part, the problem was the converging of several regiments in unprepared towns like Bloemfontein. There, in a span of seven weeks over four thousand cases of typhoid exploded, and Simpson found that the water supply had been infected. Previous to British occupation, locals used a filtered supply, and few cases of typhoid were recorded, but during the British siege of the town the filters had been destroyed, and water was subsequently pumped and distributed without filtration. With multiple regiments camped around the town, soldiers had been negligent about excremental disposal and officers had not provided efficient sanitary oversight. "Polluted water supplies, filthy latrines covered with swarms of flies and uncovered with earth, excrement, polluted soil, manure heaps and dead horses," the report observed, "have been the usual accompaniments of camps."[122] The movement of troops across the country, particularly via railroads, intensified the process. While British military units were provided with Berkefeld water filters and boiling apparatus, Simpson found that very few actually carried out proper filtration. And, in a similar indictment from the royal commission on hospitals, there were too few RAMC officers, and many of them had been pushed into service quickly with only surgical and not sanitary training. The stakes were high, not just in maintaining the strength of the army and providing military might but also in cost. Simpson, using a rough estimation, calculated that the cost of typhoid alone during the war totaled upwards of four million pounds.

Notter, a leading figure in the RAMC, was outraged at the way in which Simpson conducted the investigation. He narrowed in on the RAMC and on the waterborne causation of the disease. Notter had been professor of military hygiene at Netley from 1876 and instrumental in teaching a generation of RAMC and IMS medics. Simpson had "grossly exaggerated" the unsanitary state of the military camps, he fumed, and had not even investigated most of them, instead relying on hearsay after he returned from Cape

---

121 Hamilton, "Enteric Fever in india," 788.

122 *Report of the Commission on the Nature, Pathology, Causation, and Prevention of Dysentery, and its Relationship to Enteric Fever,* 86.

Town studying plague. Many of the base camps and stationary hospitals, he argued, were in excellent sanitary condition. The Portland Hospital, for example, had taken every reasonable precaution in preventing the spread of typhoid in Bloemfontein. Tooth and Bowlby had specifically designed the camp to isolate typhoid patients (figure 5.3), carefully overseen disinfection of linens, clothing, and excreta (figure 5.4), and boiled and filtered water. But Notter was skeptical of many field hospitals and camps on the march, information on which was woefully inadequate.

Notter's chief problem with Simpson was that much of what ended up in the latter's report had occurred before the commission even arrived in South Africa and so was not the result of personal outbreak investigation. In part three of the report Notter was willing to concede that both contaminated water and inadequate RAMC staff had been central to the high incidence of typhoid, but they were not the only factors. Notter's epidemiological gaze, no doubt braced by his wealth of experience at home and internationally, was wider than Simpson's. Notter listed twelve points that must be considered to investigated to understand the typhoid outbreak in South Africa:

- The general endemic prevalence of this class of disease in South Africa before the War
- The age and constitution of our forces
- The composition of the Army
- Flies as carriers of disease
- Liability of Kaffirs to dysentery
- Food supplies
- Water supplies
- Milk supplies
- Disposal of excreta
- Soil pollution
- Density of population in camps and personal infection
- Present state of our knowledge regarding Etiology of Enteric Fever and Dysentery.[123]

It was a wide-ranging summary of a methodological approach to understanding typhoid that had been developed for three decades. Notter even cited the

123 *Report of the Commission on the Nature, Pathology, Causation, and Prevention of Dysentery, and its Relationship to Enteric Fever,* 131.

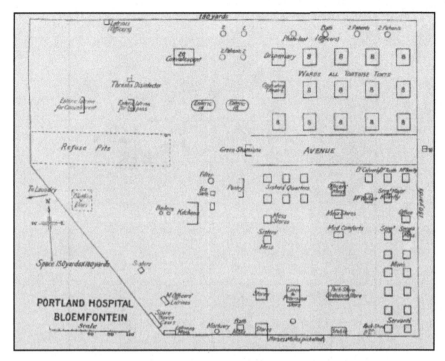

Figure 5.3 Plan of Portland Hospital, Bloemfontein. From Report of the Royal Commission Appointed to Consider and Report Upon the Care and Treatment of the Sick and Wounded during the South African Campaign, 61. House of Commons Parliamentary Papers, Crown Copyright.

collective research of epidemiologists at home, including Charles Cameron in Dublin and Bulstrode and Low at the Medical Department. Simpson had ignored most of these points, Notter argued, particularly neglecting to take into consideration the excremental pollution of the soil and the distribution of typhoid via flies. Moreover, the problem was not a lack of sanitary organization. Simpson had called for a complete reorganization of the RAMC and the creation of an Army Health Corps, which Notter, an RAMC man, had found offensive. Notter agreed that more sanitary officers and conservancy staff might be employed by the RAMC, but they had to fit into the existing military structure and not be based on the civilian scheme Simpson had advocated. "From the personal inspection of most of the camps in South Africa," Notter concluded, in a clear jab at Simpson, "I am convinced there

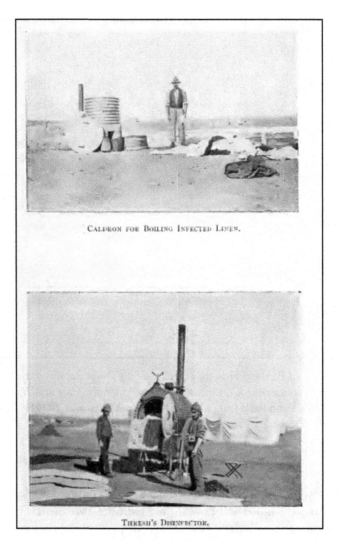

CALDRON FOR BOILING INFECTED LINEN.

THRESH'S DISINFECTOR.

Figure 5.4 Disinfection at the Portland Hospital,
Bloemfontein. From Report of the Royal Commission
Appointed to Consider and Report Upon the Care and
Treatment of the Sick and Wounded during the South
African Campaign, 40. House of Commons Parliamentary
Papers, Crown Copyright.

has not been such a complete neglect of sanitary precautions as this report would seem imply."[124]

The feud between Simpson and Notter was only in part an etiological disagreement over the cause or communication of typhoid. Simpson blamed nearly every outbreak of typhoid during the war on contaminated water, while Notter was willing to consider a wide range of etiological factors. But in their respective published work on typhoid both men shared up-to-date, progressive views on the disease consistent with elite epidemiologists at home. Both had also embraced bacteriology in fortifying epidemiological work. Simpson's *The Maintenance of Health in the Tropics* (1905) echoed the views on the etiological aspects and prevention of typhoid in the 1900 second edition of Notter and Firth's *The Theory and Practice of Hygiene,* which replaced Parkes's manual as probably the most important sanitary publication at home and abroad for health officers.[125] The intensity of the disagreement was more likely over professional identity and methodology. Simpson was forthright in his critique of the RAMC and in his suggestions to change sanitary policy gleaned from his experience in India. Notter, on the other hand, was not.

Quick to leap to Simpson's defense was George Turner, former MOH for Portsmouth who had moved to South Africa in the late 1880s and served as MOH for both Cape Town and later the Transvaal. Turner wrote to the *Lancet* shortly after the publication of the commission's report to defend Simpson. Turner had accompanied Notter and Simpson early in their investigation at the camps between Pretoria and Komatiport and noted that "so far from being exaggerated" Simpson's report on the unsanitary location of military camps "is under-stated." From six years' experience studying typhoid in South Africa, Turner, like Simpson, believed that water was the chief means of spreading the disease during the war. He and Simpson, meanwhile, had not meant to incite Notter and the RAMC: "We quarrel with the system," he argued, "or want of system, and not with the officers." [126] But the damage had been done, in spite of the *Lancet* saying that the "sturdy differences of opinion between two such recognised authorities . . . do not lessen the

124 *Report of the Commission on the Nature, Pathology, Causation, and Prevention of Dysentery, and its Relationship to Enteric Fever,* 5.

125 Simpson, *The Maintenance of Health in the Tropics.*

126 "The Report of the Commission on the Nature, Pathology, Causation, and Prevention of Dysentery and its Relation to Typhoid Fever," *Lancet* (December 13, 1903): 1750–52; Turner, "Typhoid Fever in South Africa," 381.

interest of a most valuable report."[127] The feud lingered in the press and especially with Notter. In a lecture before the Public Health Laboratory at the University of Manchester, a year after the report was published, he elaborated on his South African experience studying typhoid, providing a proto-ecological view of the disease as it spread among the soldiers during the war.

Where Notter, Simpson, and Bruce found agreement, if any was to be had, was in the pitfalls of outbreak investigation during the war. Bruce had disparaged the lack of clinical and pathological material, despite the overwhelming number of cases of typhoid and dysentery. And it had proven difficult to collect statistics from field hospitals. The reports from base hospitals and from city officials had not always noted the right kind of data (e.g., morbidity records). Field hospitals often simply listed the name and illness of an individual and not their regiment. With the near constant movement of troops, tracing an epidemic of typhoid in the tropics along well-established lines in Victorian epidemiology was nearly impossible.

The South African War marked the end of a distinctly Victorian discourse on the filth disease. The unprecedented outbreak of typhoid among British troops in three years in South Africa had led to yet another public outcry against the disease, which as the Edwardian period began was threatening the strength of an empire. We can see the response to the typhoid epidemic in South Africa as distinctly Victorian as well, as it put in sharp relief growing tensions over the success of curbing typhoid in England vis-à-vis the policies of military medicine. The appointment of a series of typhoid-centered, government-sponsored commissions also illustrates the methodological divergence in approaching and "knowing" typhoid that had culminated at the end of the Victorian period. Wright's antityphoid inoculation drew on the promises of the new laboratory science of bacteriology, but it was also frustrated by government and military red tape, public distrust, and too singular an approach by Wright himself. In tackling typhoid on the veldt, Wright's sometime opponent David Bruce had shown the inherent difficulty of practicing the new science of bacteriology during warfare, and Notter and Simpson's feud over the institutional identity of epidemiology demonstrated the uneven way in which civilian methods of outbreak investigation were integrated into military and tropical medicine.

---

127 "Report of the Commission on the Nature, Pathology, Causation, and Prevention of Dysentery and its Relationship to Enteric Fever," *Lancet* (August 29, 1903): 626.

Indeed, in many ways the experience of typhoid during the South African War had thrust to the center of British public health a protracted debate about constructing "tropical typhoid" and making it a global disease. The war, converging the experiences of British medics at home, in India, and South Africa, practically ended the localist debates about typhoid's unique status that had been rife throughout India from the mid-nineteenth century. From the war onward typhoid was understood as a global disease, a process that drew on clinical medicine, military surgery, epidemiology, and bacteriology. And it was inexorably tied to British colonialism. This suggests both an uneven process of the global understanding of disease, epidemiological knowledge making, and the new public health. As Warwick Anderson has observed, the framing and implementation of western European and North American concepts of the new public health in colonial spaces were bound up with racialized visions of indigenous culpability. As the focus of Western public health increasingly focused on bodies, it was African and Indian bodies that were especially met with epidemiological and bacteriological gazes. Well before Typhoid Mary, moreover, in turn-of-the-century British colonial spaces the modernizing discourse was one of racialized index cases. Decades of typhoid denialism had narrowed the gaze of an earlier generation of British military medics, especially in India, to focus on white European male bodies, ignoring and rejecting the filth disease in indigenous bodies. And just as the product of such a belief might be the realization that typhoid was a product of imperialism, tropical typhoid morphed into a singularly global disease. But the bringing of epidemiological and bacteriological clarity on the global nature of the disease only served to increase racialized tensions; individual responsibility narrowed to index cases of unscrupulous Indians in the bazaar and Africans on the veldt. Chakrabarti has recently shown that the promise of the germ theory engendered and intensified the morality of tropical bacteriology. A similar process was at work with tropical epidemiology.[128]

But the late Victorian approach to typhoid during the South African War, however much a failure, had at least shown a path forward. One arm of prevention was an improved version of Wright's vaccine. By 1906 Alfred Keogh, leading RAMC official, could say with satisfaction that "the results, although subjected to some adverse criticism, are now generally held to have been satisfactory."[129] And as Hardy and Linton have shown, Leishman's improved

128 Chakrabarti, *Bacteriology in British India*, 13.
129 Alfred Keogh to A. E. Widdows, May 7, 1906, National Archives, Kew WO 138/12/Almroth Wright personnel files.

typhoid vaccine played a critical role in preventing the disease among British troops in World War I.[130] The other key lesson suggested by the failures of the South African campaign were epidemiological, chiefly focused on protecting food and water supplies and the proper disposal of excreta. The experience in India and South Africa in the 1890s proved that such lessons could not be directly applied in colonial settings and were often at odds with imperial aims to control, profit, and civilize.

In the years following the South African War, the Victorian notion of and approach to the filth disease came to an end. Leading up to World War I, typhoid, as the Victorians knew it, morphed and in some ways disappeared. This was true epidemiologically, in a decrease in the incidence of the disease, and epistemologically, in the cultural ways of knowing the disease and its impact on the social body of both England and the broader British Empire. It was the end of an era, one marked by a series of critically important advances in the scientific understanding of the disease but also marred by bureaucratic obstruction and intraprofessional conflict.

---

130 Linton, "Was Typhoid Inoculation Safe and Effective during World War I?"

Conclusion

The Afterlife of Victorian Typhoid

In the fall of 1937 typhoid again reared its ugly head, exploding to epidemic proportions in the south London town of Croydon. In a few months, local officials noted nearly three hundred typhoid cases, and by the end of the outbreak forty-three local residents had died of the disease. Early in November Croydon's MOH, Oscar Holden, reached out to the Ministry of Health, who sent inspector Ernest T. Conybeare. Working with local officials, Conybeare plotted typhoid cases onto a map of the town's water supply (supplied by five wells) and instantly saw that most of the early cases were supplied with water from the high-level supply from the Addington well. A few days later the supply was cut off. Subsequent sleuthing showed that prior to the outbreak the well in question was being worked on, chlorination had stopped, and one worker—a positive typhoid carrier—had contaminated the supply.[1] While hardly the only or last fulminating outbreak of typhoid in twentieth-century Britain, Croydon became, as Anne Hardy has argued, "a cause célèbre in the preventive community."[2] In important ways the legacy of Victorian public health reformers like John Simon lived on; typhoid continued to serve as a litmus test of the "sanitary civilisation" of an area long after the disease had declined and the typhoid of the Victorians had been forgotten. We should rightly situate the Croydon outbreak, as some scholars have done, in the context of a specific set of interwar British public-health debates. These debates centered on the accidental contamination of water supplies, the question

1   Murphy, *Report on a Public Local Inquiry into an Outbreak of Typhoid Fever at Croydon.* The fascinating outbreak at Croydon has been covered by numerous historians. See Luckin, *Death and Survival in Urban Britain,* 170–88; Wall, *Bacteria in Britain, 1880–1939,* chapter 6.

2   Hardy, *Salmonella Infections,* 37. For a broad survey of typhoid epidemics in twentieth-century Britain see Smallman-Raynon and Cliff, *Atlas of Epidemic Britain,* chapter 5.

of whether local rate payers were due compensation for lapses in technical know-how, inadequate educational campaigns on personal hygiene, and the role played by chronic typhoid carriers. Yet, placed in the longer framework that stretches back to the Victorian period, the Croydon outbreak resonates with the major themes of this book: the growth and constraints of bureaucracy, the broader political attempts at preventive medicine, and the everyday practices of epidemiology.

The 1937 Croydon case, like scores of other localized outbreaks of typhoid in the twentieth century, reveals the historically contingent ways that epidemiological outbreak investigation persisted as a central feature of public health practice well into the twentieth century.[3] Even today, the Centers for Disease Control and Prevention, in their *Principles of Epidemiology in Public Health Practice,* describe the steps of outbreak investigation in ways that are remarkably different than many of the studies explored in this book.[4] Epidemiological experts working in government, investigating local outbreaks, and searching for index cases were as common in the 1870s as they are today. Disease surveillance more broadly remains central to the enterprise of modern governments and systems of public health. A 2019 study published in the *Lancet,* for example, on the global burden of typhoid fever, called for "better data and better surveillance" as central priorities.[5] Another 2019 article in *Clinical Infectious Diseases,* this one on the "invisible burden" of typhoid in the Global South, argues that what is needed is "a surveillance infrastructure that is currently lacking in many endemic countries."[6] The link to the Victorians is pretty clear in this respect structurally, even if the public health solutions are still anything but straightforward. What we can say is that the practices of disease surveillance rarely follow the rationalized vision of state medicine laid out long ago by John Simon and his cadre of later Victorian supporters. Clashes of scientific expertise in identifying public

---

3   Debate over the role of state medicine continued into the twentieth century and the creation of the Ministry of Health and the NHS. See "Discussion on the Proper Sphere of State Medicine," *Proceedings of the Royal Society of Medicine* 32 (May 1939): 729–34.

4   Centers for Disease Control and Prevention, *Principles of Epidemiology in Public Health Practice,* https://www.cdc.gov/csels/dsepd/ss1978/lesson6/section2.html

5   Typhoid and Paratyphoid Collaborators, "The Global Burden of Typhoid and Paratyphoid."

6   Pitzer et al., "The Invisible Burden."

health problems, the assignment of blame for epidemics, and the reaching of a consensus on viable solutions are inherent political problems in public health both then and now.

Although outbreak investigation remained a vital part of the Medical Department and later the Ministry of Health (as the Croydon case shows), much had changed within British epidemiology in the period from the end of Queen Victoria's reign to the interwar years. Epidemiologists continued to work in local and central government, but after World War I, as Olga Amsterdamska has argued, a new disciplinary awareness emerged, one that sought to "demarcate" epidemiology as a science vis-à-vis a number of allied fields.[7] Outspoken discipline builders in British epidemiology such as Major Greenwood, William Hamer, and F. C. Crookshank, defended new kinds of epidemiology—academic and experimental epidemiology—against would-be rivals the bacteriologists, the biometricians, and the eugenicists. By the 1930s, Hamer was able to confidently state, for example, that there were clear academic, theoretical, and practical distinctions between clinical medicine, epidemiology, and bacteriology.[8] Such a view helps us to understand the rhetorical strategies interwar epidemiologists used to bolster their cultural authority in a period when, unlike the late Victorian era, epidemiology was no longer viewed as the chief science of public health. Post-1930s formulaic definitions of academic epidemiology left little room for the kind of outbreak investigation practiced by the Victorians, though there were echoes that spoke to a continuity of practice, like William Norman Pickles's classic 1939 study *Epidemiology in Country Practice*.[9]

Central to the discipline building of the interwar period were accounts by British epidemiologists of the history of their discipline. Interestingly, epidemiologists of the 1920s and 1930s recognized Radcliffe, Ballard, Thorne, Buchanan, and Bulstrode as "household words," Robert Reece noted in 1923.[10] But by the second half of the twentieth century, the Victorian epidemiologists were mostly forgotten. This process of forgetting is central to the history of modern epidemiology and is perhaps one reason epidemiologists today, even those interested in the history of their discipline, know little about the actual practices of Victorian epidemiology or its discipline builders. As the discipline's priorities changed in the 1940s, so too did the ways in

---

7   Amsterdamska, "Demarcating Epidemiology."
8   Hamer, "The Crux of Epidemiology."
9   Pickles, *Epidemiology in Country Practice*.
10   Reece, "Progress and Problems in Epidemiology."

which epidemiologists wrote about their own history. No doubt the decline of the major infectious diseases, the rise of chronic diseases, and the emergence of risk-factor epidemiology all contributed to a waning interest in the Victorians.[11] By 1950 heart disease and cancer were leading causes of death. What mostly remains today of the Victorians in epidemiological textbooks are old myths.[12] The 2019 edition of the *CDC Field Epidemiology Manual*, for example, invokes two Victorians: William Farr, who "developed a disease classification system that ushered in the era of modern vital statistics," and John Snow "the father of modern epidemiology."[13] This book provides a very different history of Victorian epidemiology, offering a different narrative about the path from Farr and Snow in the 1850s to bacteriological clarity in the early twentieth century.[14] But the historical myths in epidemiology today are deep seated. Students who take my History of Public Health course have often already taken an introductory public health module and can almost always tell me something about John Snow (it's usually a chestnut about his heroics at the Broad Street Pump). But when I introduce them to Ballard's Islington investigation, Radcliffe's Marylebone study, or the methodical work of Barry in the Tees Valley, they come away with a more complicated picture of how epidemiology was actually practiced in the past. And while the incidence of typhoid fever in Victorian Britain was fundamental to the development of epidemiology, there was also a host of other diseases that historians have given short shrift to outside of cholera and tuberculosis. *The Filth Disease* in this regard presents a kind of test case for future historians of medicine.

My broader point here is not to unfairly pick on today's epidemiologists as bad historians but rather to think reflexively about how and why some Victorian epidemiologists and types of epidemiology are invoked instead of others when we write about the history of epidemiology. While the central figures in *The Filth Disease* have been disremembered, the practices they developed remain central. Victorian epidemiological methods of outbreak investigation, in other words, lived on well past the Victorians who pioneered them. Statistical analysis, case tracing, interviewing, mapmaking,

---

11   Parascandola, "Epidemiology in Transition"; Mendelsohn, "From Eradication to Equilibrium."

12   Fos, *Epidemiology Foundations;* Bhopal, *Concepts of Epidemiology.*

13   Rasmussen and Goodman, eds., *CDC Field Epidemiology Manual,* 58.

14   Parodi, et al., "Environment, Population, and Biology"; Halliday, *The Great Filth.*

and experimentation all remain central to epidemiological practice. The way these practices continued in the twentieth century, however, is less clear and needs addressing. We have some clues. The final question on the examination for the diploma in public health in 1900, for example, was to make a sanitary inspection of any town or village, take notes, and return to the examination hall to write up the report, including rough visual sketches.[15] It was exactly the kind of work that had originated at the Medical Department in the 1860s. But we still know much less about the role that the methods of outbreak investigation—what I have in this book called "everyday epidemiology"—played in twentieth-century Britain. Hardy's *Salmonella Infections*, which examines transnational networks of twentieth-century research on food poisoning, provides the starting point for such research. Hardy's new book picks up where *The Filth Disease* ends, and I encourage readers to think about the two in tandem.

But there is an epistemological challenge in continuing the story of Victorian typhoid far beyond the early twentieth century. What we know about typhoid today, as the most virulent of a group of *Salmonella* infections, is a scientific and cultural frame not shared by the Victorians. What was called "typhoid" or "enteric fever" in the period 1830–1900 surely encompasses what twenty-first-century biologists call "typhoid," but it almost definitely included a host of other gastrointestinal and febrile diseases. And while figuring out, biologically speaking, what typhoid "actually was" in the Victorian period might interest clinicians bent on retrospective diagnosis and historical epidemiologists, as a social and cultural historian of medicine I have focused on what typhoid meant to the Victorians. They named, perceived, and responded to a disease they called "typhoid" in historically contingent ways that do not easily translate to twentieth- or twenty-first-century definitions or attitudes.[16] Subsequent historians might find the historical analysis of typhoid in the twentieth century fruitful, but I suspect they will find very different typhoid cultures than the ones explored in this book. *The Filth Disease* in this way provides another salient example of Charles Rosenberg's framing disease metaphor, and in meaningful ways the typhoid I study in this book did not exist before the 1830s or last much longer than the early 1900s. Rosenberg's thinking about culturally situating

---

15   Examination Papers for Diploma in Public Health (1900), Wellcome Collection, MS.6807/17–23. Few scholars have studied the history of public health education. See Fee and Acheson, *A History of Education in Public Health*.

16   Rosenberg, "Disease in History," 1.

disease in its historical context has guided a generation of scholarship and has certainly influenced my approach in this book. But as *The Filth Disease* has shown, there were multiple ways of perceiving, conflicts of naming, and a lack of uniformity in responding to typhoid in Victorian Britain. In critical ways the typhoid of the Victorians resisted discipline and instead was a wedge for health reformers like John Simon, George Buchanan, and Richard Thorne Thorne to pursue the agenda of a centralized system of preventive public health. That typhoid served as a mediator, however shifting, between a broader cultural understanding of infectious disease and the everyday research of a smaller group of epidemiologists and bacteriologists, provides insight into the deep-seated ways that outbreaks of disease and the work of those that study them are inherently political activities.

For a brief historical period, from the 1860s to the early 1900s, a particular kind of epidemiological culture led public health approaches in understanding the disease. Typhoid was a wedge, in other words, that Victorian epidemiologists used to produce knowledge about disease, debate methods and theories, defend their findings, and outline their discipline. But epidemiological research did not, and still does not, develop in a cultural vacuum. Victorian epidemiologists, I explain in this book, associated typhoid with the middle and upper classes, literally their homes and their bodies, but also with middle-class anxieties in the Victorian period. It was a disease intimately tied to bourgeois respectability, citizenship, and the progressive sanitary technologies of piped water supply, drains, and water closets. It was also yoked in important ways to culturally in-demand foods like fresh cow's milk, which by the 1870s brought rural dairy farmers and urban-rural food pathways into the epidemiological gaze of governmental inspection. By the 1890s, with a nascent ecological understanding of the disease, typhoid was at the center of the realization that the health of urban dwellers, despite seemingly progressive sanitary technologies, often very much depended on the sanitary practices of those in rural areas. Typhoid, I argue, proved an index for public health authorities to understand the environmental and political boundaries urban versus rural locations.

But Victorian epidemiology represented just one, albeit influential, way of knowing the filth disease. Even by the end of the century there were still viable alternatives for explaining typhoid. Charles Creighton, in his well-known 1894 study, *A History of Epidemics in Britain,* for example, still clung to a Murchison-like theory that most cases of typhoid were caused by miasmas rising from the soil or leaking through drainpipes.[17] Such a stance seemed retrograde to the mainstream group of British epidemiologists who had built a discipline studying typhoid as a fecal-oral disease. But Creighton's insistence suggests the protean nature of typhoid in the Victorian period. And the debate over the disease shifted again in the twentieth century as the typhoid of the Victorians morphed into the *Salmonella* group. By the 1937 Croydon outbreak typhoid was just the typhoid as we know it now, and the controversy was over.

The Filth Disease ends with a kind of optimism not unique to the Victorians but certainly emblematic of their age. For a brief period in the early twentieth century doctors and public health officials believed they understood typhoid better than any other infectious disease. There was unbridled faith that the tools of epidemiology, bolstered by the new science of bacteriology had uncovered the truth of the filth disease. In a paper given at the Epidemiological Society of London in 1899, titled "Ten Years' Experience of Enteric Fever in a Midland Town, and its Lessons," Philip Boobbyer made this view quite clear. "For all practical purposes of Public Health administration and reform," he declared, "we have already as much knowledge as we want concerning the life-history and etiology of enteric fever." He added: "There is probably no chapter in the history of epidemiology more full of interest and importance to the human race than this."[18] Nowhere was Boobbyer's confidence more clearly displayed than in American sanitary engineer George Whipple's well-known 1908 study, *Typhoid Fever: Its Causation, Transmission and Prevention*. Whipple there produced a typhoid diagram that visualized the coming together of fifty years' worth of epidemiological research on typhoid; it represented a model of typhoid prevention driven by outbreak investigation and the search for disease media—food, water, people—at the center of preventive medicine. There were practical reasons for the confidence of early twentieth-century observers, not least was the decline of typhoid in Britain.

The Filth Disease helps to contextualize why early twentieth-century public health officials were so optimistic about understanding and preventing typhoid. As we have seen, typhoid fever was a model disease for weighing etiological debates and for substantiating the bureaucratic strategies of disease surveillance and municipal sanitation. Typhoid was a disease without a name before 1829 and hotly debated in clinical and pathological circles

---

17   Creighton, *A History of Epidemics in Britain*.
18   Boobbyer, "Ten Years' Experience of Enteric Fever," 89.

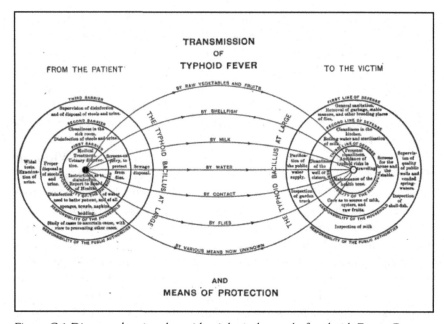

Figure C.1 Diagram showing the epidemiological spread of typhoid. From, George Whipple, Typhoid Fever: Its Causation, Transmission and Prevention (New York: John Wiley & Sons, 1908). Image used with Permission, Courtesy of Medical Heritage Library.

for more three decades. By the 1860s, when this book begins, public health authorities were driven to answer the question of why typhoid was so ubiquitous, sudden, and fulminating. The stakes, we have seen, were high. No doubt the typhoid attacks on the British monarchy, explored in chapter 1, killing Queen Victoria's husband, Albert, in 1861 and nearly killing their son, Prince Albert Edward, in 1871 were an important popular impetus. Typhoid emerged as the central target for public health reformers like John Simon as a result of changes in medical science as well: the disease began to stabilize as an ontological concept, it was separately listed from typhus and continued fever on death certificates, and statisticians like William Farr at the GRO began to analyze the disease statistically on a nationwide scale. The fight against the filth disease, in other words, was a calculated political attack at a moment of public outcry. In the period 1860–80 typhoid riveted the British public, and as we saw in chapter 2 a unique typhoid culture emerged at the Medical Department and among medical officers of health, who sought to use typhoid as a model disease of state medicine to orchestrate a nationwide system of public health infrastructure and disease surveillance. This impetus epitomized the late Victorian approach to public health and coincided with landmark administrative changes in parliamentary law that first sought to push local authorities to provide municipal sanitation schemes and monitor the health of local populations. Local outbreaks of typhoid were battlegrounds and opportunities for Simon and his followers to implore local authorities to undertake sanitary reform; implement sewerage, drainage, waterworks; or fix earlier failed attempts at sanitary technology.

Scholars have been hesitant in recent years to give too much weight to the work of central authorities such as Simon; many conclude, as Simon Szreter has recently, that while "central government provided concessionary grants-in-aid and technical advice if requested . . . it was primarily local government that initiated, staffed, sometimes devised and most funded the enormous expansion in urban infrastructure and social services."[19] The general story is one of a weak central government in the last third of the nineteenth century but a burgeoning local spirit of preventive medicine, one shaped by the work of medical officers of health and a new civic activism in ushering in municipal sanitation and health education. This book provides a more complicated picture. Christopher Hamlin has shown that the massive public works implemented in the course of the nineteenth century, sewerage, drainage, and a filtered public water supply were often accomplished in spite of conflicts within sanitary science.[20] Epidemiological investigations of typhoid from 1860 to 1900 often showed how and when such modernizing systems failed, on the one hand, and how they might be improved on the other. Municipal sanitation, in other words, came to depend on the science of epidemiology, sometimes for its findings but often for its methods. Establishing differential mortality and morbidity, using contact tracing, finding index cases, and discovering faults with domestic and municipal sanitary systems became the hallmark of practical methods in public health that were pioneered in the late Victorian period. But as we have seen, sometimes local officials followed epidemiological advice begrudgingly. In an era where central and local government relations were often strained, the core of epidemiological practice was routine inspection of local communities while investigating outbreaks of infectious disease. The methods of outbreak investigation, pioneered at

---

19   Szreter, *Health and Wealth*, 287.
20   Hamlin, *A Science of Impurity*.

the Medical Department, and the networks of epidemiologists practicing as MOsH and as epidemiologists in the British colonies, actively contributed to cajoling local officials into sanitary action. After all, in practice, as in theory, public health then as now is inherently a political activity.

The two decades between 1860 and 1880, explored in chapter 2, saw the emergence and consolidation of epidemiological methods of outbreak investigation. Learning through the everyday epidemiology of outbreak investigation, and forging networks across a range of professional societies, British epidemiologists began to think of themselves and their work as a distinct field. Inspectors at the Medical Department and local MOsH who studied typhoid in this period revealed some painful truths about the growth of public health infrastructure. The earliest adopters—middle- and upper-class Britons—of a Chadwickian dream of houses with drains and water closets, not to mention entire pipe-bound cities, were more frequently succumbing to typhoid, mostly through the contamination of water supplies. In an inversion of Chadwick's vision of sanitary engineers guiding public health practice, it was epidemiologists who sleuthed outbreaks to index cases and identified leaks in drains and untrapped toilets. Where epidemiologically research took place, both geographically and demographically, was critical to understanding this story, and what we might think of as the space and place of epidemiological research needs more historical attention.

With the methods of outbreak investigation starting to standardize, from the 1870s the role of outbreak investigation expanded due to the discovery that food also spread typhoid fever. Several high-profile milk-borne outbreaks in metropolitan London raised a new red flag, as we saw in chapter 3. Epidemiological outbreak investigation in these examples ushered in new fears of sick cows, unscrupulous dairymen, and the most dangerous realization of all: that cow's milk, which was idealized as a bourgeois nutritional staple, could spread a deadly disease that was undetectable by sight or smell. The epidemiological finding that milk could spread disease heightened the awareness of British epidemiologists that other media might also be at fault, and without much of a logical jump shellfish, ice-cream, and watercress came under the auspices of the epidemiological gaze.

In the 1880s a new lot of disease researchers—bacteriologists—came armed with microscopes, slides, stains, and Koch's postulates, and they made important inroads into linking typhoid with a specific bacillus, *B. typhosus*. We might see such laboratory findings as the aha moment in the story of typhoid, but the British epidemiologists who had become typhoid experts in the previous two decades argued that bacteriological evidence only served to confirm what they had been saying all along. A. C. Houston for example, in a lecture before the Section of State Medicine at the Sixty-Ninth Annual Meeting of the British Medical Association, in 1901, noted that he was "forcibly struck by the fact that the discoveries of recent times" on the bacteriology of typhoid "have only confirmed the wisdom of the teaching of epidemiologists at a time when the science of bacteriology was unknown, or only in its infancy."[21] As we saw in chapter 4, epidemiological methods of outbreak investigation continued to dominate the approach to understanding typhoid in the 1880s and early 1890s, and only slowly did British epidemiologists begin to team up with bacteriologists. Central to the new model of a combined field and laboratory approach was the finding that *B. typhosus* could live outside of the human body in soils, which linked epidemiology and bacteriology to the emerging science of ecology in important ways in the twentieth century. By 1900, with a nascent ecological understanding of the disease, typhoid was at the center of the realization that the health of urban dwellers, despite seemingly progressive sanitary technologies, often depended on the sanitary practices of those in rural areas.[22]

With the cultural authority of epidemiology at what was perhaps its peak, and with rates of typhoid waning at home in Britain, the single largest outbreak of typhoid occurred during the South African War. Massive losses of British soldiers to typhoid presented new opportunities for studying the disease, as explored in chapter 5, and brought to a popular and wider professional audience a central question that colonial doctors had been asking for decades—was the typhoid in Britain the same disease across the globe? Disease and warfare wrought opportunities for testing the new typhoid identification and prevention technologies of the Widal Test and Almroth Wright's antityphoid vaccine. But in the end, both bacteriology and epidemiology failed to make a significant mark on preventing typhoid abroad. Neither were perfected but instead became shining examples of a new hope in fighting the filth disease. In the first decade of the twentieth century the typhoid picture seemed to be coming into even sharper relief; the local outbreaks that continued were probably due to healthy (or chronic typhoid)

---

21   Houston, "A Discussion on Enteric Fever in its Public Health Aspects," 395.
22   British epidemiologist Sheldon Dudley in the 1930s argued that epidemiology is perforce ecological. See Dudley, "The Ecological Outlook on Epidemiology."

carriers, although some British epidemiologists such as William Hamer famously and stubbornly denied their role in the spread of the disease.[23]

Which brings us back to Boobbyer's optimism and Whipple's typhoid diagram. Municipal sanitation, the local efforts of medical officers of health, routine disease surveillance by the central authorities, hygienic education, the Widal Test, and a new promise of a vaccine were seen as the clear path forward. The late Victorians and early Edwardians thought they knew typhoid and believed they could prevent the disease. And except for the disastrous events in South Africa, typhoid rates were plummeting. And at that cultural moment the typhoid of the Victorians disappeared, splintering into the new category of the *Salmonellas*, morphing by the interwar period—with outbreaks such as those at Croydon—into the typhoid that is recognizable to us today.

So, what can we say about the typhoid of the Victorians? In the course of the twentieth century typhoid disappeared as a model disease in Britain and North America. Typhoid even largely disappeared in popular discourse in the West, to the extent that in the course of researching and writing this book I interacted with dozens of people in Europe and North America who either had never heard of typhoid or who asked me how my book on "typhus" was coming along. If folks had heard of typhoid it was usually by association with the salient story of Typhoid Mary. All this cultural memory, even the amnesia, has given me some pause. A popular story in the history of public health is that the nineteenth-century public health reformers focused on environments as the foci of disease, whereas twentieth-century public health reformers focused on individual people. Typhoid Mary fits that model really well, although my research on Victorian typhoid shows that the model is far too simplistic, and Mary Mallon was part of a long line of index cases such as "J. K.," the Caterham construction worker in 1878. Talking to people today about typhoid has led to some amusing and peculiar moments. Benjamin Ward Richardson was right that calling the disease "typhoid" has led to "the absurdest confusion, particularly by the ordinary people."[24] But more than anything else, my anecdotal interactions are powerful reminders that public health interests change. The next big disease to overtake typhoid in the

23 Davies and Hall, "A Discussion on the Etiology and Epidemiology of Typhoid,"191. For a broader discussion on typhoid carriers, see Wall's *Bacteria in Britain,* chapter 5; Gradmann, "Robert Koch and the Invention of the Carrier State." For a comparative discussion of work on carriers between America and Britain see McKay, *Patient Zero,* chapter 1.

24 Richardson, *Vita Medica,* 88

British consciousness was probably influenza, but then it, too, faded and was replaced around 1950 by an emphasis on heart disease and cancer. An interest and a fear of emerging and reemerging infectious diseases have perhaps tilted the scales back to thinking about epidemics, something HIV/AIDS did in the 1980s and 1990s.

As this book goes to press, we are in the middle of a new pandemic of coronavirus, COVID-19, which supposedly emerged out of Wuhan Province in central China. Students in my History of Medicine course want to know three things: Where did it start? Will it spread to us? And what measures are being adopted to contain the disease? Framing, naming, blaming: these seem almost universals now in thinking about how populations understand infectious disease. But we should also include forgetting. In real ways that were not just epistemological, typhoid disappeared in the West, only to be replaced by new fears. But this is not the case in the Global South, where typhoid surges endemically in Asia, Africa, and Latin America. Shifting the story of the filth disease to a global scale is a story yet to be told, but it is an important one that awaits scholarly attention.

Bibliography

National Archives, Kew (NA)
Wellcome Library
London Metropolitan Archives (LMA)
Archives of the Royal College of Physicians of London
Archives of the Royal College of Surgeons of London

Acland, T. D. *A Collection of the Published Writings of William Withey Gull.* London: New Sydenham Society, 1896.

"The Addresses to their Constituents Sent Out." *Times*, September 21, 1900, 7.

Adler, Richard. *Victor Vaughan: A Biography of the Pioneering Bacteriologist, 1851–1929.* Jefferson, NC: McFarland, 2015.

"The Adulteration Act." *Pharmaceutical Journal* 3 (June 7, 1873): 979–80.

"The Adulteration of Food in Marylebone." *Food, Water, & Air* 1 (November 1871): 91.

"Agglutination in Typhoid Fever and "Anti-Typhoid' Vaccination." *Lancet* 151 (March 19, 1898): 805.

Airy, Hubert. "Report to the Local Government Board on an Outbreak of Enteric Fever in Chichester" in *Annual Report of the Medical Officer of the Local Government Board for 1878* (London: Spottiswoode, 1879).

Aisenberg, Andrew. *Contagion: Disease, Government, and the "Social Question" in Nineteenth-Century France.* Stanford, CA: Stanford University Press, 1999.

Aitken, William. *The Science and Practice of Medicine.* Vol. 1. London: Charles Griffin and Company, 1864.

Allbutt, Clifford T. "On the Propagation of Enteric Fever." *British Medical Journal* 482 (March 26, 1870): 308–9.

Allen, Michelle. *Cleansing the City: Sanitary Geographies in Victorian London.* Athens: Ohio University Press, 2008.

Amsterdamska, Olga. "Demarcating Epidemiology." *Science, Technology, & Human Values* 30 (Winter 2005):17–51.

Anderson, Benedict. *Imagined Communities: Reflections on the Origins and Spread of Nationalism.* London: Verso, 1983.

———. "'Where Every Prospect Pleases and Only Man is Vile': Laboratory Medicine and Colonial Discourse." *Critical Inquiry* 18 (1992): 506–29.

"The Annus Medicus." *Lancet* 98 (December 30, 1871): 925.

Armstrong, David. "Medical Surveillance of Normal Populations." In *Technologies of Modern Medicine: Proceedings of a Seminar Held at the Science Museum, London, March 1993*, edited by Ghislaine Lawrence, 73–87. London: Science Museum, 1994.

———. "The Rise of Surveillance Medicine." *Sociology of Health and Illness* 17 (1995): 393–404.

Arnold, David. "Cholera and Colonialism in British India." *Past & Present* 113, no. 1 (November 1986): 118–51.

———. *The Tropics and the Traveling Gaze: India, Landscape, and Science, 1800–1856*. Seattle: University of Washington Press, 2006.

Arnold-Forster, Agnes. "Mapmaking and Mapthinking: Cancer as a Problem of Place in Nineteenth-Century England." *Social History of Medicine* (October 2018): 1–26.

Asph, A. G. "The South African Hospitals Enquiry." *National Review* 37 (1901): 39–44.

Atkins, Peter. *Liquid Materialities: A History of Milk, Science and the Law*. Farnham, UK: Ashgate, 2010.

Babington, Benjamin Guy. "Objects of the Epidemiological Society." *Transactions of the Epidemiological Society of London* 1 (London: John W. Davies, 1863): 1–8.

Baldwin, Peter. *Contagion and the State in Europe, 1830–1930*. Cambridge: Cambridge University Press, 1999.

———. "The Victorian State in Comparative Perspective." In *Liberty and Authority in Victorian Britain*, edited by Peter Mandler, 51–70. Oxford: Oxford University Press, 2006.

Ballard, Edward. "Observations of Some of the Ways in Which Drinking-Water May Become Polluted." *British Medical Journal* 994 (1880): 82–84.

———. "On a Localised Outbreak of Typhoid Fever in Islington." *Medical Times and Gazette* 2 (1870): 611–17.

———*On a Localised Outbreak of Typhoid Fever in Islington, Traced to the Use of Impure Milk*. London: J&A Churchill, 1871.

———. "On Some Sanitary Aspects of Cowkeeping, and the Trade in Milk in London." *The Milk Journal* 1 (London, 1871): 6–8.

———. *Report on the Sanitary Condition of the Parish of Saint Mary, Islington During the Year 1870*. London: J&L Tirebuck, 1871.

———. *What to Observe at the Bed-Side and After Death in Medical Cases*. London: John Churchill, 1854.

"Barnard Castle." *Teesdale Mercury*, November 5, 1890, 4.

"Barnard Castle." *Teesdale Mercury*, January 31, 1894, 4.

"Barnard Castle." *Teesdale Mercury*, June 28, 1893, 4.

Barnes, David. *The Great Stink of Paris and the Nineteenth Century Struggle Against Filth*. Baltimore: Johns Hopkins University Press, 2006.

Barr, James. *The Treatment of Typhoid Fever*. London: H. K. Lewis, 1892.

Barry, Frederick. "Interim Report on an Epidemic Prevalence of Enteric Fever in the Valley of the River Tees." In *Annual Report of the Medical Officer of the Local Government Board for 1890.* Parliamentary Papers. London: Spottiswoode, 1891.

———. "Report on Enteric Fever in the Tees Valley During 1890–91." In *Annual Report of the Medical Officer of the Local Government Board for 1891.* Parliamentary Papers. London: Spottiswoode, 1893.

Bashford, Alison. *Purity and Pollution: Gender, Embodiment and Victorian Medicine.* Basingstoke, UK: Macmillan, 1998.

Bellamy, Christine. *Administering Central-Local Relations, 1871–1919: The Local Government Board in its Fiscal and Cultural Context.* Manchester: Manchester University Press, 1988.

Bhopal, Raj S. *Concepts of Epidemiology: Integrating the Ideas, Theories, Principles, and Methods of Epidemiology.* Oxford: Oxford University Press, 2016.

Bingham, P., et al. "John Snow, William Farr and the 1849 Outbreak of Cholera that Affected London." *Public Health* 118 (2004): 387–94.

Blaxall, Frank. "The Relations of Bacteriology to Epidemiology." *Transactions of the Epidemiological Society of London* 18 (1899): 153–72.

Blyth, Alexander Wynter. *A Manual of Public Health.* London: Macmillan, 1890.

Boddice, Rob. *The History of Emotions.* Manchester: Manchester University Press, 2018.

Boobbyer, Philip. "Ten Years' Experience of Enteric Fever in a Midland Town, and its Lessons." *Transactions of the Epidemiological Society of London* 18 (1899): 88–110.

Bourdieu, Pierre. *Outline of a Theory of Practice.* Cambridge: Cambridge University Press, 1977.

Brand, Jeanne. *Doctors and the State: The British Medical Profession and Government Action in Public Health, 1870–1912.* Baltimore: Johns Hopkins University Press, 1965.

———. "John Simon and the Local Government Board Bureaucrats, 1871–1876." *Bulletin of the History of Medicine* 37 (March–April 1963): 184–94.

Brieger, Gert. "The Historiography of Medicine." In *Companion Encyclopedia of the History of Medicine,* edited by William Bynum and Roy Porter, 22–44. London: Routledge, 1993.

Briggs, Asa. "Cholera and Society in the Nineteenth Century." *Past and Present* 119 (April 1961): 76–96.

"British Medical Association." *The Veterinary Journal* 11 (1880): 349.

Brown, Michael. "Surgery, Identity and Embodied Emotion: John Bell, James Gregory and the Edinburgh 'Medical War.'" *History* 104 (January 2019): 19–41.

———. "From Foetid Air to Filth: The Cultural Transformation of British Epidemiological Thought, ca.1780–1848." *Bulletin of the History of Medicine* 82, no. 3 (2008): 515–44.

Brown, Samuel Sneade. *A Lay Lecture on Sanitary Matters, with a Paper on Sewer Ventilation.* London: Kerby and Endean, 1873.

Bruce, David. "Analysis of the Results of Professor Wright's Method of Anti-Typhoid Inoculation." *Journal of the Royal Army Medical Corps* 4 (1905): 244–55.

Brumberg, Joan Jacobs. *Fasting Girls: The Emergence of Anorexia Nervosa as a Modern Disease.* Cambridge, MA: Harvard University Press, 1988.

Brunton, Deborah. *The Politics of Vaccination.* Rochester, NY: University of Rochester Press, 2008.

Brunton, T. Lauder. "Enteric Fever: A Crucial Instance of its Spread Through the Medium of Drinking Water." *Practitioner* 22 (January–June 1879): 473–80.

———. "Dr. Klein and the Pathology of Small-Pox and Typhoid Fever." *Practitioner* 14 (1875): 5–10.

———. "Another Aspect of the Tyndall Typhoid Controversy." *Practitioner* 14 (1875): 62–67.

Bryden, J. L. *On Age and Length of Service as affecting the Sickness, Mortality, and Invaliding of the European Army.* Calcutta: Superintendent of Government Printing, 1874.

Buchanan, George. "Aids to Epidemiological Knowledge." *Transactions of the Epidemiological Society of London* 1 (1883): 1–14.

———. *Annual Report of the Medical Officer of the Local Government Board for 1879.* Parliamentary Papers. London: Eyre and Spottiswoode, 1880.

———. *Annual Report of Medical Officer for Local Government Board for 1881.* Parliamentary Papers. London: Eyre and Spottiswoode, 1882.

———. *Annual Report of the Medical Officer of the Local Government Board for 1887.* Parliamentary Papers. London: Eyre and Spottiswoode, 1888.

———. *Annual Report of the Medical Officer of the Local Government Board for 1888.* Parliamentary Papers. London: Eyre and Spottiswoode, 1889.

———. "Cholera in Europe." In *Annual Report of the Medical Officer of the Local Government Board for 1884.* Parliamentary Papers. London: Eyre and Spottiswoode, 1885.

———. "Citizenship in Sanitary Work," *Practitioner* 17 (1876): 384–400.

———. "On an Outbreak of Typhoid Fever at Guildford." In *Annual Report of the Medical Officer of the Privy Council for 1867.* Parliamentary Papers. London: Eyre and Spottiswoode, 1868.

———. "On Some Recent Inquiries Under the Public Health Act, 1858." *In Annual Report of the Medical Officer of the Local Government Board for 1873.* Parliamentary Papers. London: Eyre and Spottiswoode, 1874.

———. "On the Dry Earth System of Dealing with Excrement." In *Annual Report of the Medical Officer of the Privy Council for 1870.* Parliamentary Papers. London: Eyre and Spottiswoode, 1871.

———. "Report on the Results which have hitherto been gained in Various parts of England by Works and Regulations Designed to Promote the Public Health." In *Annual Report of the Medical Officer of the Privy Council for 1866.* Parliamentary Papers. London: Eyre and Spottiswoode, 1867.

Buchanan, George and John Netten Radcliffe. "On the Construction and use of Midden Closets." In *Annual Report of the Medical Officer of the Privy Council for 1870.* Parliamentary Papers. London: Eyre and Spottiswoode, 1871.

Buckle, George Earle. *The Letters of Queen Victoria. Volume 5 (1870–1878)* Cambridge: Cambridge University Press, 1926.

Budd, William. *Typhoid Fever: Its Nature, Mode of Spreading, and Prevention.* London: Longmans, Green, and Co., 1873.

———. *The Siberian Cattle-Plague, or the Typhoid Fever of the Ox.* Bristol: Kerslake and Co., 1865.

Bulstrode, H. Timbrell. "Report Upon Prevalence of Enteric Fever in the City of Chichester." In *Annual Report of the Medical Officer of the Local Government Board for 1896–97.* Parliamentary Papers. London: Spottiswoode, 1897.

Burdett-Coutts, William. "Our Wars and Our Wounded." *Times,* June 27, 1900, 4.

———. *The Sick and Wounded in South Africa: What I Saw and Said of Them.* London: Cassell & Co., 1900.

——— "The South African Hospitals." *Times,* February 13, 1901, 11.

Burney, Ian. *Bodies of Evidence: Medicine and the Politics of the English Inquest, 1830–1926.* Baltimore: Johns Hopkins University Press, 2000.

Bynum, W. F. "The Evolution of Germs and the Evolution of Disease: Some British Debates, 1870–1900." *History and Philosophy of Science of the Life Sciences* 24 (2002): 53–68.

——— "Hospital, Disease and Community: The London Fever Hospital, 1801–1850." In *Healing and History: Essays for George Rosen,* edited by Charles E. Rosenberg, 97–115. New York: Science History Publications, 1979.

Bynum, W. F., and Helen Bynum. "Object Lessons: Fever Chart." *Lancet* 389 (January 28, 2017): 859.

Cameron, Charles. "Half-Yearly Report on Public Health." *Dublin Quarterly Journal of Medical Science* 51 (1871): 475–98.

———. *Lectures on the Preservation of Health.* London: Cassell, Petter, and Galpin, 1868.

———. *A Manual of Hygiene.* Dublin: Hodges, Foster, & Co., 1874.

Carpenter, Mary Wilson. *Health, Medicine, and Society in Victorian England.* Santa Barbara, CA: ABC CLIO, 2010.

Carpenter, Alfred. "Typhoid Fever." *Times,* November 13, 1874, 3.

———. "A Consideration of Some of the Fallacies Which are Based Upon a Narrow View of the Germ-Theory." *British Medical Journal* 994 (1880): 79–81.

———. *Some Points in the Physiological and Medical Aspects of Sewage Irrigation.* London: Hardwicke, 1870.

Casper, Stephen and Rick Welsh. "British Romantic Generalism in the Age of Specialism, 1870–1990." *Social History of Medicine* 1 (February 29, 2016): 154–74.

Cassal, Charles and B. A. Whitelegge. "Remarks on the Examination of Water for Sanitary Purposes." *Sanitary Record* 5 (April 15, 1884): 479–82.

Cassedy, James H. "Hygeia: A Mid-Victorian Dream of a City of Health." *Journal of the History of Medicine and Allied Sciences* 17, no. 2 (1962): 217–28.

"The Cause of the Illness of H.R.H. The Prince of Wales." *Lancet* 98 (December 16, 1871): 857.

Cayley, Henry. "A Note on the Value of Inoculation Against Enteric Fever." *British Medical Journal* (January 12, 1901): 84.

Cayley, William. *On Some Points in the Pathology and Treatment of Typhoid Fever.* London: J&A Churchill, 1880.

Chakrabarti, Pratik. *Bacteriology in British India.* Rochester: University of Rochester Press, 2012.

Charnley, Berris. "Arguing over Adulteration: The Success of the Analytical Sanitary Commission." *Endeavour* 32, no. 4 (November 30, 2008): 129–33.

Christison, Robert. "President's Address in the Public Health Department of the Social Science Association." *British Medical Journal* 147 (October 24, 1863): 437–45.

Cirillo, Vincent. *Bullets and Bacilli: The Spanish American War and Military Medicine.* New Brunswick, NJ: Rutgers University Press, 2004.

Cohen, William A., and Ryan Johnson. *Filth: Dirt, Disgust, and Modern Life.* Minneapolis: University of Minnesota Press, 2005.

Coleman, William. *Yellow Fever in the North: The Method of Early Epidemiology.* Madison: University of Wisconsin Press, 1987.

Collie, Alexander. "The Etiology of Enteric Fever." *British Medical Journal* 994 (January 17, 1880): 84–87.

Corbin, Alain. *The Foul and the Fragrant: Odor and the French Social Imagination.* Cambridge, MA: Harvard University Press, 1986.

Conan-Doyle, Arthur. "The War in South Africa." *British Medical Journal* 2062 (July 7, 1900): 49.

"Conference on National Water Supply, Sewerage and Health." *Journal of the Society of Arts* 28 (June 20, 1879): 662.

"The Convalescence of the Prince of Wales." *Illustrated London News*, January 20, 1872, 54.

Corfield, William Henry. "On the Alleged Spontaneous Production of the Poison of Enteric Fever." *Transactions of the Epidemiological Society of London* 3 (1876): 493–502.

———. *Disease and Defective House Sanitation.* London: H. K. Lewis, 1896.

———. *Dwelling Houses: Their Sanitary Construction and Arrangements.* London: H. K. Lewis, 1885.

———. *The Etiology of Typhoid Fever and its Prevention.* London: H. K. Lewis, 1902.

———. *Foul Air in Houses.* London: William Clowes & Sons, 1884.

———. *The Laws of Health.* London: Longmans, 1896.

———. "Londesborough Lodge." *Times*, January 22, 1872, 4.

———. "The Progress of Sanitary Science." *British Medical Journal* 669 (October 25, 1873): 480–81.

———. "The Source of Infection." *British Medical Journal* 659 (August 16, 1873): 207–8.

———. *The Treatment and Utilisation of Sewage.* London: Macmillan, 1887.

———. "Typhoid Fever in Marylebone." *The Times,* August 14, 1873, 7.

Cory, Robert. "On the Results of the Examination of Certain Samples of Water Purposely Polluted with Excrements from Fever Patients, and with Other Matters." In *Eleventh Annual Report of the Medical Officer of the Local Government Board, 1881.*

"Court Circular." *Times,* November 19, 1871, 7.

Crawford, Thomas. "Inaugural Address." *Transactions of the Epidemiological Society of London* 9 (1891): 1–22.

Creighton, Charles. "Note on Certain Unusual Coagulation Appearances Found in Mucus and other Abdominal Fluids." *Proceedings of the Royal Society of London* 25 (1876–77): 140–41.

———. *A History of Epidemics in Britain.* Vol. 2. Cambridge: Cambridge University Press, 1894.

Crook, Tom. "Danger in the Drains: Sewer Gas, Sewerage Systems and the Home, 1850–1900." In *Governing Risks in Modern Britain: Danger, Safety, and Accidents, c.1800–2000,* edited by Tom Crook and Mike Esbester, 105–26. London: Palgrave, 2016.

———. *Governing Systems: Modernity and the Making of Public Health in England, 1830–1910.* Oakland: University of California Press, 2016.

Cunningham, J. M. "The Sanitary Lessons of Indian Epidemics." *Transactions of the Epidemiological Society of London* 2 (1883): 102–18.

Curtin, Philip. *Disease and Empire: The Health of European Troops in the Conquest of Africa.* Cambridge: Cambridge University Press, 1998.

"The Dairy Reform Company and the Typhoid Outbreak in London." *British Medical Journal* 663 (September 13, 1873): 336.

"The Dairy Reform Company and the Epidemic of Typhoid Fever in London." *British Medical Journal* 663 (September 20, 1873): 358–61.

"Dairy Reform Company." *Milk Journal* 1 (1871): 6.

"The Dairy Reform Company" *Milk Journal* 3 (1871): 30.

Dale, George P., John W. M. Taylor, Stewart and Bury, William Peacock, J. H. Carroll, and Septimus Bland. "Londesborough Lodge." *Times,* December 11, 1871, 5.

Davidson, Randall T., and William Benham. *Life of Archibald Campbell Tait, Archbishop of Canterbury.* London: Macmillan, 1891.

Davey, Alexander G. "The Prevention of Enteric Fever." *British Medical Journal* 1082 (September 24, 1881): 509.

Davies, David S. "On an Outbreak of Milk-Borne Enteric Fever in Clifton." *Transactions of the Epidemiological Society of London* 17 (1898): 78–103.

———. "The Trials and Difficulties of a Health Officer." *British Medical Journal* 561 (September 30, 1871): 377–78.

Davies D. S., and I. Walker Hall. "A Discussion on the Etiology and Epidemiology of Typhoid (Enteric) Fever: Typhoid Carriers, with an Account of Two Institution Outbreaks Traced to the Same Carrier." *Proceedings of the Royal Society of Medicine* 1 (1908): 175–91.

Day, Carolyn A. *Consumptive Chic: A History of Beauty, Fashion, and Disease.* London: Bloomsbury, 2017.

Deb Roy, Rohan. *Malarial Subjects: Empire, Medicine, and Nonhumans in British India, 1820–1909.* Cambridge: Cambridge University Press, 2017.

"Detection of Adulteration of Milk." *British Medical Journal* 647 (May 24, 1873): 594.

DeRenzy, A. C. C. "The Sanitary State of the British Troops in Northern India." *Transactions of the Epidemiological Society of London* 2 (1883): 21–45.

Dilke, Charles. *On the Cost of the Crown.* London: G. Shield, 1871.

"Discussion on the Proper Sphere of State Medicine." *Proceedings of the Royal Society of Medicine* 32 (May 1939): 729–34.

Doll, Richard. "Proof of Causality: Deduction from Epidemiological Observation." *Perspectives in Biology and Medicine* 45 (Autumn 2002): 499–515.

Downs, James. *Empire's Laboratory: How Colonialism, War and Slavery Transformed Medicine. Cambridge, MA:* Harvard University Press, forthcoming.

"Dr. Klein On the Pathology of Small-pox and Typhoid Fever. " *Practitioner* 14 (1875): 10.

Dudley, Sheldon. "The Ecological Outlook on Epidemiology." *Proceedings of the Royal Society of Medicine* 30 (1936): 57–70.

Dunnill, M. S. *William Budd: Bristol's Most Famous Physician.* Bristol, UK: Redcliffe, 2006.

Dyke, T. J. "The Work of a Medical Officer of Health, and How to Do It." *British Medical Journal* 620 (November 16, 1872): 543–45.

"The Epidemic of Fever at Terling." *Builder* 26 (February 15, 1868): 106.

"Editorial" *Times,* August 27, 1873, 7.

"Editorial." *Times,* November 30, 1871, 9.

"Editorial." *Illustrated London News,* December 16, 1871, 570.

Englemann, Lukas, John Henderson, Christos Lynteris. *Plague and the City.* London: Routledge, 2018.

"Enteric Fever in the Tees Valley." *Dublin Journal of Medical Science* 97 (1894): 49–53.

"The Epidemiological Society." *Medical Times and Gazette* 2 (November 20, 1875): 580–81.

Eyler, John. *Sir Arthur Newsholme and State Medicine, 1885–1935*. Cambridge: Cambridge University Press, 1997.

———. "The Changing Assessments of John Snow's and William Farr's Cholera Studies." *Social and Preventive Medicine* 46 (2001): 225–32.

———. *Victorian Social Medicine: The Ideas and Methods of William Farr*. Baltimore: Johns Hopkins University Press, 1979.

Ewald, Paul. *Plague Time: How Stealth infections Cause Cancers, Heart Disease, and Other Deadly Ailments*. London: Free Press, 2000.

Ewart, Joseph. "Enteric Fever in India, with some Observations on its Probable Etiology in that Country." *Transactions of the Epidemiological Society of London* 4 (1880): 285–98.

———. *The Sanitary Condition and Discipline of Indian Jails*. London: Smith, Elder and Co., 1860.

Farr, William. "Report on the Cholera Epidemic of 1866 in England." *Supplement to the Twenty-Ninth Annual Report of the Registrar-General*. Parliamentary Papers. London: Eyre and Spottiswoode, 1868.

Fayrer, Joseph. "Inaugural Address." *Transactions of the Epidemiological Society of London* 4 (1880): 263–84.

———. *On the Climate and Fevers of India*. London: J&A Churchill, 1882.

Fee, Elizabeth and Roy Acheson. *A History of Education in Public Health: Health That Mocks the Doctors' Rules*. Oxford: Oxford University Press, 1991.

Fergus, Andrew. "Excremental Pollution as a Cause of Disease, with Hints to Remedial Measures." *Transactions of the National Association for the Promotion of Social Science* (1872): 450–58.

"The Fever at Terling." *Medical Times and Gazette* 36 (January 11, 1868): 36.

"The Fever at Terling." *Medical Times and Gazette* 36 (February 8, 1868): 152.

"The Fever at Terling." *Medical Times and Gazette* 36 (February 22, 1868): 209.

Finer, S. E. *The Life and Times of Sir Edwin Chadwick*. London: Methuen, 1952.

First Report of the Royal Sanitary Commission. London: Eyre and Spottiswoode, 1869.

Fisher, John R. "Professor Gamgee and the Farmers." *Veterinary History* 1 (1979–81): 47–63.

Foucault, Michel. *The Birth of the Clinic*. London: Routledge, 1989.

Forth, Aidan. *Barbed-Wire Imperialism: Britain's Empire of Camps, 1876–1903*. Oakland: University of California Press, 2017.

Fos, Peter J. *Epidemiology Foundations: The Science of Public Health*. San Francisco, CA: John Wiley, 2011.

Fox, Cornelius B. "Is Enteric Fever Ever Spontaneously Generated." *British Medical Journal* 795 (March 25, 1876): 374–77.

Frankel, Oz. *States of Inquiry: Social Investigations and Print Culture in Nineteenth Century Britain and the United States*. Baltimore: Johns Hopkins University Press, 2006.

Frankland, Edward. *Experimental Researches in Pure, Applied, and Physical Chemistry.* London: John Van Voorst, 1877.

Frankland, Percy F. "The Behaviour of the Typhoid Bacillus and of the Bacillus Coli Commune in Potable Waters." *Proceedings of the Royal Society of London* 56 (1894): 315–556.

Gamgee, John. *The Cattle Plague and Diseased Meat, in Their Relation with the Public Health.* London: T. Richards, 1857.

———. "Country Versus Town Milk." *Medical Times and Gazette* 1 (1871): 38–39, 67–68.

Garcia, M. "Typhoid Fever in Nineteenth-Century Colombia: Between Medical Geography and Bacteriology." *Medical History* 58 (2014): 27–45.

"General Memorandum of the Proceedings Which are Advisable in Places Attacked or Threatened by Epidemic Disease." *Daily News,* July 24, 1865, 6.

"General French's Mounted Infantry Crossing The Vaal at Viljoen's Drift." *Sphere,* September 15, 1900, 328.

Gilbert, Pamela. *Cholera and Nation: Doctoring the Social Body in Victorian England.* Albany: State University of New York Press, 2008.

Goldman, Lawrence. *Science, Reform, and Politics in Victorian Britain: The Social Science Association.* Cambridge: Cambridge University Press, 2002.

Goodall, E. W. "Introduction to a Discussion on the Infectivity of Enteric Fever," *Transactions of the Epidemiological Society of London* 19 (April 20, 1900): 164–98.

———. "William Budd: A Forgotten Epidemiologist." *Proceedings of the Royal Society of Medicine* 25, no. 3 (1932): 277–94.

Gordon, C. A. "On Certain Views Regarding Fever in India." *Transactions of the Epidemiological Society of London* 4 (1880): 313–37.

———. "Enteric Fever in India." *British Medical Journal* 1366 (March 5, 1887): 540.

———. "Enteric or Typhoid Fever in India." *Medical Times and Gazette* 2 (July 24, 1880): 97–98.

———. "Prize For Essay on Fevers." *Medical Times and Gazette* 2 (December 13, 1879): 673.

———. *Report on Typhoid or Enteric Fever in Relation to British Troops in the Madras Command.* Madras: Government Press, 1878.

Gradmann, Christoph. "Robert Koch and the Invention of the Carrier State: Tropical Medicine, Veterinary Infections and Epidemiology around 1900." *Studies in History and Philosophy of Biological and Biomedical Science* 41 (2010): 232-40.

Greenhow, E. H. "On the Different Prevalences of Certain Diseases in Different Districts of England and Wales. In *Papers Relating to the Sanitary State of the People of England. Report to the General Board of Health.* Parliamentary Papers. London: Eyre and Spottiswoode, 1858.

Greenwood, Major. "President's Address: The General Register Office." *Proceedings of the Royal Society of Medicine* 25 (November 1931): 1–6.

Gresswell, D. A. "Report on the Sanitary Condition of Cradley, and on Enteric Fever There." In *Annual Report of the Medical Officer of the Local Government Board*. Parliamentary Papers. London: Eyre and Spottiswoode, 1889.

Gull, William W. "An Address on the Collective Investigation of Disease." *British Medical Journal* 1152 (January 27, 1883): 141–44.

———. "A Lecture on Typhoid Fever, Delivered at Guy's Hospital." *Lancet* 2548 (1872): 896–98.

———. "On Typhoid Fever." *The Retrospect of Medicine and Surgery* 66 (January 1873): 17.

Hall, Sherwin A. "John Gamgee and the Edinburgh New Veterinary College." *Veterinary Record* 87 (1965): 1237–41.

Halliday, Steven. *The Great Filth: Disease, Death, and the Victorian City*. Stroud, UK: History Press, 2011.

Haffkine, W. M. "Discussion on Preventive Inoculation." *British Medical Journal* 2009 (July 1, 1899): 11–15.

Hamer, William H. "A Bird's Eye View of Typhoid Fever in London During the last Seventy Years." *Public Health* 35 (October 1921): 57–64.

———. "The Crux of Epidemiology." *Proceedings of the Royal Society of Medicine* 10 (August 1931): 1425–40.

Hamilton, J. B. "Enteric Fever in Tropical and Sub-Tropical Climates." *South African Medical Journal* (August 1894): 95.

———. "Enteric Fever in India." *British Medical Journal* 1553 (October 4, 1890): 787–89.

Hamlin, Christopher. "'Cholera Forcing'; The Myth of the Good Epidemic and the Coming of Water." *American Journal of Public Health* 99 (2009): 1946–54.

———. *More Than Hot: A Short History of Fever*. Baltimore: Johns Hopkins University Press, 2014.

——— "Muddling in Bumbledom: On the Enormity of Large Sanitary Improvements in Four British Towns, 1855–1885." *Victorian Studies* 32, no. 1 (Autumn 1988): 55–83.

——— "Politics and Germ Theories in Victorian Britain: The Metropolitan Water Commissions of 1867–9 and 1892–3." In *Government and Expertise: Specialists, Administrators and Professionals, 1860–1919*, edited by Roy MacLeod, 111–23. Cambridge: Cambridge University Press, 1988.

———. *Public Health and Social Justice in the Age of Chadwick*. Cambridge: Cambridge University Press, 1998.

———. "Public Sphere to Public Health: The Transformation of 'Nuisance.'" In *Medicine, Health, and the Public Sphere in Britain, 1600–2000*, edited by Steve Sturdy, 189–204. Abingdon, UK: Routledge, 2002.

———. "Sir John Simon, 1816–1904." Oxford Dictionary of National Biography. Oxford: Oxford University Press, 2004.

————. "State Medicine in Great Britain." in *The History of Public Health and the Modern State*, edited by Dorothy Porter. Amsterdam: Rodopi, 1994.

Hanley, James G. *Healthy Boundaries: Property, Law, and Public Health in England and Wales, 1815–1872*. Rochester, NY: University of Rochester Press, 2016.

————. "Parliament, Physicians, and Nuisances: The Demedicalization of Nuisance Law, 1831–1855." *Bulletin of the History of Medicine* 80, no. 4 (2006): 702–32.

Hardy, Anne. "Cholera, Quarantine, and the English Preventive System." *Medical History* 37 (1993): 250–69.

————. *Epidemic Streets: Infectious Disease and the Rise of Preventive Medicine, 1856–1900*. Oxford: Clarendon, 1993.

————. *Health and Medicine in Britain Since 1860*. Basingstoke, UK: Palgrave, 2001.

————. "On the Cusp: Epidemiology and Bacteriology at the Local Government Board, 1890–1905." *Medical History* 42 (1998): 328–46.

————. "Methods of Outbreak Investigation in the 'Era of Bacteriology,' 188–920." In *A History of Epidemiologic Methods and Concepts*, edited by A. Morabia, 199–206. Berlin: Birkhauser Verlag, 2004.

————. "Public Health and the Expert: The London Medical Officers of Health, 1856–1900." In *Government and Expertise: Specialists, Administrators, and Professionals, 1860–1919*, edited by R. M. MacLeod, 128–42. Cambridge: Cambridge University Press, 1988.

————. *Salmonella Infections, Networks of Knowledge, and Public Health in Britain, 1880–1975*. Oxford: Oxford University Press, 2015.

————. "Straight Back to Barbarism: Antityphoid Inoculation and the Great War, 1914." *Bulletin of the History of Medicine* 74 (2000): 265–90.

Harling, Philip. "The Powers of the Victorian State." In *Liberty and Authority in Victorian Britain*, edited by Peter Mandler, 25–50. Oxford: Oxford University Press, 2006.

Harrison, *Public Health in British India: Anglo-Indian Preventive Medicine*. Cambridge: Cambridge University Press, 1994.

————. "A Question of Locality: The Identity of Cholera in British India, 1860–1890." In *Warm Climates and Western Medicine: the Emergence of Tropical Medicine, 1500-1900*, edited by David Arnold, 133–59. Amsterdam: Rodolpi, 1996.

————. "Tropical Medicine in Nineteenth Century India." *British Journal for the History of Science* 25 (1992): 299–318.

Hart, Ernest. "The Dairy Reform Company." *British Medical Journal* 663 (September 13, 1873): 337–39.

————. "The Decadence of the Medical Department of the Local Government Board." *British Medical Journal* 928 (October 12, 1878): 565.

————. "Dr. Klein's Researches on the Typhoid Germ." *London Medical Record*, November 11, 1874, 720.

————. "The Influence of Milk in Spreading Zymotic Disease." *Transactions of the Seventh Session of the International Medical Congress* (1881): 491–544.

————. "The Outbreak of Typhoid Fever from the Distribution of Infected Milk." *British Medical Journal* 659 (August 16, 1873): 206–7.

————. "On the Bacillus of Typhoid Fever." *British Medical Journal* 1091 (November 26, 1881): 877.

————. "Public Health Legislation and the Needs of India." *British Medical Journal* 1805 (August 3, 1895): 287–91.

————. "The Recent Epidemic of Enteric Fever in the Caterham Valley." *British Medical Journal* 957 (May 3, 1879): 669–70.

————. *A Report on the Influence of Milk in Spreading Zymotic Disease.* London: Smith, Elder & Co., 1897.

————. "Waterborne Typhoid: A Historic Summary of Local Outbreaks in Great Britain and Ireland." *British Medical Journal* 1800 (June 29, 1895): 1446–47.

————. "Typhoid Fever." *British Medical Journal* 724 (November 14, 1874): 621.

Haviland, Alfred. "The Geographical Distribution of Typhoid Fever in England and Wales." *British Medical Journal* 580 (February 10, 1872): 148–49.

————. "The Geographical Distribution of Typhoid Fever in England and Wales." *British Medical Journal* 583 (March 2, 1872): 232–34.

————. "Special Report on the Epidemic at Terling." *Medical Times and Gazette* (January 11, 1868): 40–41.

Heggie, Vanessa. "Lies, Damn Lies, and Manchester's Recruiting Statistics: Degeneration as an 'Urban Legend' in Victorian and Edwardian Britain." *Journal of the History of Medicine and Allied Sciences* 63, no. 2 (April 2008): 178–216.

Hobsbawm, Eric. "Language, Culture, and National Identity." *Social Research* 63, no. 4 (1996): 1065–80.

Hope, William. "The Dairy Reform Company." *British Medical Journal* 663 (September 13, 1873): 337–39.

Homans, Margaret. *Royal Representations: Queen Victoria and British Culture, 1837–1876.* Chicago: University of Chicago Press, 1998.

Houston, A. C. "A Discussion on Enteric Fever in its Public Health Aspects." *British Medical Journal* 2120 (August 17, 1901): 389–400.

————. "Enteric Fever in its Public Health Aspects." *Lancet* 158 (August 17, 1901): 468v69.

————. "Report on the Chemical and Bacteriological Examination of Tunbridge Wells Deep Well Water." In *Annual Report of the Medical Officer of the Local Government Board for 1902–1903.* Parliamentary Papers. London: Spottiswoode, 1904.

"The Hospital Scandals in South Africa." *Sphere*, September 8, 1900, 287.

Howell, Joel. *Technology in the Hospital.* Baltimore: Johns Hopkins University Press, 1995.

Hudson, Robert. "The Germ-Theory of Enteric Fever." *British Medical Journal* 859 (June 16, 1877): 740–41.

———. "Facts Illustrative of the Spread of Enteric Fever and Diarrhoea, by the Agency of Polluted Drinking-Water." *British Medical Journal* 994 (January 17, 1880): 88–89.

"Illness of the Prince of Wales." *Illustrated London News*, December 16, 1871, 597.

"The Illness of H.R.H. The Prince of Wales." *British Medical Journal* 572 (December 16, 1871): 699.

"The Illness of H.R.H. The Prince of Wales." *Lancet* 2519 (December 9, 1871): 671–73.

Jackson, Lee. *Dirty Old London: The Victorian Fight Against Filth.* New Haven, CT: Yale University Press, 2014.

Jalland, Pat. *Death in the Victorian Family.* Oxford: Oxford University Press, 1996.

———. "Victorian Death and its Decline, 1850–1918." In *Death in England: An Illustrated History,* edited by Peter C. Jupp and Claire Gittings, 230–55. Manchester: Manchester University Press, 1999.

Jenner, William. "An Address on the Treatment of Typhoid Fever." *Lancet* 2933 (November 15, 1879): 715–20.

Jones, Susan. *Death in a Small Package: A Short History of Anthrax.* Baltimore: Johns Hopkins University Press, 2010.

Joyce, Patrick. *The Rule of Freedom: Liberalism and the Modern City.* London: Verso, 2003.

Kearns, Gerry. "Biology, Class, and the Urban Penalty." In *Urbanising Britain: Essays on Class and the Community in the Nineteenth Century,* edited by Gerry Kearns and Charles W. J. Withers, 12–31. Cambridge: Cambridge University Press, 1991.

———. "Cholera, Nuisances, and Environmental Management in Islington, 1830–1855." In *Living and Dying in London,* edited by William Bynum and Roy Porter, 94–125. *Medical History,* Supplement, 11. London: Wellcome Institute for the History of Medicine, 1991.

Kennedy, Dane. *The Magic Mountains: Hill Stations and the British Raj.* Berkeley: University of California Press, 1996.

Kerr, Norman. "Enteric Fever, Diarrhoea, Diphtheria, and Scarlatina, Originating from Drinking-Water." *British Medical Journal* 994 (January 17, 1880): 88.

"Killed in the Service of the State." *British Medical Journal* 672 (November 15, 1873): 578.

Klein, Edward. "On the Abilities of Certain Pathogenic Microbes to Maintain their Existence in Water." In *Annual Report of the Medical Officer of the Local Government Board for 1894–95.* Parliamentary Papers. London: Eyre and Spottiswoode, 1896.

———. "Further Report on the Etiology of Typhoid Fever." In *Annual Report of the Medical Officer of the Local Government Board for 1893–94*. Parliamentary Papers. London: Eyre and Spottiswoode, 1894.

———. "Further Observations on the Influence of Perchloride of Mercury on Pathogenic Organisms Growing in Nutritive Gelatine." In *Annual Report of the Medical Officer of the Local Government Board*. Parliamentary Papers. London: Eyre and Spottiswoode, 1886.

———. *Microorganisms and Disease*. London: Clay and Sons, 1886.

———. "On the Minute Pathology of Enteric Fever: Preliminary Notice." *British Medical Journal* 727 (5 December 1874): 699–700.

———. "Report of Bacteriological Analysis of the Chichester Public Water Supply." In *Annual Report of the Medical Officer of the Local Government Board for 1896–97*. Parliamentary Papers. London: Spottiswoode, 1897.

———. "Report on the Fate of Pathogenic and other Infective Microbes in the Dead Animal Body." In *Annual Report of the Medical Officer of the Local Government Board for 1898–99*. Parliamentary Papers. London: Spottiswoode, 1899.

———. "Report on the Influence of Heat upon Microorganisms." In *Annual Report of the Medical Officer of the Local Government Board*. Parliamentary Papers. London: Eyre and Spottiswoode, 1889.

———. "Report on the Intimate Anatomical Changes in Enteric or Typhoid Fever." In *Annual Report of the Medical Officer of the Local Government Board*. Parliamentary Papers. London: Eyre and Spottiswoode, 1875.

———. "Report on the So-Called Enteric or Typhoid Fever of the Pig." In *Annual Report of the Medical Officer of the Local Government Board for 1875*. Parliamentary Papers. London: Eyre and Spottiswoode, 1876.

———. "Research on the Smallpox of Sheep." *Proceedings of the Royal Society of London* 22 (1874): 388–91.

———. "Zur Kenntniss der feineren Pathologie des Abdominaltyphus," *Centralblatt für die medicinischen Wissenschaften* 692 (December 5, 1874): 706.

Koch, Robert. "An Address on Cholera and its Bacillus." *British Medical Journal* 1235 (August 30, 1884): 40307.

Koch, Tom. *Disease Maps: Epidemics on the Ground*. Chicago: University of Chicago Press, 2011.

Kudlick, Catherine J. *Cholera in Post-Revolutionary Paris*. Berkeley: University of California Press, 1996.

La Berge, Ann F. "Medical Statistics at the Paris School: What was at Stake?" In *Body Counts: Medical Quantification in Historical and Sociological Perspective*, edited by Gerard Jorland, Annick Opinel, and George Weisz, 89–109. Montreal: McGill-Queen's University Press, 2005.

Lambert, Royston. *Sir John Simon and English Social Administration, 1816–1904*. London: MacGibbon and Fee, 1963.

"The Late Epidemic of Enteric Fever at Caterham and Redhill." *Medical Times and Gazette* (May 10, 1879): 507.

Lawrence, Christopher. "Incommunicable Knowledge: Science, Technology and the Clinical Art in Britain, 1850–1914." *Journal of Contemporary History* 20, no. 4 (October 1985): 503–20.

Laxton, Paul. "Fighting for Public Health: Dr. Duncan and His Adversaries, 1847–1863." In *Body and City: Histories of Urban Public Health,* edited by Sally Sheard and Helen Power, 59–88. Aldershot, UK: Ashgate, 2000.

Leavitt, Judith Walzer. *Typhoid Mary: Captive to the Public's Health.* Boston: Beacon, 1996.

Letheby, Henry. "Cows in Cow-Houses, and Their Milk." *British Medical Journal* 59 (February 15, 1862): 185.

———. *Report to the Honorable Commissioners of Sewers of the City of London on Sewage and Sewer Gases, and on the Ventilation of Sewers.* London: M. Lownds, 1858.

Lilienfeld, David E. "Celebration: William Farr—An Appreciation on the 200th Anniversary of His Birth." *International Journal of Epidemiology* 36 (October 2007): 985–87.

———. "The Greening of Epidemiology: Sanitary Physicians and the London Epidemiological Society (1830–1870)." *Bulletin of the History of Medicine* 52 (1978): 503–28.

Linton, Derek S. "Was Typhoid Inoculation Safe and Effective during World War I? Debates within German Military Medicine." *Journal of the History of Medicine and Allied Sciences* 55 (2000): 101–33.

"On a Localised Outbreak of Typhoid Fever in Islington during the Months of July and August, 1870." *Lancet* 2474 (January 28, 1871): 120–21.

Low, Bruce R. "The Origin of Enteric Fever in Isolated Rural Districts." *British Medical Journal* 1036 (November 6, 1880): 733–36.

Lowy, Ilana. "From Guinea Pigs to Man: The Development of Haffkine's Anti-cholera Vaccine." *Journal of the History of Medicine and Allied Sciences* 47 (1992): 270–309.

Luckin, Bill. *Death and Survival in Urban Britain: Disease, Pollution, and Environment, 1800–1950.* London: I. B. Tauris, 2015.

———. "The Final Catastrophe- Cholera in London, 1866." *Medical History* 21 (1977): 32–42.

———. "Revisiting the Idea of Degeneration in Urban Britain, 1830–1900." *Urban History* 33, no. 2 (2006): 234–52.

MacDonagh, Oliver. "The Nineteenth Century Revolution in Government: A Reappraisal." *Historical Journal* 1 (1958): 52–67.

Maclean, W. C. "On the Prevalence of Enteric Fever among Young Soldiers in India: its Causes, and the Most Rational Means of Prevention." *Transactions of the Seventh Session of the International Medical Congress* (1881): 528–33.

MacLeod, Roy M. "The Anatomy of State Medicine: Concept and Application." In *Medicine and Science in the 1860s,* edited by F. N. L. Poynter, 199–277. London, Wellcome Institute for the History of Medicine, 1968.

———. *Government and Expertise: Specialists, Administrators, and Professionals, 1860–1919.* Cambridge: Cambridge University Press, 2003.

———. "The Frustration of State Medicine, 1880-1899." *Medical History* 11 (1967): 15–40.

McKay, Richard. *Patient Zero and the Making of the AIDS Epidemic.* Chicago: University of Chicago Press, 2017.

Mukharji, Projit Bihari. "Cat and Mouse: Animal Technologies, Trans-imperial Networks and Public Health from Below, British India, c. 1907–1918." *Social History of Medicine* 31 (August 2018): 510–32.

MacNamara, Nottidge Charles. *A History of Asiatic Cholera.* London: Macmillan, 1876.

MacLagan, T. J. *Fever: A Clinical Study.* London: J&A Churchill, 1888.

MacNalty, Arthur Salusbury. *The History of State Medicine in England.* London: Royal Institute of Public Health and Hygiene, 1947.

Maconochie, D. "The Late Typhoid Epidemic." *Times,* August 26, 1873, 8.

———. "Dr. Murchison and the Dairy Reform Company." *Times,* September 3, 1873, 3.

Manson, Patrick. *Tropical Diseases: A Manual of Diseases of Warm Climates.* London: Cassell and Company, 1898.

Marks, Harry. "Until the Sun of Science . . . the True Apollo of Medicine Has Risen: Collective Investigation in Britain and America, 1880–1910." *Medical History* 50, no. 2 (April 2006): 147–66.

Martin, Sidney. "Preliminary Report on the Growth of the Typhoid Bacillus in Soil." In *Annual Report of the Medical Officer of the Local Government Board for 1896–97.* Parliamentary Papers. London: Spottiswoode, 1897.

———. "The Growth of the Typhoid Bacillus in Soil." In *Annual Report of the Medical Officer of the Local Government Board for 1898–99.* Parliamentary Papers. London: Spottiswoode, 1899.

———. "Further Report on the Growth of the Typhoid Bacillus in Soil." In *Annual Report of the Medical Officer of the Local Government Board for 1899–1900.* Parliamentary Papers. London: Spottiswoode, 1900.

Matthews, J. Rosser. "Major Greenwood versus Almroth Wright: Contrasting Visions of 'Scientific' Medicine in Edwardian Britain." *Bulletin of the History of Medicine* 69, no. 1 (1995): 30–43.

Maulitz Russell. *Morbid Appearances: The Anatomy of Pathology in the Early Nineteenth Century.* Cambridge: Cambridge University Press, 1987.

Mayo, Charles. "Typhoid Fever." *Times,* December 6, 1871, 3.

McBridge, John. "Report on Cases of Contagion of the Foot-and-Mouth Exanthema to the Human Subject." *British Medical Journal* 463 (November 13, 1869): 536–37.

McLeod, Kari. "Our Sense of Snow: The Myth of John Snow in Medical Geography." *Social Science and Medicine* 50 (2000): 923–35.

McNeill, J. "A Contribution to the Etiology of Typhoid Fever." *British Medical Journal* 1036 (November 6, 1880): 739–40.

"Medical Annotations." *Lancet* 2280 (May 11, 1867): 575–76.

"Medical Aspects of the War." *British Medical Journal* 2062 (July 7, 1900): 51.

Meli, Domenico Bertoloni. *Visualizing Disease: The Art and History of Pathological Illustration* Chicago: University of Chicago Press, 2017.

Mendelsohn, J. A. "A Bacteriological Approach to Controlling Typhoid." In *Health, Disease, and Society in Europe, 1800–1930,* edited by Deborah Brunton, 185–88. Manchester: Manchester University Press, 2004.

———. "From Eradication to Equilibrium: How Epidemics Became Complex after World War I." In *Greater than the Parts: Holism in Biomedicine, 1920–1950,* edited by C. Lawrence and George Weisz, 303–31. Oxford: Oxford University Press, 1998.

Mercer, Alex. *Infections, Chronic Disease, and the Epidemiological Transition: A New Perspective.* Rochester, NY: University of Rochester Press, 2014.

Metropolitan Board of Works. *Return Showing the Number of Persons Employed in the Board's Sewers and the Number Attacked by Fever.* Judd & Co., 1872.

Mooney, Graham. *Intrusive Interventions: Public Health, Domestic Space, and Infectious Disease Surveillance in England, 1840–1914.* Rochester, NY: University of Rochester Press, 2015.

———. "Professionalisation in Public Health and the Measurement of Sanitary Progress in Nineteenth Century England and Wales." *Social History of Medicine* 10 (1997): 53–78.

Mooney, Graham, and Andrea Tanner. "Infant Mortality, a Spatial Problem: Notting Dale Special Area in George Newman's London." In *Infant Mortality: A Continuing Social Problem,* edited by Eilidh Garrett, Chris Galley, Nicola Shelton, and Robert Woods, 169–90. Aldershot, UK: Ashgate, 2007.

Morabia, Alfredo. *Enigmas of Health and Disease: How Epidemiology Helps Unravel Scientific Mysteries.* New York: Columbia University Press, 2014.

———. "Epidemiology and Bacteriology in 1900: Who is the Handmaid of Whom? *Journal of Epidemiology and Community Health* 52 (1998): 617–18.

Morabia, Alfredo, and Anne Hardy. "The Pioneering Use of a Questionnaire to Investigate a Food-Borne Disease Outbreak in Early 20th-Century Britain." *Journal of Epidemiology and Community Health* 59, no. 2 (February 2005): 94–99.

Morehead, Charles. *Clinical Researches on Disease in India.* London: Longman, Brown, Green, and Longmans, 1856.

Morgan, Kenneth O. "The Boer War and the Media (1899–1902)." *Twentieth Century British History* 12 (2002): 1–16.

Mortimer, P. P. "Mr. N. the Milker, and Dr. Koch's Concept of the Healthy Carrier." *Lancet* 353 (April 17, 1999): 1354–56.

Morris, Frankie. "The Illustrated Press and the Republican Crisis of 1871–72." *Victorian Periodicals Review* 25, no. 3 (Fall 1992): 114–26.

"Mr. Radcliffe's Report on the London Cholera Epidemic." *Lancet* 2305 (November 2, 1867): 558–59.

Mullin, Robert Bruce. "Science, Miracles, and the Prayer-Gauge Debate." In *When Science & Christianity Meet,* edited by David Lindberg and Ronald Numbers, 203–24. Chicago: University of Chicago Press, 2003.

Murchison, Charles. "The Dairy Reform Company." *Times*, August 30, 1873, 7.

———. "The Germ-Theory of Disease." *British Medical Journal* 749 (May 8, 1875): 621–27.

———. *A Treatise on the Continued Fevers of Great Britain.* London; Parker, Son, and Bourn, 1862.

———. *A Treatise on the Continued Fevers of Great Britain.* London: Spottiswoode, 1873.

———. *A Treatise on the Continued Fevers of Great Britain.* London: Spottiswoode, 1884.

———. "Typhoid Fever and the Public Health." *Times,* September 2, 1873, 5.

"The Murchison Address and Testimonial." *British Medical Journal* 695 (April 25, 1874): 555.

Murphy, Harold L. *Report on a Public Local Inquiry into an Outbreak of Typhoid Fever at Croydon.* London: His Majesty's Stationery Office, 1938.

Murphy, Shirley F. "On the Study of Epidemiology." *Transactions of the Epidemiological Society of London* 14 (1895): 1–24.

———. "The Etiology of Enteric Fever." *British Medical Journal* 955 (April 19, 1879): 581–83.

Nash, Linda. *Inescapable Ecologies: A History of Environment, Disease, and Knowledge.* Berkeley: University of California Press, 2004.

Newsholme, Arthur. "Enteric Fever in the Tees Valley." *Public Health* 6 (1894): 144–47.

———. *The Last Thirty Years in Public Health.* London: George Allen & Unwin, 1936.

Newsom Kerr, Matthew. *Contagion, Isolation, and Biopower in Victorian London.* Cham, Switzerland: Palgrave Macmillan, 2018.

Nolte, Karen. "Protestant Nursing Care in Germany in the 19th Century." In *Routledge Handbook on the Global History of Nursing,* edited by Patricia D'Antonio and Julie Fairman, 167–83. Oxon, UK: Routledge, 2013.

"Notes." *Sanitary Record* 20 (October 15, 1897): 407.

Notter, J. Lane. "The Influence of Soil as a Factor in the Production of Disease, Especially in Hot Climates." *Transactions of the Epidemiological Society of London* 14 (1895): 96–112.

———. "International Sanitary Conferences of the Victorian Era." *Transactions of the Epidemiological Society of London 17* (1898): 1–14.

"Obituary for Almroth Edward Wright." *Biographical Memoirs of Fellows of the Royal Society* 17 (November 30, 1948): 297–314.

"Obituary of Dr. F. W. Barry." *Lancet* 150 (October 16, 1897): 1016–17.

"Obituary for Edward Ballard." *British Medical Journal* 1883 (January 30, 1897): 281–82.

"Obituary for John Simon." *Transactions of the Epidemiological Society of London* 23 (1904): 253–58.

"Obituary for Michael Waistell Taylor." *British Medical Journal* 1667 (December 10, 1892): 1315.

"Obituary for Robert Cory." *St. Thomas's Hospital Reports.* London: J.&A Churchill, 1902.

"Obituary for Thomas Godart." *British Medical Journal* (January 28, 1888): 220.

"Obituary for William Henry Corfield." *Lancet* 162 (September 12, 1903): 778–81.

"Obituary for William Henry Corfield." *Transactions of the Epidemiological Society of London* 22 (1903): 160–63.

"Obituary for William Miller." *Lancet* 96 (October 8, 1870): 523.

"Obituary for William Withey Gull." *Guy's Hospital Reports* 47 (1890): xxv–xliii.

Orland, Barbara. "Enlightened Milk: Reshaping a Bodily Substance into a Chemical Object." In *Materials and Expertise in Early Modern Europe: Between Market and Laboratory*, edited by Ursula Klein and Emma C. Spray, 163–98. Chicago and London: University of Chicago Press, 2010.

Oshinsky, David. *Polio: An American Story.* Oxford: Oxford University Press, 2005.

Otter, Chris. "The Vital City: Public Analysis, Dairies and Slaughterhouses in Nineteenth-Century Britain." *Cultural Geographies* 13 (2006): 517–37.

"The Outbreak of Typhoid Fever in London." *British Medical Journal* 660 (August 23, 1873): 229–30.

Packard, Randall M. *White Plague, Black Labor: Tuberculosis and the Political Economy of Health and Disease in South Africa.* Berkeley: University of California Press, 1989.

Parascandola, Mark. "Epidemiology in Transition: Tobacco and Lung Cancer in the 1950s." In *Body Counts: Medical Quantification in Historical and Sociological Perspective*, edited by Gerard Jorland, Annick Opinel, and George Weisz, 226–48. Montreal: McGill-Queen's University Press, 2005.

Parkes, E. A. *A Manual of Practical Hygiene.* London: J&A Churchill, 1873.

———. "Report on the Outbreak of Cholera in and about Southampton in September and October 1865." In *Annual Report of the Medical Officer of the Privy Council for 1865.* Parliamentary Papers. London: Eyre and William Spottiswoode, 1866.

Parkes, Louis. "Reviews of Books." *Journal of the Sanitary Institute of Great Britain* 16 (1896): 143–52.

Parodi, A., D. Neasham, and P. Vineis. "Environment, Population, and Biology: A Short History of Modern Epidemiology." *Perspectives in Biology and Medicine* 49, no. 3 (Summer 2006): 357–68.

Parsons, H. Franklin. "On the Comparative Mortality of English Districts." *Transactions of the Epidemiological Society of London* 19 (1900): 1–24.

Pelling, Margaret. *Cholera, Fever, and English Medicine, 1825–1865.* Oxford: Oxford University Press, 1978.

Penner, Barbara. "The Prince's Water Closet: Sewer Gas and the City." *Journal of Architecture* 19, no. 2 (2014): 249–71.

Pettenkofer, Max von. "Boden and Grundwasser in ihren Beziehungen zu Cholera und Typhus." *Zeitschrift fur Biologie* 2 (1869): 171–310.

Pickles, William Norman. *Epidemiology in Country Practice.* Bristol, UK: John Wright and Sons, 1939.

Pickstone, John. *Ways of Knowing: A New History of Science, Technology, and Medicine.* Manchester: Manchester University Press, 2000.

———. "Dearth, Dirt and Fever Epidemics: Rewriting the History of British 'Public Health', 1780–1850." In *Epidemics and Ideas: Essays on the Historical Perception of Pestilence,* edited by Terence Ranger and Paul Slack, 125–48. Cambridge: Cambridge University Press, 1992.

Pitzer Virginia, James Meiring, Frederick Martineau, Conall Watson, Gagandeep Kang, Buddah Basnyat, Stephen Baker. "The Invisible Burden: Diagnosing and Combatting Typhoid Fever in Asia and Africa." *Clinical Infectious Diseases* 69 (November 2019): 395–401.

Playfair, Lyon. *Subjects of Social Welfare: Public Health.* London: Cassell & Company, 1889.

Plunkett, Harriette. *Women, Plumbers, and Doctors, or Household Sanitation.* New York: D. Appleton and Co., 1885.

Poore, G. Vivian. "Milk and its Relation to Health and Disease." *Clinical Journal* 19 (January 8, 1908): 177–83.

Poovey, Mary. *Making a Social Body: British Cultural Formation, 1830–1864.* Chicago: University of Chicago Press, 1995.

Porter, Bernard. *Critics of Empire: British Radicals and the Imperial Challenge.* London: Macmillan, 1968.

Porter, Dorothy. *Health, Civilization, and the State: A History of Public Health From Ancient to Modern Times.* London: Routledge, 1999.

Porter, Roy. *Bodies Politic: Disease, Death, and Doctors in Britain, 1650–1900.* London: Reaktion, 2001.

———. *The Greatest Benefit to Mankind: A Medical History of Humanity.* New York: HarperCollins, 1997.

Porter, Theodore. *The Rise of Statistical Thinking*. Princeton, NJ: Princeton University Press, 1988.

Power, William Henry. "Obituary Notice for Edward Ballard." *Proceedings of the Royal Society of London* 62 (1898): iii–v.

———. "Report to the Local Government Board on an Epidemic of Enteric Fever Occurring at Eagley," In *Annual Report of the Medical Officer of the Local Government Board for 1875*. Parliamentary Papers. London: Eyre and Spottiswoode, 1876.

Prest, John M. *Liberty and Locality: Parliament, Permissive Legislation, and Ratepayers' Democracies in the Nineteenth Century*. Oxford: Clarendon, 1990.

Price, Kim. *Medical Negligence in Victorian Britain: The Crisis of Care Under the English Poor Law, c.1834–1900*. London: Bloomsbury, 2015.

"The Prince of Wales." *John Bull*, December 30, 1871, 908.

"The Prince of Wales." *John Bull*, December 23, 1871, 881.

"The Prince of Wales." *Lancet* 98 (December 2, 1871): 790.

"The Prince of Wales." *Lancet* 98 (December 9, 1871): 824.

"The Prince of Wales' Physicians." *Illustrated London News*, December 16, 1871, 597.

"The Prince of Wales." *Illustrated London News*, December 16, 1871, 567.

"The Prince's Physicians." *Lancet* 98 (December 23, 1871): 893–94.

Pringle, Robert. "Enteric Fever in India: Its Increase, Causes, Remedies, and Probable Consequences." *Transactions of the Epidemiological Society of London* 9 (1891): 111–32.

"Proceedings of the Incorporated Society of Medical Officers of Health." *Public Health* 6 (1894): 130–36.

"The Progress of Cholera in Egypt." *Era* 1400 (July 23, 1865): 9.

"The Progress of H.R.H. The Prince of Wales." *Lancet* 98 (December 16, 1871): 857.

"Public Companies and the Public Health." *Lancet* 92 (August 1, 1868): 150–51.

Radcliffe, John Netten. "Report on the Sources and Development of the Present Diffusion of Cholera in Europe." In *Annual Report of the Medical Officer of the Privy Council for 1865*. Parliamentary Papers. London: George Eyre and William Spottiswoode, 1866.

———. "On the Outbreak of Cholera at Theydon Bois Essex in 1865, with Special Reference to the Propagation of Cholera by Water as a Medium." *Transactions of the Epidemiological Society of London* 3 (1869): 85–98.

———. "Preliminary Report on the Present Prevalence of Enteric Fever in Marylebone and Adjoining Metropolitan Districts." In *Annual Report of the Medical Officer of the Local Government Board for 1873*. Parliamentary Papers. London: George Eyre and William Spottiswoode, 1874.

———. "Report on the Recent Epidemic of Cholera, 1865–1866." *Transactions of the Epidemiological Society of London* 3 (1869): 232–45.

————. "Report on Cholera in London, and Especially in the Eastern Districts." In *Annual Report of the Medical Officer of the Privy Council for 1866–7.* Parliamentary Papers. London: Eyre and Spottiswoode, 1867.

————. "On the Recent Progress of Epidemiology in England." *Practitioner* 15 (1875): 459–80.

Radcliffe, John Netten, and W. H. Power, "Report on an Outbreak of Enteric Fever in Marylebone and the Adjoining Parts of London." In *Annual Report of the Medical Officer of the Local Government Board for 1872.* Parliamentary Papers. London: Eyre and Spottiswoode, 1873.

Rasmussen, Sonja A., and Richard A. Goodman. *CDC Field Epidemiology Manual.* Oxford: Oxford University Press, 2019.

Reece, Robert. "Progress and Problems in Epidemiology." *Proceedings of the Royal Society of Medicine* 16 (1923): 35–48.

"The Regulation of the Sale of Milk." *Sanitary Record* 3 (September 18, 1875): 199–200.

"The Religious Press on the Thanksgiving at St. Paul's." *Public Opinion* 21 (March 2, 1872): 262–63.

"Remarks on the Epidemic of Enteric Fever in the Tees Valley During 1890–91." *Practitioner* 52 (1894): 55–67.

"The Report on Enteric Fever in the Tees Valley." *British Medical Journal* 1725 (January 20, 1894): 132–38.

"The Report of the Lancet Sanitary Commission." *Times*, December 9, 1871, 9.

"Report of the Lancet Sanitary Commission on the State of Londesborough Lodge and Sandringham, in Relation to the Illness of H.R.H. The Prince of Wales." *Lancet* 98 (December 9, 1871): 828–31.

Report on the Sanitary Measures in India in 1894–95. London: Eyre and Spottiswoode, 1896.

Report of the Commission on the Nature, Pathology, Causation, and Prevention of Dysentery, and Its Relationship to Enteric Fever. London: Harrison and Sons, 1903.

Report of the Royal Commission Appointed to Consider and Report Upon the Care and Treatment of the Sick and Wounded. London: Eyre and Spottiswoode, 1901.

"The Report of the Commission on the Nature, Pathology, Causation, and Prevention of Dysentery and Its Relation to Typhoid Fever." *Lancet* 162 (December 19, 1903): 1750–52.

"Report of the Commission on the Nature, Pathology, Causation, and Prevention of Dysentery and Its Relationship to Enteric Fever." *Lancet* 162 (August 29, 1903): 626–27.

"Review of William Budd's *Typhoid Fever.*" *Edinburgh Medical Journal* 19 (1874): 820–22.

Richardson, Benjamin Ward. *Hygeia: A City of Health.* London: Macmillan, 1876.

————. "The Present Position and Prospects of Epidemiological Science." *Transactions of the Epidemiological Society of London* 2 (1865): 119–33.

————. *Vita Medica: Chapters of Medical Life and Work*. London: Longmans, Green, 1897.

Richardson, Nigel. *Typhoid in Uppingham: Analysis of a Victorian Town and School in Crisis, 1875–77*. London: Pickering & Chatto, 2008.

Ritch, Alistair. *Sickness in the Workhouse*. Rochester, NY: University of Rochester Press, 2019.

Robinson, M. K. "The Cause of the Contagion of Typhoid Fever." *British Medical Journal* 692 (1874): 451–52.

Roechling, H. Alfred. *Sewer Gas and its Influence Upon Health*. London: Biggs, 1898.

Romano, Terrie. "The Cattle Plague of 1865 and the Reception of 'The Germ Theory' in Mid-Victorian Britain." *Journal of the History of Medicine and Allied Sciences* 52, no. 1 (1997): 51–80.

Rosenberg, Charles. "Disease in History: Frames and Framers." *Millbank Quarterly* 67, no. 1 (1989): 1–15.

————. *The Cholera Years: The United States in 1832, 1849, and 1866*. Chicago: University of Chicago Press, 1962.

————. "Framing Disease: Illness, Society, and History." In *Framing Disease: Studies in Cultural History*, edited by Charles Rosenberg and Janet Golden, xiii–xxvi. New Brunswick, NJ: Rutgers University Press, 1992.

Ross, George. *Report on the Sanitary Conditions of the St. Giles District, During the Year 1869 to Vestry of St. Giles District*. London: Those, Penny, 1870.

Royal College of Physicians. *The Nomenclature of Disease*. London: Spottiswoode, 1869.

Royal Commission to Inquire Into the Water Supply of the Metropolis. Parliamentary Papers. London. Eyre and Spottiswoode, 1893.

Rugg, H. Hodson. *Observations on London Milk*. London: Bailey and Moon, 1850.

Rumsey, Henry Wyldebore. *Essays on State Medicine*. London: John Churchill, 1856.

Russell, James. *Lectures on the Theory and General Prevention and Control of Infectious Diseases*. Glasgow: James Maclehose, 1879.

Ryle, J. C. *What Good Will it Do? A Question About the Disestablishment of the Church of England, Examined and Answered*. London: William Hunt and Co., 1872.

Sanderson, John Burdon. "Intimate Pathology of Contagion." In *Annual Report of the Medical Officer of the Privy Council for the Year 1870*. Parliamentary Papers. London: Spottiswoode, 1871.

"Sanitary Science and the Milk Panic." *Engineer* 36 (August 29, 1873): 137–38.

Santa, Prosper De Pietra. "An Address on Typhoid Fever in Paris During the Years 1875–1882." *British Medical Journal* 1168 (May 19, 1883): 947–50.

"Scarborough & Sandringham." *Lancet* 98 (December 9, 1871): 821.

Schneider, Dona, and David E. Lillienfeld. *Foundations of Epidemiology*. Oxford and New York: Oxford University Press, 2015.

"The Scientific Aspects of Epidemics." *Sanitary Record* 2 (June 19, 1875): 404.

"The Sherlockian Method in Epidemiology." *Lancet* 228 (September 12, 1936): 639.

Secord, James. "Knowledge in Transit." *Isis* 95 (2004): 654–72.

Seaton, Edward Cox. "A Discussion on the Etiology and Epidemiology of Typhoid (Enteric) Fever." *Proceedings of the Royal Society of Medicine* 1 (1908): 169–75.

———. "Impure Water as a Cause of Typhoid Fever." *Lancet* 88 (October 20, 1866): 448–49.

———. *Infectious Diseases and their Prevention*. London: University of London Press, 1911.

Seaton, Edward. "Report on Circumstances Endangering the Public Health of Chichester." In *Annual Report of the Medical Officer of the Privy Council for 1865*. Parliamentary Papers. London: Eyre and Spottiswoode, 1866.

———. "Evolution of Sanitary Administration in the Victorian Era." *British Medical Journal* 1903 (June 19, 1897): 1636–40.

Sedgwick, William T., George R. Taylor, and J. Scott MacNutt. "Is Typhoid Fever a 'Rural' Disease?" *Journal of Infectious Disease* 2 (September 1912): 141–92.

Sedgwick, William T. *Principles of Sanitary Science and Public Health*. London: Macmillan, 1922.

Shapin, Steven. *Never Pure: Historical Studies of Science As If It Was Produced by People with Bodies, Situated in Times, Space, Culture, and Society, and Struggling for Credibility and Authority*. Baltimore: Johns Hopkins University Press, 2010.

Sheppard, Edgar. *George Duke of Cambridge*. London: Longman, Green, 1906.

Siena, Kevin. *Rotten Bodies: Class and Contagion in Eighteenth Century Britain*. New Haven, CT: Yale University Press, 2019.

Sigsworth, Michael, and Michael Worboys. "The Public's View of Public Health in Mid-Victorian Britain." *Urban History* 21, no. 2 (October 1994): 237–50.

Simon, John. "Address Delivered at the Opening of the Section of Public Medicine." *British Medical Journal* 1075 (August 6, 1881): 219–23.

———. *Annual Report of the Medical Officer of the Privy Council for 1865*. Parliamentary Papers. London: Eyre and Spottiswoode, 1866.

———. *Annual Report of the Medical Officer of the Privy Council for 1866*. Parliamentary Papers. London: Eyre and Spottiswoode, 1867.

———. *Annual Report of the Medical Officer of the Privy Council for 1867*. Parliamentary Papers. London: Eyre and Spottiswoode, 1868.

———. *Annual Report to the Medical Officer of the Privy Council* for 1869. Parliamentary Papers. London: Eyre and Spottiswoode, 1870.

———. *Annual Report of the Medical Officer of the Local Government Board for 1874*. Parliamentary Papers. London: Eyre and Spottiswoode, 1875.

———. *Annual Report of the Medical Officer of the Local Government Board for 1875*. Parliamentary Papers. London: Eyre and Spottiswoode, 1876.

———. *English Sanitary Institutions: Reviewed in their Course of Development and in Some of Their Political and Social Relations*. London: John Murray, 1890.

———. "An Essay on Contagion: its Nature and Mode of Action." *British Medical Journal* 990 (December 20, 1879): 973–75.

————. *Filth-Diseases and Their Prevention: Supplementary Report to the Local Government Board.* London: George Eyre and William Spottiswoode, 1874.

————. *Filth-Diseases and Their Prevention.* London: Churchill, 1875.

————. *Filth-Diseases and Their Prevention.* Boston: James Campbell, 1876.

————. "Windsor." *Annual Report of the Medical Officer of the Privy Council for the Year 1858.* Parliamentary Papers. London: Eyre and Spottiswoode, 1859.

Simpson, W. J. *The Maintenance of Health in the Tropics.* New York: Wood and Co., 1905.

Sinnema, Peter. "Anxiously Managing Mourning: Wellington's Funeral and the Press." *Victorian Review* 24, no. 2 (Winter 2000): 30–60.

Sixth Report of the Commissioners Appointed in 1868 to Inquire into the Best Means of Preventing the Pollution of Rivers. London: Eyre and Spottiswoode, 1874.

Smallman-Raynon, Matthew, and Andrew Cliff. *Atlas Of Epidemic Britain: A Twentieth Century Picture.* Oxford: Oxford University Press, 2012.

Smart, W. R. E. "Introductory Address." *Transactions of the Epidemiological Society of London* 3 (1876): 455–73.

Smee, Alfred. *Milk, Typhoid Fever, and Sewage: A Series of Letters.* London: W. H. & L. Collingridge, 1873.

————. *Sewage, Sewage Produce, and Disease.* London: W. H. & L. Collingridge, 1873.

Smith, Dale C. "The Rise and Fall of Typhomalarial Fever." *Journal of the History of Medicine and Allied Sciences* 37 (1982): 182–200.

Smith, P. Horton. "On the Respective Parts Taken by the Urine and the Feces in the Dissemination of Typhoid Fever." *Lancet* 153 (May 20, 1899): 1346–52.

Smith, M. Van Wyk. *Drummer Hodge: The Poetry of the Anglo-Boer War.* Oxford: Oxford University Press, 1978.

Smocovitis, Vassiliki Betty. *Unifying Biology: The Evolutionary Synthesis and Evolutionary Biology.* Princeton, NJ: Princeton University Press, 1996.

Spear, John. "The Dangers of Water-Contamination during Distribution in Mains and Service Pipes." *Transactions of the Epidemiological Society of London* 7 (1889): 134–52.

————. "Report on Appearances of Typhus Fever in Various Parts of England during the Year 1886–87." In *Annual Report of the Medical Officer of the Local Government Board for 1886.* Parliamentary Papers. London: Eyre and Spottiswoode, 1887.

————. "Report on an Epidemic of Typhoid Fever in the Mountain Ash Urban Sanitary District." In *Annual Report of the Medical Officer of the Local Government Board for 1887.* Parliamentary Papers. London: Eyre and Spottiswoode, 1888.

Stallybrass, C. O. *The Principles of Epidemiology.* London: George Routledge & Son, 1931.

Stark, James F. *The Making of Modern Anthrax, 1875–1920.* London: Pickering & Chatto, 2014.

Statement Exhibiting the Moral and Material Progress and Condition of India during the Year 1894–1895. London: Eyre and Spottiswoode, 1896.

Stewart, Alexander P. "Some Considerations on the Nature and Pathology of Typhus and Typhoid Fever." *The Edinburgh Medical and Surgical Journal* 54 (1840): 289–339.

Stewart, W. "A New Theory of the Origin of Typhoid Fever." *British Medical Journal* 845 (March 10, 1877): 289–90.

Stevenson, Lloyd. "Exemplary Disease: The Typhoid Pattern." *Journal of the History of Medicine and Allied Sciences* 37, no. 2 (April 1982): 159–81.

———. "A Pox on the Ileum: Typhoid Fever Among the Exanthemata." *Bulletin of the History of Medicine* 51, no. 3 (Fall 1977): 496–504.

Strange, Julie-Marie. *Death, Grief and Poverty in Britain, 1870–1914*. Cambridge: Cambridge University Press, 2005.

Strange, William. "Notes on the Origin and Diffusion of Enteric Fever and of Diphtheria." *British Medical Journal* 1082 (September 24, 1881): 507–9.

"Stray Arrows." *Teesdale Mercury*, October 29, 1890, 4.

"Stray Arrows." *Teesdale Mercury*, October 4, 1893, 5.

Steere-Williams, Jacob. "A Conflict of Analysis: Analytical Chemistry and Milk Adulteration in Victorian Britain." *Ambix* 61, no.3 (August 2014): 279–98.

———. "Milking Science for Its Worth: The Reform of the British Milk Trade in the Late Nineteenth Century." *Agricultural History* 89, no. 2 (Spring 2015): 263–88.

"Surgeon-General Gordon on Enteric Fever in the European Army of Madras." *Indian Medical Gazette* 13, no. 10 (October 1878): 276.

Susser, Mervyn, and Zena Stein. *Eras in Epidemiology: The Evolution of Ideas*. Oxford: Oxford University Press, 2009.

Swithinbank, Harold, and George Newman. *The Bacteriology of Milk*. London: John Murray, 1903.

Szreter, Simon. *Fertility, Class and Gender in Britain, 1860–1940*. Cambridge: Cambridge University Press, 1996.

———. *Health and Wealth: Studies in History and Policy*. Rochester, NY: University of Rochester Press, 2005.

———. "The Importance of Social Intervention in Britain's Mortality Decline, c. 1850–1914: A Re-Interpretation of the Role of Public Health." *Social History of Medicine* (1988): 1–37.

Tait, Lawson. "The Influence of Milk in the Propagation of Contagious Disease." *British Medical Journal* 508 (September 24, 1870): 344.

Taylor, Michael W. "On the Communication of the Infection of Fever by Ingesta." *Edinburgh Medical Journal* 3 (1858): 993–1004.

———. "Notes of a Recent Epidemic of Typhoid Fever, and its Mode of Propagation." *Edinburgh Medical Journal* 18 (1872): 124–33.

————. "On the Transmission of the Infection of Fevers by Means of Fluids." *British Medical Journal* 519 (December 10, 1870): 623–25.

"The Thanksgiving Day." *Illustrated London News*, March 2, 1872, 206.

Tew, J. S. "The Agglutinative Reaction in Typhoid Fever and 'Anti-Typhoid' Vaccination." *Public Health* 10 (1898): 183–91.

Thomson, William. "Typhoid Fever: Contagious, Infectious, and Communicable." *British Medical Journal* 949 (March 8, 1879): 343–45.

Thomson, Theodore, and Col. J. T. Marsh. "Enteric Fever in the City of Chichester." In *Annual Report of the Medical Officer of the Local Government Board for 1899–1900*. Parliamentary Papers. London: Spottiswoode, 1900.

Thorne Thorne, Richard. *Annual Report of the Medical Officer of the Local Government Board for 1896–1897*. Parliamentary Papers. London: Eyre & Spottiswoode, 1897.

————. "Effects Produced on the Human Subject by Consumption of Milk from Cows Having Foot-and-Mouth Disease." In *Annual Report of the Medical Officer of the Privy Council for 1868*. Parliamentary Papers. London: Eyre and Spottiswoode, 1869.

————. "On an Extensive Epidemic of Enteric Fever at Red Hill, Caterham, and Other Adjoining Places." In *Annual Report of the Local Government Board for 1879*. Parliamentary Papers. London: Spottiswoode, 1880.

————. *On the Progress of Preventive Medicine During the Victorian Age*. London: Shaw & Sons, 1888.

————. "The Propagation of Enteric Fever." *British Medical Journal* 486 (April 23, 1870): 426.

————. "The Recent Outbreak of Enteric Fever at Caterham and Redhill." *Royal Society of Arts* 28 (1879): 117–19.

————. "Remarks on the Origin of Infection." *Transactions of the Epidemiological Society of London* 4 (1879): 234–46.

————. "Reports on an Epidemic of Typhoid Fever at Terling." In *Annual Report of the Medical Officer of the Privy Council for 1865*. Parliamentary Papers. London: Eyre and Spottiswoode, 1867.

————. "Report on Epidemic Typhoid Fever at Winterton." In *Annual Report of the Medical Officer of the Privy Council for 1867*. Parliamentary Papers. London: Eyre and Spottiswoode, 1868.

Tomes, Nancy. "The Private Side of Public Health: Sanitary Science, Domestic Hygiene, and the Germ Theory, 1870–1900." *Bulletin of the History of Medicine* 64, no. 4 (1990): 509–39.

Tooth, Howard. "The Recent Epidemic of Typhoid Fever in South Africa." *British Medical Journal* 2098 (March 16, 1901): 642–48.

Turner, Frank. *Contesting Cultural Authority: Essays in Victorian Intellectual Life*. Cambridge: Cambridge University Press, 1993.

Turner, George. "Typhoid Fever in South Africa: Its Cause and Prevention." *British Medical Journal* 2146 (February 15, 1902): 381–83.

Tyndall, John. "Cholera and Disinfection." *Daily News*, 1883, 6.

———. *The Prayer-Gauge Debate*. Boston: Congregational Publishing Society, 1876.

———. "Typhoid Fever." *Times*, November 9, 1874, 7.

"Typhoid Fever." *Lancet* 98 (December 2, 1871): 788.

Typhoid and Paratyphoid Collaborators. "The Global Burden of Typhoid and Paratyphoid." *Lancet* 19, no. 4 (April 2019): 369–81.

"Typhoid at Guildford." *Lancet* 2306 (November 9, 1867): 587.

"Typhoid at Terling." *Lancet* 94 (February 8, 1868): 204.

"Typhoid Fever at Winterton." *Lancet* 2312 (December 21, 1867): 772.

"Typhoid Fever Spread by Water." *Bristol Mercury and Daily Post*, 1897, 3.

"Typhoid Fever in Islington." *British and Foreign Medico-Chirurgical Review* 48 (July to October 1871): 25–26.

Vacher, Francis. "The Influence of Various Articles of Food in Spreading Parasitic, Zymotic, Tubercular and other Diseases." *Transactions of the International Medical Congress* 3 (1881): 489–90.

Vandersloot, Samantha, et al. "Water and Filth: Reevaluating the First Era of Sanitary Typhoid Intervention (1840–1940)." *Clinical Infectious Disease* 69, no. 5 (November 2019): 377–84.

Vickerman, F. L. "The Sanitary State of Nelson." *Nelson Examiner* 46 (April 16, 1868): 2.

"A Village in Arcadia." *Punch* 54 (February 22, 1868): 87–88.

"Villa Residences and Typhoid Fever." *Times*, December 12, 1871, 12.

Vinten-Johansen, Peter, et al. *Cholera, Chloroform, and the Science of Medicine*. Oxford: Oxford University Press, 2003.

Waddington, Keir. *Bovine Scourge: Meat, Tuberculosis, and Public Health, 1850–1914*. Woodbridge, UK: Boydell, 2006.

———. "It Might Not be a Nuisance in a Country Cottage: Sanitary Conditions and Images of Health in Victorian Rural Wales." *Rural History* 23, no. 2 (October 2012): 185–204.

Wall, Rosemary. *Bacteria in Britain: 1880–1939*. London: Pickering & Chatto, 2013.

Wanklyn, J. Alfred. *Milk Analysis: A Practical Treatise on the Examination of Milk and Its Derivatives*. London: Trubner and Co., 1874.

Warner, John Harley. *The Therapeutic Perspective: Medical Practice, Knowledge, and Identity in America, 1820–1885*. Cambridge: Harvard University Press, 1986.

———. "The Uses of Patient Records by Historians: Patterns, Possibilities and Perplexities." *Health and History* 1, no. 2/3 (1999): 101–11.

"Water and Sanitary Affairs." *Gas Journal* 62 (July 4, 1893): 11.

Watkins, Dorothy. "The English Revolution in Social Medicine, 1889–1911." PhD diss., University College London, 1984.

Welshman, John. *Municipal Medicine: Public Health in Twentieth-Century Britain.* New York: Peter Lang, 2000.

"Sir William Withey Gull." *Punch* 82 (February 25, 1882): 94.

Whitaker, William. *The Geology of London.* London: Eyre and Spottiswoode, 1889.

Wilson, George. *A Handbook of Hygiene and Sanitary Science.* London: J&A Churchill, 1883.

———. "Sanitary Work in Rural Districts." *Sanitary Record* 4 (March 4, 1876): 155–59.

Wintroub, Michael. "Taking a Bow in the Theatre of Things." *Isis* 101 (2010): 779–93.

Weisz, George. *Divide and Conquer: A Comparative History of Medical Specialization.* Oxford: Oxford University Press, 2006.

White, Alexandre I. R. "Global Risks, Divergent Pandemics: Contrasting Responses to Bubonic Plague and Smallpox in 1901 Cape Town." *Social Science History* 42, no. 1 (Spring 2018): 135–58.

Whitehead, H. R. "Tropical Typhoid Fever." In *Hygiene & Diseases of Warm Climates,* edited by Andrew Davidson, 217–65. Edinburgh: Young J. Pentland, 1893.

Whitmore, John. *Report on the Adulteration of Milk and Other Articles of Food: Report of the Medical Officer of Health for St. Marylebone.* London: Vestry of St. Marylebone, 1873.

Williamson, Stanley. *The Vaccination Controversy: The Rise, Reign, and Fall of Compulsory Vaccination for Smallpox.* Liverpool: Liverpool University Press, 2007.

Wilks, Samuel and George Thomas Bettany. *A Biographical History of Guy's Hospital.* London: Ward, Lock, Bowden & Co., 1892.

Wils, Kaat, Raf de Bont, and Sokhieng Au. *Beyond Borders: Moving Anatomies, 1750–1950.* Leuven, Belgium: Leuven University Press, 2017.

Wilkinson, Lise. *Animals and Disease: An Introduction to the History of Comparative Medicine.* Cambridge: Cambridge University Press, 1992.

Wilson, Leonard. "The Historical Riddle of Milk-Borne Scarlet Fever." *Bulletin of the History of Medicine* 60 (1986): 321–42.

Winslow, Charles Edward-Amory. *The Conquest of Epidemic Disease: A Chapter in the History of Ideas.* Madison: University of Wisconsin Press, 1943.

Wohl, Anthony S. *Endangered Lives: Public Health in Victorian Britain.* Cambridge: Cambridge University Press, 1983.

Woods, Abigail. *A Manufactured Plague? The History of Foot and Mouth Disease in Britain.* London: Earthscan, 2004.

Woods, Robert. *The Demography of Victorian England and Wales.* Cambridge: Cambridge University Press, 2000.

Woods, Robert, and John Woodward. *Urban Disease and Mortality in Nineteenth Century England.* London: St. Martin's Press, 1984.

Worboys, Michael. "Almroth Wright at Netley: Modern Medicine and the Military in Britain, 1892–1902." In *Medicine and Modern Warfare,* edited by Roger Cooter, Mark Harrison, and Steve Sturdy, 77–97. Amsterdam: Rodopi, 1999.

———. "Practice and the Science of Medicine in the Nineteenth Century." *Isis* 102 (2011): 109–15.

———. *Spreading Germs: Disease Theories and Medical Practice in Britain, 1865–1900.* New York: Cambridge University Press, 2000.

———. "Was There a Bacteriological Revolution in Late Nineteenth-Century Medicine?" *Studies in History and Philosophy of Science* 38, no. 1 (March 2007): 20–42.

Wright, A. E., and D. Bruce. "On Haffkine's Method of Vaccination against Asiatic Cholera." *British Medical Journal* 1675 (February 4, 1893): 227–31.

Wright, A. E., and D. Semple. "On the Presence of Typhoid Bacilli in the Urine of Patients Suffering from Typhoid Fever." *Lancet* 146 (July 27, 1895): 196–99.

——— "Remarks on Vaccination Against Typhoid Fever." *British Medical Journal* 1 (January 30, 1897): 256.

Wright, A. E. and F. Smith, "On the Application of the Serum Test to the Differential Diagnosis of Typhoid and Malta Fever." *TLancet* (March 6, 1897): 656.

Wright, A. E. *A Short Treatise on Anti-Typhoid Inoculation.* Westminster, UK: Archibald Constable & Co., 1904.

Index

Addison, Thomas, 34
Airy, Hubert, 74, 188, 210
Aitken, William, 108–9
Albert, Prince Consort, 11, 33
Albert, Prince Edward (later King
  Edward VII), 11, 26, 30–32, 35–36,
  123, 128–30; recovery, 32, , 37–38,
  50–53, 76, 170, 178; sickness, 33,
  38–49, 53, 66, 71, 75, 77–78, 170,
  225, 278; visit to Londesborough
  Lodge, 63–64, 75–76
Allbutt, Clifford, 41, 90, 106
Allen, Alfred, 201
analytical chemistry,11, 16, 81, 115,
  118–19, 124, 144–45, 150, 152–53,
  164, 185–86, 200
Analytical Sanitary Commission of *The
  Lancet*, 135
anthrax, 181, 184, 187–88, 190,
  219n121
anti-typhoid inoculation, 28, 223, 228;
  development by Almroth Wright,
  242–246; testing in India, 246–50;
  use during South African War,
  250–254
Army Medical Department (Royal
  Army Medical Corps), 229, 231,
  235, 238n47, 239, 241, 243, 248–
  53, 254, 256, 258–67, 269
Association of Metropolitan Medical
  Officers of Health (later Society of
  Medical Officers of Health), 2n4,
  7, 88n34, 136, 137n29, 139–40,
  141n43, 145, 196n66, 244

Axe, J. Wortley, 181

Babington, Benjamin Guy, 34,
  116n136
bacteriological revolution, 27, 201
bacteriology, 11, 13n53, 14–16, 26–28,
  74–75, 108, 118, 123–24, 171–73,
  176–78, 186–87, 191, 195, 206–9,
  212–13, 214, 218, 221–22, 228,
  240, 250, 267–69, 273, 278; of
  B.typhosus, 171, 176–77, 182–183,
  194, 201–2, 205–8, 220, 223, 236,
  239–244, 260, 280–81; of milk, 134
Ballard, Edward, 66, 91, 116n139, 122,
  125, 127, 137, 168, 188–89, 210,
  214, 219, 232, 273–74; investigation of food poisoning at Welbeck,
  181–83; investigation of typhoid
  at Islington, 130–31, 136, 138–48,
  151, 164–65, 169; investigation of
  typhoid at Leeds, 150; views on milk
  adulteration, 148–50
Barry, Frederick, 17, 177, 219; investigation of typhoid in the Tees Valley:
  190–206, 213, 214, 219, 222, 274
Bazalgette, Joseph, 72
Blaxall, Frank H., 13n53, 188,195;
  investigation of typhoid at Sherborne, 74–75
Blyth, Alexander Wynter, 87, 88n30
biostatistics, 15, 273
Boobbyer, Philip, 278, 282
Bowditch, Henry, 10
Bowlby, Anthony, 250–51, 253, 264

Bristowe, J. S., 136; investigation of
   typhoid at Grantham, 69
British Medical Association, 36, 122,
   132, 133n11, 181, 196n66, 204,
   219n122, 240–41, 281
Brown, Samuel Sneade, 32
Brown Animal Sanatory Institution,
   172n1, 175n4, 177, 180–81, 243
Bruce, David, 245n65, 246n71, 253;
   research on South African Royal
   Commission, 258–68
Brunton, T. Lauder, 122n162,
   124n173, 175n6, 179
Bryden, James L., 230–34, 238
Bubonic plague, 246–47, 259–60, 264
Buchanan, George, 5, 7n30, 10n43, 19,
   28, 29n109, 67, 75, 85n22, 107,
   148, 189, 210, 219, 232, 234, 273,
   276; as Chief Medical Officer of
   the Medical Department, 112, 115,
   120, 126, 137n30, 185–88, 190,
   192, 195; investigation of typhoid
   at Cambridge, 73–74, 76; investigation of typhoid at Guildford, 91,
   94–96, 119; investigation of typhoid
   at Worthing, 70; work as Medical
   Officer of Health for St. Giles, London, 69
Budd, William, 14, 25, 66, 72–75,
   78–80, 83, 107–13, 115, 125,
   132–33, 140, 146, 151, 170, 173,
   176–80, 231, 234, 244; research on
   comparative pathology: 180–82
Bulloch, William, 177, 254
Bulstrode, H. T., 17, 126, 176–77,
   191, 210, 265, 273; investigation of
   typhoid at Chichester, 208–23
Burdett-Coutts, William, 224–27,
   254–58

Cameron, Charles, 23, 135, 146, 264
cancer, 101, 180, 274, 283

Carpenter, Alfred, 179, 219n120
Cassal, Charles, 186
cattle plague of 1865, 131, 134–38
Cayley, William H., 106n89, 117n140,
   252–53
Centers for Disease Control and Prevention, 272, 274
Chadwick, Edwin, 2, 13–14, 21,
   61–62, 67, 108, 114–15, 126, 280
Chevers, Norman, 233
cholera, 8n32, 12, 14n56, 16, 17n71,
   19, 32, 34, 75, 76n155, 78, 90,
   107–8, 110–11, 122n166, 139,
   141, 178, 182, 187–88, 191, 202,
   232, 236–37, 241, 243, 248, 245,
   259–60, 274; outbreak at Theydon
   Bois, Essex, 79–85, 88–89; outbreak
   in London in 1865–66, 84–89
Church, William, 255
cinchona bark, 230
civic gospel of cleanliness, 6, 279
Clark, James, 33, 67
Clinical Society of London, 34
Contagious Diseases (Animals) Acts,
   137, 167
Conybeare, Ernest T., 271
Corfield, William H., 70, 72–73, 76,
   79, 90n42, 130, 190, 213; inves-
   tigation of Londesborough Lodge,
   65–66; investigation of typhoid in
   St. Marylebone, London, 155–167
Cory, Robert, 184–86
COVID-19, 283
Cowsheds, 135–39, 142, 149
Crawford, Thomas, 233, 236–37
Creighton, Charles, 176, 180, 186,
   276–77
Crimean War, 48, 80
Crookshank, F. C., 273
Croydon, 74, 131, 179, 219; 1852
   typhoid outbreak, 67–69; 1937
   typhoid outbreak, 271–73, 277, 282

Cunningham, D. D., 237–38
Cunningham, D. J., 255
Cunningham, J. M., 232, 237n43

Dairies, Cow-Sheds, and Milk-Shops Order, 167
Dairy Reformed Company, 130, 205; involvement in the outbreak of typhoid in St. Marylebone, London, 151–67
Darwin, Charles, 173, 175, 180, 220n126
Davidson, Andrew, 238
Davies, David, 2n4, 244, 282n23
delirium, as a symptom of typhoid, 20, 22, 33, 40–41, 48, 226
DeRenzy, C. C., 236
diphtheria, 20, 111, 139, 168, 188
Diploma in Public Health, 106n89, 168, 192, 207, 259, 275
disinfection, 63, 96, 98, 100, 121, 122n166, 158, 183, 187, 214, 219, 224, 239, 242, 259, 264–66
Dodgson, R. W., 252–54
domestic sanitation; drains, 9,11, 13, 17, 20, 24, 26, 61, 66–70, 74–76, 82, 84, 90, 98, 107, 113, 129, 140, 142–43, 165, 170, 189, 197, 276, 280; cesspools, 9, 20, 21, 64, 66, 70–71, 81, 84, 90–92, 95, 98, 100, 103, 108, 113, 119, 143, 149, 195, 211–12; privies, 62, 84, 91–92, 109, 113, 157–58, 188, 194, 197, 211–13; ventilation, 64, 66, 67–70; water-closets, 13, 20, 26, 61–62, 64, 68–71, 74, 76, 82, 92, 109, 129, 143, 170, 276, 280
Doyle, Arthur Conan, 227n11, 251
Druitt, Robert, 145
Duguid, William, 181
Dupre, August, 81, 158n91, 185–86
Durham, Herbert, 243

East India Company, 24, 231
Eberth, Karl, 176, 182–83, 185
ecology of disease, 28, 85, 150, 139, 177, 191, 195, 204, 213, 268, 276, 281
emotions: of typhoid patients and clinicians, 38–39, 41–42, 45–46, 48, 51; of epidemiological outbreak investigation, 92, 113, 194
enteric fever. See also typhoid fever
environmental contamination, 78, 81, 95–96, 103–4, 107, 113, 126, 141, 156–58, 188–89, 220, 264; of rivers; 13, 85, 155, 157, 160, 188, 192–206, 208; of wells, 13, 17, 20, 27–28, 78, 81–82, 84, 90–100, 102–3, 115–16, 119, 121, 157–60, 193, 195, 206–9, 211, 251, 261, 271–72
epidemiological gaze, 2, 18, 26, 69–70, 76, 78, 86, 102, 112, 119, 121, 123, 146, 148, 160, 169–70, 190–91, 196, 203, 230, 233, 235, 240, 242, 258, 264, 269, 276, 280. See also outbreak investigation
Epidemiological Society of London, 7, 14, 34, 38, 66, 69, 73, 80, 82, 84, 89, 111n116, 116, 118, 139, 156, 214, 222, 228, 232, 236, 238, 278
epidemiological transition, 6, 8n34, 274
etiology, of infectious disease; 8, 15, 19n82, 20, 21, 25, 31, 36, 40, 61, 63, 67, 72–73, 75, 77–78, 82–84, 89–90, 94, 96, 98, 106n90, 108–9, 112–13, 118, 126, 131, 133, 137–40, 146, 158, 167–68, 173, 176, 178–83, 187–88, 191, 203, 213, 219–22, 276; debates about disease in colonial environments; 230–242, 258–267. See also germ theory
eugenics, 273
Ewart, Joseph, 229, 233–36

excrement removal, 9, 19n80, 24,
28, 67–69, 73, 78, 87n29, 90, 92,
94–95, 103, 107, 113, 124–26, 130,
184, 188, 194–95, 201, 208, 220,
235, 239, 261, 265–66. *See also*
environmental contamination
Exham, R., 256

Farr, William, 4, 14, 25, 85–86, 88–89,
110–11, 139, 274, 278
Fayrer, Joseph, 233–37, 240
fever chart, 41–43, 46
fever dens, 61, 108
filth, moral notions of, 1–2, 9–11, 21,
22, 32, 61, 68, 70, 72, 76–77, 95,
98, 102, 107–12, 124, 129, 183,
189, 213, 226; in colonial environments; 223, 225, 227, 232–43. *See
also* middle class respectability
Fleming, George, 114
food pathways, 13, 27, 66, 113, 126,
131, 135, 148, 181, 222, 239
food poisoning, 28, 182, 275
Foot and mouth disease, 136–37
Foucault, Michel, 18. *See also* epidemiological gaze
Fox, Cornelius, 106
Frankland, Edward, 86, 88–89, 155,
184–85, 195, 201, 204, 207–8
Frankland, Percy, 201, 207–8
Franks, Kendal, 257

Gaffky, Georg, 176, 182–83
Gamgee, John, 135–37, 139, 148–50,
180
General Board of Health, 2, 67
General Registrar's Office, 4, 9n35,
14–15, 21, 22, 31, 69–70, 80, 156,
210, 278
germ theory, 15, 25, 27, 31, 71, 77–78,
89, 123–25, 136, 140, 149, 168,

173–83, 194, 219–23, 240–41. *See
also* bacteriological revolution
Gladstone, William, 50, 59, 60n101
Godart, Thomas, 22–24
Gordon, C. A., 231–35, 238
Grant Medical College, Bombay, 229
Greenwood, Major, 4n18, 248n77, 273
Gresswell, D. A, 189
Grunbaum, Albert, 243
Gull, William Withey; treatment of the
Prince of Wales, 33–49, 50, 52, 66;
views on the etiology of typhoid,
77–78, 109, 127, 235
Guy's Hospital, 34, 43n38, 77

Haffkine, Waldemar, 245, 248, 259
Hamer, William H., 132n8, 134, 176,
186, 273, 282
Hamilton, George, 241–42, 247–48
Hamilton, J. B., 236–40, 263
Hankin, Ernest Hanbury, 240
Hart, Ernest, 6, 120, 130, 151, 169,
179, 182–83, 204–5, 241; investiga-
tion of typhoid at St. Marylebone,
London, 162–67
Hassall, Arthur Hill, 135, 148, 150
Haviland, Alfred, 26, 76, 101–2, 110,
112, 130
Hinton, Joseph, 261–62
HIV/AIDS, 283
Holden, Oscar, 271
Hope, William, 154–67. *See also* Dairy
Reformed Company
Houston, A. C., 176, 209, 219–20,
281

index case, the search for during outbreak investigation, 16, 25, 73,
80, 82–83, 85–86, 89, 94, 97–98,
102–3, 116–20, 125, 132, 156–57,
160, 189, 194–96, 197, 203, 235,
261, 269, 272, 279–80, 282

Indian Medical Service, 233, 237, 241, 243, 263
Indian Mutiny/Rebellion, 48
India Plague Commission, 246–47, 250
industrial health, 2, 131, 139–40
influenza, 244, 283
International Medical Congress, 169, 187, 235–36

Jameson, James, 249
Jenner, William, 66, 76, 229; early distinction between typhoid and typhus; 33–44; investigation of typhoid at St. Marylebone, London, 130, 151, 162–67, 205; treatment of the Prince of Wales, 33–44, 49, 66, 76, 205, 229
jingoism, 60, 226

Keogh, Alfred, 253–54, 269
Kipling, Rudyard, 251
Kitasato, Shibasaburo, 260
Klein, Edward Emmanuel, 28, 81, 122n166, 206, 225, 240, 243–44, 260; animal research on comparative pathology, 178–82, 223–24; experimentation during the outbreak of typhoid at Chichester, 208, 212–13, 220, 222–23; laboratory research on B.coli, 206–8; laboratory research on B.typhosus, 183–84, 186–87, 194, 206–9; supposed discovery of the "germ" of typhoid, 172–80
Koch, Robert, 178, 181–83, 187, 237, 260, 280, 282n23

Lambert, John, 113n128, 114
Lancet Sanitary Commission, 63–66
Lankester, E. Ray, 201
Lansdowne, Lord, 246–29
Latham, Baldwin, 123
Lawley, William, 53–56

Leishman, William, 253, 269–70
Letheby, Henry, 67, 88n34, 137, 201n74
Liebig, Justus von, 88
Linnean Society, 178
Lister, Joseph, 71, 250
London Fever Hospital, 20, 24, 38, 61, 117n140, 128–29, 162
London School of Hygiene and Tropical Medicine, 180n18, 259
Louis, Pierre, 20
Low, R. Bruce, 3n11, 112, 191n53, 206, 258, 265
Lowe, John, 40, 49

Macdonald, J. D., 236
Maclean, William Campbell, 235–238
Maconochie, D.S.S, 152–65. See also Dairy Reformed Company
malaria, 231
malta fever, 243
Manson, Patrick, 228–29
Martin, Sidney, 176; investigation of typhoid in soils at Chichester, 208, 218–21
Mayo, Charles, 62
McNaulty, Arthur S., 186
McPherson, R. H., 240
methods, epidemiological: case-fatality, as a statistical measure, 140–41; case-tracing, 16, 34, 75, 80–83, 86, 89, 95, 98, 103, 113, 116–19, 130, 132, 142, 146–48, 152, 156, 160–62, 168–69, 182, 188–89, 191–94, 206, 235, 244–45, 274; charts, 17, 81–82, 191, 196, 198, 203; diagrams, 17, 79, 92–93, 98–99, 103, 142, 144–45, 148, 158–62, 189, 196, 198, 277–78; experimentation, 4, 16, 66, 79, 82–85, 90, 95, 116–21, 124, 143, 188, 191, 274; interviewing, 79, 92, 97–98, 103,

methods, epidemiological: interviewing (*continued*) 117–18, 124, 142, 154, 156–58, 160–62, 182, 191, 211, 274; maps, 16–17, 74, 79, 86–87, 98, 101, 103–5, 124, 139, 144, 156, 189, 191n53, 197, 199, 203, 213–18, 222, 271, 274; photography, 27, 200, 202, 204; questionnaires, 210
Metropolitan Asylums Board, 174
miasma theory, 63, 67, 107–8, 133, 140, 276. *See also* disease etiology; sewer gas
military hygiene, 24, 28, 80, 196, 225, 228–23, 268; in cantonments, 230, 235–40, 242; in hill stations, 230
milk, as a medium of disease, 13, 20, 27, 62, 73–75, 77–78, 97–98, 102, 108, 113, 117, 126–27, 188, 210, 244, 280; as medicine; 37, 134; middle class notions of, 20, 130–31, 135, 148, 153, 165, 276; milk adulteration, 135, 143–144, 148, 154, 164, 168, 170; milk-borne outbreak in Islington, London, 130, 138–48, 150; milk-borne outbreak in St. Marylebone, London, 128–30
Miller, William Allen, 81–82, 95, 103, 119. *See also* water analysis
Milroy, Gavin, 233
Milroy lecture, Royal College of Physicians, 66
Ministry of Health, 3, 5, 271–73
Morehead, Charles, 229
Morton, J. Chalmers, investigation of typhoid in St. Marylebone, London, 155–167
municipal sanitation, 1, 6–7, 9, 11–12, 27, 29, 60, 71, 88–89, 96, 124, 126, 188–90, 193–94, 211–12, 226, 278–80, 282; water filtration, 84, 193–95, 197–206, 263–65

Murchison, Charles, 20–21, 23–26, 37–38, 68–69, 72–73, 83–84, 109, 111–13, 140, 176–79, 205, 219, 231, 234–35, 276; investigation of typhoid in St. Marylebone, London, 128–30, 151–67
Murphy, Shirley, 19, 188, 125n177, 202, 222, 271

National Thanksgiving Day, 17, 26, 30–32, 46, 50, 53–60
Newman, George, 27, 134, 170
Newsholme, Arthur, 6, 126, 134, 205
Notification of Infectious Diseases Act, 18, 104, 193, 203, 206, 222
Notter, J. Lane, 29, 214, 233, 258; investigation of typhoid in South Africa on Royal Commission, 258–68
nuisance removal, 97, 100, 107, 135, 139, 194, 209. *See also* filth

Panum, Peter, 110
pathology, 8, 11, 22, 25, 36, 41, 115, 118n145, 172, 175, 177–78, 180, 227, 234, 243, 250, 254 Pathological Society of London, 179
parasitology, 229
Parkes, Edmund Alexander, 75n153, 80, 146, 154n80, 231–32, 267
Parsons, Franklin, 111, 189
Pasteur, Louis, 71, 245
performance, public health strategies of, 5, 7, 10, 12–13, 17, 51, 119–22, 124, 144, 163, 170, 175, 209, 212–13, 214, 220–21, 247
Pettenkofer, Max von, 98, 219
Pickles, William Norman, 273
Playfair, Lyon, 183
pleuro-pneumonia, 136–37
Poor Law Medical Officers, 95, 104, 138

Poore, George Vivian, 147
popular press, 30, 47, 53, 84n18, 101
Portland Hospital, 250–251, 264–66
Power, William Henry, 5, 115, 130,
147–48, 158n91, 168; investigation
of typhoid at St. Marylebone, London, 161–67
prayer-gauge debate, 51–52, 112n121,
178–79
Pringle, Robert, 238, 241
professionalization of public health,
6–7, 11, 14–18, 38, 72, 88, 122,
139, 147. *See also* Association of
Medical Officers of Health; Epidemiological Society of London
Metropolitan
Public Health Act, 1858, 69
Public Health Act 1872, 1, 2n4, 10, 60,
114, 153, 191
Public Health Act 1875, 1, 60, 104,
137, 150, 167
public prayer, 31, 48–53, 61, 178. *See
also* prayer-gauge debate
pythogenic theory of typhoid fever,
21, 23, 68–69, 72, 83–84, 129n5,
151, 231, 235–36. *See also* disease
etiology; germ theory; Murchison,
Charles

Radcliffe, John Netten, 38, 67, 72–73,
78–79, 89–90, 107, 122, 127, 148,
168, 188–89, 193, 195, 202, 205,
209–10, 219, 232, 234, 273; investigation of cholera in London, 84–89;
investigation of cholera at Theydon
Bois, Essex, 79–85, 187, 191; investigation of typhoid at Forest Hill, 71;
investigation of typhoid at Stamford,
103–6; investigation of typhoid at
St. Marylebone, London, 155–67,
191, 214
Rawlinson, Robert, 129

Reece, Robert, 273
relapsing fever, 34, 38
respectability, middle class notions of,
18, 23, 26, 31, 51, 62, 170, 276
Richardson, Benjamin Ward, 21, 108,
164, 282
Richardson, J., 237
Ross, George, 135
Ross, Ronald, 229
Royal Army Medical Corps (RAMC),
248, 250, 253–54, 256, 258, 260,
261, 263–67, 269
Royal College of Physicians of London,
21, 34, 66, 91, 117n140, 139, 233,
255
Royal Commission on the Care and
Treatment of the Sick and Wounded,
227, 255–58
Royal Commission on Rinderpest, 139
Royal Commission on the Nature,
Pathology, Causation, and Preven-
tion of Dysentery and its Relation-
ship to Enteric Fever, 227, 251,
258–70
Royal Medical and Chirurgical Society,
34, 139
Royal Reception Committee, 53–59
Royal Sanitary Commission, 101, 107,
119
Royal Victoria Military Hospital, Netley,
228, 235–36, 242–47, 253, 255, 263
Rugg, H. Hodson, 135
Russell, James, 146, 173, 220n126

Sanderson, John Burdon, 71, 81, 103,
118n145, 136, 172–73, 177, 186–
87, 220
Sandringham, 33, 40, 44–46, 50, 64,
77
Sanitary Act 1866, 2n3, 10, 70, 99–100
sanitary engineering, 8, 15, 61, 63–65,
95, 123, 129, 170, 255, 278, 280

sanitary surveillance, 1, 3, 5, 11–12, 18, 29, 138, 149, 164, 272, 279, 282

scarlet fever, 111, 133–134, 139, 168, 188, 190

Scriven, J. B., 229, 236

Seaton, Edward Cator, 5, 85n22, 115, 127, 186, 209–10, 232

Seaton, Edward Cox, 19, 82n13, 115–16, 126–27, 168, 189, 222

Semple, David, 243–46

sewer gas, 20, 26, 31, 40, 61–69, 71–77, 102, 126–27, 129, 143n50, 165, 170, 188, 203, 235. *See also* disease etiology; household sanitation

shellfish, as a medium of disease, 66, 113, 126, 168, 171, 210, 280. *See also* disease etiology

Shiga, Kiyoshi, 260–62

Simon, John, 1–6, 9–13, 65, 67–71, 73, 79–82, 84, 87, 91, 96, 100, 102–3, 121, 127, 137, 139, 144, 147, 154–55, 161, 169, 210, 232, 239, 271–72, 276, 278–79; administrative tensions at the Local Government Board, 113–15; rhetorical crusade against filth, 22, 107–15, 225; support of bacteriological research, 172, 175–80, 186–187

Simonds, James Beart, 137, 181

Simpson, Benjamin, 237

Simpson, W. J., 251; research on South African Royal Commission, 258–70

smallpox, 139, 185, 188

Smee, Alfred, 131, 219

Smith, Thomas Southwood, 108

Snow, John, 14, 16, 34, 80, 83–85, 87n28, 110, 125, 133, 139, 274

Social Science Association, 7, 183

Society of Public Analysts, 150, 201

soil, as a medium of typhoid fever, 9, 20, 24, 26, 28, 63–67, 70, 75, 95,

103, 109, 117, 121, 171, 177, 179, 189, 194–95, 206–9, 211–13, 214, 218–23, 261, 263, 265–66, 277. *See also* disease etiology

South African War, 28–29, 32, 60, 223–28, 241, 250–70, 281

Spear, John, 188–90

spontaneous generation, 22–25, 31, 72–73, 78, 83, 94, 106, 112, 178, 219, 231. *See also* disease etiology

St. Thomas's Hospital, 2, 20, 26, 37, 101–2, 110, 168, 185, 189

St. Bartholomew's Hospital, 22–24, 91, 177, 212, 250

Stallybrass, C. O., 75

Stansfeld, James, 114

state medicine, 2–7, 11, 88, 114–15, 124–25, 130, 144, 214, 218, 272, 279, 281

Stewart, Alexander, 22

Stewart, William, 32

Stock, W. F. K, 201

Stockwell Fever Hospital, 174

Swete, Horace, 106

Swithinbank, Harold, 134

Tait, Lawson, 138

Tait, Archibald Campbell, 50–51, 59

Taylor, Michael, 131–134, 141–142, 147, 150

Tew, J. S., 244, 246

therapeutic skepticism, 37–38, 46

thermometer, 41–43, 46, 48

Thomson, Theodore, 125n177, 191, 206, 208n95, 213

Thorne Thorne, Richard, 5, 72n144, 75, 81, 107, 148, 189, 195, 203, 210, 213, 214, 232, 273, 276; as Chief Medical Officer of the Medical Department, 75, 115, 176, 210, 213, 214, 218–21; investigation of typhoid at Caterham, 115–25, 144,

186, 200, 202, 204, 209, 213, 214, 222; investigation of typhoid at Terling, 96–102, 119, 134, 142, 191; investigation of typhoid at Winterton, 91–94, 119, 142

Thudichum, J. L. W., 81, 186

Thursfield, W. N., 45

Tooth, Howard, 247n76, 249n85, 250–53, 264

tuberculosis, 8, 20, 101, 181, 188, 274

Turner, George, 267–268

Tyndall, John, 52, 71, 112n121, 122n166; involvement in Tyndall-Typhoid Controversy, 177–80

typhoid fever; clinical descriptions of, 22, 24, 33, 38–47; diagnosis of, 8, 104, 190, 230, 237, 245, 275; endemic nature, 12, 20, 26, 32, 94, 110, 205, 208–9, 212–13, 221–22, 226, 231–32, 239, 264, 272, 283; healthy carrier state, 29, 113, 125, 223, 271–72, 281–82; incubation period, 41, 98, 117, 194, 212, 219 ; infectious typhoid corpses, 224–28, 255–56; laboratory research on, 176–77, 222–23; morbidity rates, 4, 64, 91, 95, 97, 103–4, 268, 279; nursing typhoid patients, 245–46, 258; perambulatory, 124–25; racial attitudes of, 227–42; relationship to paratyphoid, 244, 252, 272; relationship to typho-malarial fever, 231; saprophytic existence of outside the human body, 177, 219–23; *Salmonella* family, 14, 21, 29, 183, 222, 244–45, 275, 277, 282; urban versus rural incidence, 9, 13, 27, 32, 73, 78–79, 81, 89, 96, 101–6, 109–13, 115, 117, 124–26, 131–32, 160–61, 169–70, 177, 190–91, 193, 218, 281; tropical typhoid, 28, 228–31, 269. *See also* enteric fever

Typhoid Mary, 20, 125, 223, 269, 282

typhus, 20–21, 31–34, 38, 61, 101, 106, 132, 190, 278, 282

University College London, 65, 139, 218

Vacher, Francis, 168, 181

vaccination, 3, 60, 140, 185, 245n65, 248n81

Victoria, Queen, 11, 26, 30–34, 40–41, 44–46, 50–51, 53, 55–56, 58–60, 67, 151, 224, 226, 273, 278

vital statistics, 4, 11, 14, 15, 22, 24, 85, 88, 104, 139, 141, 163, 210, 274. *See also* General Registrar's Office

veterinary public health, 8, 11, 131, 135–38, 164, 167, 169, 180–81

Wakley, Thomas, 135, 146

Wanklyn, James Alfred, 144, 150, 153, 184–85

water analysis, 81, 86, 88, 92, 118–19, 123, 175–76, 182–186, 188, 197–206, 212

Watson, Thomas, 108, 151

Whipple, George, 277–78, 282

Whitaker, William, 86, 94, 117

Whitehead, H. R., 229, 239

Whitelegge, B. A., 186

Whitmore, John, investigation of typhoid at St. Marylebone, London, 152–167, 169

Widal test, 28, 106; development of, 243–44; testing in India, 246–250; use in South Africa, 252, 261

Wright, Almroth, 28–29, 223, 228, 242, 268–69; antityphoid inoculation testing in India, 245–50; antityphoid inoculation testing in South Africa, 250–54, 261; background,

Wright, Almroth: background
　　(*continued*)
　　243–44; experiments on the Widal
　　test, 243–45. *See also* antityphoid
　　inoculation; Widal test
Wilson, A. C., 201
Wilson, David Doull, 201–5
Wilson, George, 82–83 91, 98
Williamson, Alexander, 66

Windsor, and 1858 typhoid outbreak,
　　67–69, 76
Woodhead, G. S., 201
World War I, 253–54, 256, 270, 273

zoonotic spread of disease, 131, 136–37
zymotic theory, 25, 169, 181. *See also*
　　etiology of disease; Farr, William

Printed in the United States
by Baker & Taylor Publisher Services